Critical Care for Postgraduate Trainees

Critical Care for Postgraduate Trainees

Adam Brooks, Keith Girling, Bernard Riley & Brian Rowlands

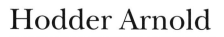

Hodder Arnold

A MEMBER OF THE HODDER HEADLINE GROUP

First published in Great Britain in 2005 by
Hodder Arnold, a member of the Hodder Headline Group,
338 Euston Road, London NW1 3BH

http://www.hoddereducation.com

Distributed in the United States of America by
Oxford University Press Inc.,
198 Madison Avenue, New York, NY10016
Oxford is a registered trademark of Oxford University Press

Whilst the advice and information in this book are believed to be true and
accurate at the date of going to press, neither the author[s] nor the publisher
can accept any legal responsibility or liability for any errors or omissions
that may be made. In particular (but without limiting the generality of the
preceding disclaimer) every effort has been made to check drug dosages;
however it is still possible that errors have been missed. Furthermore,
dosage schedules are constantly being revised and new side-effects
recognized. For these reasons the reader is strongly urged to consult the
drug companies' printed instructions before administering any of the drugs
recommended in this book.

British Library Cataloguing in Publication Data
A catalogue record for this book is available from the British Library

Library of Congress Cataloging-in-Publication Data
A catalog record for this book is available from the Library of Congress

ISBN-10:   0 340 80967 1
ISBN-13:   978 0 340 80967 9

1 2 3 4 5 6 7 8 9 10

Commissioning Editor: Sarah Burrows
Development Editor: Layla Vandenbergh
Project Editor: Dan Edwards
Production Controller: Lindsay Smith
Cover Design: Sarah Rees

Typeset in 9 pts Minion by Charon Tec Pvt. Ltd, Chennai, India
Printed and bound in Great Britain by CPI Bath

What do you think about this book? Or any other Hodder Arnold title?
Please visit http://www.hoddereducation.com

Contents

Contributors

Simon Allison

Professor of Clinical Nutrition, Queen's Medical Centre, University Hospital, Nottingham, UK

Adam Brooks

Fellow in Trauma and Surgical Critical Care, Hospital University of Pennsylvania, Philadelphia, USA
Specialist Registrar in General Surgery, Queen's Medical Centre, University Hospital, Nottingham, UK

Mark Ehlers

Consultant in Adult Critical Care, Queen's Medical Centre, University Hospital, Nottingham, UK

Keith Girling

Consultant in Adult Critical Care, Queen's Medical Centre, University Hospital, Nottingham, UK

Hilary Humphreys

Professor of Microbiology and Consultant Microbiologist, Department of Clinical Microbiology, RCSI Education and Research Centre, Smurfit Building, Beaumont Hospital, Dublin, Ireland

Dileep Lobo

Senior Lecturer in Gastrointestinal Surgery and Honorary Consultant Hepatopancreaticobiliary Surgeon, Queen's Medical Centre, University Hospital, Nottingham, UK

James Low

Consultant in Anaesthesia and Critical Care, Derby Hospitals NHS Foundation Trust, Derby, UK

Ravi Mahajan

Reader and Honorary Consultant in Anaesthesia and Intensive Care, University of Nottingham, Nottingham City Hospital, Nottingham, UK

Peter Mahoney

Senior Lecturer (Military), Leonard Cheshire Centre of Conflict Recovery, London, UK

Iain Moppett

Clinical Lecturer in Anaesthesia and Intensive Care, University of Nottingham, Queen's Medical Centre, University Hospital, Nottingham, UK

Roslyn Purcell

Senior Registrar, Intensive Care Unit, The Princess Alexandra Hospital, Brisbane, Queensland, Australia

Bernard Riley

Consultant in Adult Critical Care, Queen's Medical Centre, University Hospital, Nottingham, UK

Brian Rowlands

Professor of Surgery, Queen's Medical Centre, University Hospital, Nottingham, UK

C William Schwab

Director of Trauma and Surgical Critical Care, Hospital University of Pennsylvania, Philadelphia, USA

David Selwyn

Consultant in Adult Critical Care, Queen's Medical Centre, University Hospital, Nottingham, UK

David Sperry

Consultant in Adult Critical Care, Queen's Medical Centre, University Hospital, Nottingham, UK

Jonathan Thompson

Senior Lecturer and Honorary Consultant in Anaesthesia and Critical Care, Leicester Royal Infirmary, Leicester, UK

Simon Wharton

Consultant in Respiratory Medicine, Queen's Medical Centre, University Hospital, Nottingham, UK

John Williams

Specialist Registrar in Anaesthesia and Critical Care, Leicester Royal Infirmary, Leicester, UK

Robert Winter

Consultant in Adult Critical Care, Queen's Medical Centre, University Hospital, Nottingham, UK

Foreword

Twenty years or so ago there began a great expansion in the provision of intensive care medicine in the UK while the last decade has witnessed a quiet but equally significant maturation of intensive care in our hospitals. That process has seen the concept of multidisciplinary and multi-level critical care develop rapidly with the acceptance that care of the critically ill occurs in wards, emergency departments, high dependency areas and specialist units as well as on the Intensive Care Unit. Along with nursing and other colleagues, much of that critical care is delivered by anaesthetic and surgical teams, as well as by intensivists and the importance of critical care is reflected in its adoption as a central component of the training and examination of all anaesthetic and surgical trainees.

Training in critical care has evolved too with practical courses designed to complement the theory available from large textbooks but to date there have been few successful and readable textbooks designed to fill the gap between the two. This book accomplishes that admirably and will prepare the reader well for critical care practice as well as for examinations.

As one would anticipate from authors renowned both for their clinical expertise and their commitment to training, the book is pitched at an ideal level for the higher trainee. Basic sciences are covered in just the right amount of depth to provide understanding without inducing somnolence and a strong clinical focus is maintained throughout. The combination will prepare candidates (and examiners) well for exams and the clear chapter layout with learning objectives and viva topics reinforces this. The major issues of current debate are addressed with authority and the chapter references facilitate further reading.

Critically ill patients, modern clinical practice and examiners all demand that today's doctors understand how colleagues think and approach problems and the joint approach which this book offers to trainees in anaesthesia, surgery and intensive care is appropriate, timely and successful. With its clear style and systematic approach which takes readers through from the basics up to the details of critical care practice, this book is well placed to meet those needs.

Iain D Anderson MD FRCS
Consultant Surgeon
Hope Hospital
Manchester, UK
Tutor in Surgical Critical Care
The Royal College of Surgeons of England
London, UK

1 Epidemiology of critical care

DAVID SPERRY

Viva topics

- Define critical illness and a critical care unit.
- Discuss the implications of the 'Comprehensive critical care' document to UK intensive care practice.
- What does APACHE stand for and what are the uses of the APACHE scoring systems?
- How are scoring systems applied in modern intensive care practice?

INTRODUCTION

Critical care is a growing specialty offering increasingly complex care for both surgical and medical patients. Identification of patient groups requiring critical care, and the current pattern of use, is a key requirement for our understanding of the function of a modern intensive care unit. Outcome analysis in intensive care is more advanced than in any other specialty, led by the desire to identify patients in whom the extreme cost of critical care will not be justified by results. Recent changes to the requirements for critical care services set out by the UK government have broadened the scope of input for the intensivist beyond the doors of the intensive care unit to a wider view of critical illness throughout the hospital.

DEFINITION OF CRITICAL ILLNESS

Critical illness is the impairment of vital organ function or the presence of instability, or the risk of serious and potentially preventable complications. A modern intensive care unit is an area of the hospital where critically ill patients are grouped with trained personnel and equipment specific to their care.[1]

Intensive care is a specialty that deals in uncertainty. Where the patient is certain to survive the current illness there is no requirement for intensive care. Where the patient is certain to die, palliative care outside the intensive care unit offers a better quality of death. Between these two groups lies a varying degree of uncertainty, and it is the function of the intensivist to attempt to quantify both the likely prognosis and the likely impact of intensive care on that prognosis. Such categorization is obviously fraught with ethical and legal difficulties. This direct quotation from the Department of Health Expert Group demonstrates the problems:

> Management of patients who will not benefit from admission to critical care units or from continuation of treatment once admitted is difficult. It is recommended that current guidance from professional bodies such as the British Medical Association and the Royal College of Nursing and appropriate legislation including the Human Rights Act should be used when developing local policies for the care of such patients. Such guidance needs to take account of the need for a mechanism for the review of decisions made by clinicians in individual cases, for the management of the expectations of the public about the appropriateness of the deployment of critical care resources and of the likelihood of legal challenge of decisions by individual clinicians.[2]

In addition to alterations in the expectations of the public, human rights legislation and demographic changes, therapeutic advances alter the requirements and indications for intensive care admission.

The recent Department of Health publication 'Comprehensive critical care' divides critically ill patients into three levels of severity (Table 1.1). Level 1 patients are considered 'at risk'; level 2 patients have single organ impairment; and level 3 patients have two organ impairments or respiratory failure requiring mechanical ventilation. There is no mention of patient diagnosis, specialty or individual characteristics in this formula for care. Level 1 patients can continue to be cared for on the ward of origin, provided a critical care outreach team is involved. Level 2 patients are appropriate

Table 1.1 *Levels of critical illness*

Level 0	Patients whose needs can be met through normal ward care in an acute hospital.
Level 1	Patients at risk of their condition deteriorating, or those recently relocated from higher levels of care, whose needs can be met on an acute ward with additional advice and support from the critical care team.
Level 2	Patients requiring more detailed observation or intervention including support for a single failing organ system or post-operative care and those 'stepping down' from higher levels of care.
Level 3	Patients requiring advanced respiratory support alone or basic respiratory support together with support of at least two organ systems. This level includes all complex patients requiring support for multi-organ failure.

for high-dependency care, and level 3 patients can only be cared for in intensive care units. Stratification in this way – by the number of organs impaired – is based on scoring system risk assessment and is discussed in the next section. To understand which patient groups require admission to intensive care and high-dependency areas, an understanding of work on outcomes of the various patient groups is vital. A perfect assessment of the patient's outcome before or during admission is impossible to achieve, but it continues to guide general admission guidance to critical care areas in the UK.

SCORING SYSTEMS FOR PREDICTION IN CRITICAL ILLNESS

Scoring systems were designed initially to categorize patients with single, specific diagnoses into risk and prognosis groups. Well-known examples still in use today include the Burns Score (1971) and the Glasgow Coma Score (GCS) (1974). Low scores on these systems indicate a need for higher care and transfer to specialist units. Scoring systems were gradually broadened to include variables representing the whole of the patient's physiology. The applicability of the new systems to the widely varying diagnoses and conditions of critical illness did not meet with uniform acclaim, as evidenced by this quote from the Textbook of Critical Care: 'Probability estimates will never approach 100 per cent accuracy unless they are made so restrictive that they apply to very few patients and thus are rendered useless'.[3]

The new scoring systems were accepted, at least as a means of providing comparable patients, for clinical trials and to some extent for comparison of intensive care units.

Early systems included the acute physiology and chronic health evaluation system (APACHE) and simplified acute physiology scores (SAPS). In the initial systems variables to be included were chosen by panels of experts, but this soon gave way to statistical analysis of large databases of intensive care patients (e.g. APACHE II). Scoring systems can be classified according to the predominant feature that is scored.

Physiological scoring systems

APACHE II

APACHE stands for Acute Physiology and Chronic Health Evaluation. This scoring system was developed by the combination of diverse variables such as creatinine level, heart rate, patient age and previous illness. These were analysed by multivariate regression to determine both their ability to predict outcome and the levels of derangement at which the likelihood of death was increased. Variables that showed no relation to outcome were removed from the scoring system, whereas those strongly related to mortality were assigned a high weighting within the system (Figure 1.1). Variables included in APACHE II are shown in Table 1.2. The most notable feature of the score is the relative weighting attributed between the main categories. The maximum score for physiology is 60, age is 4, and chronic health is out of 5.

Very few patients qualify for points in the chronic health category because this is defined as long-term *severe* organ insufficiency. More points are added to chronic health in the event of either emergency surgery or where a patient has not had an operation. Thus, the elective surgical patient has a low mortality in intensive care. Less easy to comprehend is the higher mortality for emergency medical (non-operative) patients over that of emergency surgery patients. Presumably this is due to several factors. Emergency surgery patients have already been selected preoperatively into likely survivors who undergo surgery, and non-survivors who receive palliative care. A proportion of extremely ill surgical patients die in theatre before reaching intensive care, and the operation may already be correcting the underlying critical process, resulting in high first-day scores that improve rapidly. The ICNARC (Intensive Care National Audit And Research Centre) database found intensive care patients' hospital mortality to be 37 per cent for non-surgical patients and 19 per cent overall for surgical patients, with emergency surgery having a mortality of 30 per cent and elective surgery requiring ITU a mortality of 10 per cent.[4]

It will be noted, therefore, that the chance of dying during an episode of critical illness is related to the severity of the acute physiological derangement rather than the presence of

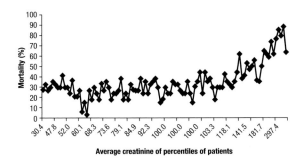

Figure 1.1 Relationship between admission creatinine and mortality for a single ITU (QMC)[2]

Table 1.2 *APACHE II scoring system*

APACHE II	Variable	Maximum score
Physiology	Temperature	4
	Mean arterial pressure	4
	Heart rate	4
	Respiratory rate	4
	Oxygenation	4
	pH	4
	Na+	4
	K+	4
	Creatinine	4
	Haemoglobin	4
	White count	4
	Glasgow Coma Score	12
Age	<44	0
	45–54	1
	55–64	2
	65–74	3
	>75	4
Chronic health	History of severe organ system insufficiency or immunocompromise AND:	
	Emergency surgery or No operation	5
	Elective operation	2

any pre-existing condition. Where more than one organ is affected by the illness process, the score is abnormal for more variables and the overall score is higher.

This statistical view was confirmed clinically in 1990 by Ridley.[5] He examined the levels of care required by patients in the year before admission to intensive care, as a predictor of outcome in intensive care. He included nursing home, rehabilitation and ward care, and found that '…chronicity, as measured by the amount of care required in the year before intensive care unit admission, does not independently influence survival'. By contrast, inpatient care in the 2 days prior to intensive care admission was a significant predictor of poor outcome. The main determinant of death is therefore the 'degree and potential reversibility of the physiologic derangement'.

POSSUM

The Physiological and Operative Severity Score for the enUmeration of Mortality and Morbidity (POSSUM) is a scoring system developed to enable comparative audit for general surgical procedures that allows for the effects of case mix. The POSSUM dataset is based on 12 preoperative factors that on multivariate analysis were independently predictive of outcome (Table 1.3). Each of these is graded and scored exponentially, with the highest values being given to the most deranged value; together these provide a POSSUM physiology score. Although this score was found to be prognostic for individual patients, it has been augmented by an operative severity score derived from 6 factors whose values depend on the size and severity of the operation (Table 1.4). The physiology and operative scores are then entered into regression analysis equations to calculate a percentage morbidity and mortality risk.

A number of criticisms have been levelled at the original equation used for the calculation of morbidity and mortality, specifically that it overpredicted mortality in certain patient groups. Hence, the Portsmouth predictor equation, or P-POSSUM, was developed. This equation, using the original POSSUM dataset, has predicted outcome in 10 000 patient episodes in general surgery.

The value of POSSUM has been demonstrated in numerous studies of general surgery and has allowed the comparison of both individual surgeons and hospitals. As subspecialty procedures are frequently those with the highest risk, POSSUM and P-POSSUM have been used by several subspecialty organizations to audit data on specialist procedures. It is likely, however, that separate equations will be required for each major procedure.

As with all scoring systems, care must be exercised in data collection and analysis and there are several aspects of the POSSUM system that require caution. Notably, it has been shown that the physiology score can be improved by preoperative resuscitation. Therefore, the timing of the data used for calculating morbidity and mortality may artificially alter the values. Other concerns include missing data, and the subjective nature of the operative score.

Table 1.3 *Physiological dataset and scores*

	Score			
	1	**2**	**4**	**8**
Age	<60	61–70	>71	
Cardiac signs	Normal	Cardiac drugs or steroids	Oedema, warfarin, borderline cardiomegaly	Raised JVP, cardiomegaly
Respiratory signs	Normal	Shortness of breath on exertion, mild COPD	Short of breath on stairs, moderate COPD	Short of breath at rest, any other
Systolic blood pressure (mmHg)	110–129	130–170 or 100–109	>170 or 90–99	<90
Pulse rate (per min)	50–80	81–100 or 40–49	101–120	>120 or <40
Glasgow Coma Score	15	12–14	9–11	<9
Serum urea (mmol/L)	<7.5	7.5–10.0	10.1–15.0	>15.0
Serum sodium (mmol/L)	>136	131–135	126–130	<126
Serum potassium (mmol/L)	3.5–5.0	3.1–3.4 or 5.1–5.3	2.9–3.1 or 5.4–5.9	<2.9 or >5.9
Haemoglobin (g/L)	13.0–16.0	11.5–12.9 or 16.1–17.0	10.0–11.4 or 17.1–18.0	<10.0 or >18.0
White cell count ($\times 10^9$/L)	4.0–10.0	10.1–20.0 or 3.1–3.9	>20.0 or <3.1	
Electrocardiogram	Normal		Atrial fibrillation (60–90 min)	Any other

Table 1.4 *Operative severity data set and scores*

	Operative score			
	1	**2**	**4**	**8**
Operation category	Minor	Intermediate	Major	Major +
No. of procedures	1	2	>2	
Total blood loss (mL)	<=100	101–500	501–999	>1000
Peritoneal soiling	None	Serous blood (<250 mL)	Local pus	Any other
Malignancy	None	Primary only	Nodal metastases	Distant metastases
Timing of operation	Elective		Urgent, within 2 hours (resuscitation possible)	Emergency, immediate (no resuscitation possible)

POSSUM has been compared against APACHE II in 117 patients and was found to be more predictive of outcome. POSSUM predicts only 30-day mortality and not long-term outcome.

SUMMARY

Physiological scoring systems have abounded since the production of APACHE II, and modern systems include APACHE III (1991), SAPS II (1993) and the Mortality Prediction Model (MPM II). The division of care into levels according to the number of organ failures as performed in 'Comprehensive critical care' is a logical step towards quantifying the threat to the individual and targeting the resources of intensive care to the patients with the most uncertain outcome.

Organ failure scoring systems

Multiple organ failure is the leading cause of mortality and morbidity in patients admitted to the intensive care unit. Several organ dysfunction scores have been developed for use in the critically ill. These include the Multiple Organ Dysfunction Score (MODS), the Sequential Organ Failure Assessment (SOFA) and the Logistic Organ Dysfunction System (LODS). MODS and SOFA remain the most commonly used and are based on very similar data collection. Details of the scores are given in Tables 1.5 and 1.6. Given the similarity of the data collected, it is not surprising that these scores result in very similar mortality predictions. Using the SOFA score, it has been shown that

Table 1.5 *The multiple organ dysfunction score (MODS)*

Organ system	Score				
	0	1	2	3	4
Respiratory: Po_2/FiO_2 ratio (mmHg)	>300	226–300	151–225	76–150	≤75
Renal: serum creatinine (mg/dL)	≤1.1	1.2–2.2	2.3–3.9	4–5.6	≥5.7
Hepatic: serum bilirubin (mg/dL)	≤1.2	1.3–3.5	3.6–7	7–14	>14
Cardiovascular: PAR	≤10	10.1–15	15.1–20	20.1–30	>30
Haematologic: platelet count ($\times10^3$/mL)	>120	81–120	51–80	21–50	≤20
Neurologic: Glasgow Coma Score	15	13–14	10–12	7–9	≤6

PAR, pressure-adjusted heart rate calculated as the product of the heart rate multiplied by the ratio of the right atrial pressure to the mean arterial pressure

Table 1.6 *The sequential organ failure assessment (SOFA)*

	0	1	2	3	4
Respiratory: P_AO_2/FiO_2 ratio (mmHg)	>400	≤400	≤300	≤200[b]	≤100[b]
Renal: creatinine (mg/dL) or urine output	<1.2	1.2–1.9	2.0–3.4	3.5–4.9 or <500 mL/day	≥5.0 or <200 mL/day
Hepatic: bilirubin (mg/dL)	<1.2	1.2–1.9	2.0–5.9	6.0–11.9	≥12.0
Cardiovascular: hypotension	No hypotension	MAP < 70 mmHg	Dopamine ≤5 or dobutamine (any dose)[a]	Dopamine >5 or epinephrine ≤0.1 or norepinephrine ≤ 0.1[a]	Dopamine >15 or epinephrine >0.1 or norepinephrine >0.1[a]
Haematologic: platelet count ($\times10^3$/mL)	150	≤150	≤100	≤50	≤20
Neurologic: Glasgow Coma Score	15	13–14	10–12	6–9	<6

[a] Adrenergic agents administered for at least 1 hour (doses given in μg/kg/min)
[b] With ventilatory support

the mortality increases as more organs fail, and approximately 9 per cent of patients with no organ failure on admission to intensive care would be expected to die, compared to 69 per cent of those with four or more organs failing. If the SOFA score totals more than 15 during the patient's admission the predicted mortality increases to 90 per cent.

Intervention-based scoring systems

The Therapeutic Intervention Scoring System (TISS) (1974) represents an alternative method of scoring based on the number of interventions performed on a patient. The theory behind this system is that as the disease process becomes more life threatening, more medical and nursing interventions are required, and this can be quantified. The original system looked at 70 variables. Examples include the

need for one-to-one nursing care, central line insertion and the presence of a catheter. The major advantage of this approach is that it allows cost assessment for an individual in addition to severity assessment. The disadvantages are differences between practice in different areas – possibly even within the same hospital – and the complexity of the data collection required. TISS 28 reduced the number of predictive variables to 28 without a great loss in predictive ability.

IMPORTANT DISEASE-SPECIFIC SCORING SYSTEMS

Several scoring systems for individual diseases or disease groups are currently in use in practice.

The assessment of burn area by the 'rule of 9s' has been around since 1944 (Figure 1.2). In 1971, Bull[6] demonstrated

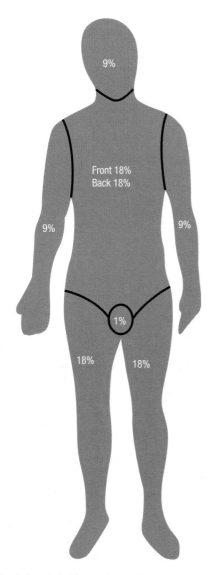

Figure 1.2 Rule of 9s for burns patients

outcomes, allowing some quantification and comparison of outcomes in an illness where prediction for an individual is poor.

A number of scoring systems have been developed and compared for the evaluation of trauma severity and to provide prognostic information on the outcome. The most widely recognized of these are the Injury Severity Score (ISS) and the Revised Trauma Score (RTS).

The ISS is an anatomical scoring system based on the severity of patients' injuries. Using the Abbreviated Injury Score, injuries that provide the highest values are scored for the six body regions (head and neck; abdomen and pelvis; bony pelvis and limbs; face; chest; body surface). The squares of the three highest scores are summed to give a final value out of a maximum of 75.

The RTS is a physiologically based system that predicts survival based on the derangement of respiratory rate, systolic blood pressure and GCS (Table 1.7).

Both purely physiological and anatomical systems have obvious drawbacks, and therefore to overcome these issues RTS and ISS have been combined to make TRISS. TRISS uses constants derived from the major trauma outcome study, ISS, RTS, the patient's age, and whether the injury was blunt or penetrating, to provide a usable measure of the probability of survival.

Pancreatitis is another disease which can be mild and self-limiting or life threatening. Several scoring systems aid the division of patients into the two groups for higher care. The Ranson criteria (1974) identify patients at 48 hours based on admission levels (age, white cell count, glucose, AST and LDH levels) and changes in physiological factors since admission (fluid sequestration, decreasing haematocrit, increasing urea, low calcium, base deficit and hypoxia). This visionary early attempt to assess both disease at the outset and the failure of initial treatment remains a good prognostic system. Imrie subsequently simplified the number of variables collected. APACHE II has also been shown to predict outcome well in this disease.[8]

Medical disease has not lagged behind. Community-acquired pneumonia is a common condition that infrequently requires intensive care therapy. Severe pneumonia carries a high mortality, so the division of patients between moderate and severe disease has outcome and resource benefits. The British Thoracic Society has produced guidelines for the assessment of patients, allowing the classification of severe pneumonia.[9] The simplified assessment tool uses just three variables: respiratory rate >30 breaths/min, diastolic pressure <60 mmHg, and urea >7 mmol/L. The presence of two or more of these factors increases mortality very significantly.

that the percentage burn from this score predicted mortality, and recommended urgent volume resuscitation in adults with more than 15 per cent burns and children with more than 10 per cent burns.

Coma scoring using the GCS is an accepted tool in head injury. It now forms the basis of neurological assessment in virtually all broader ITU scoring systems. Prediction of outcome in head injury has since been refined by dividing patients into 'bins' of defined outcome probabilities using a decision tree, the Virginia prediction tree (Figure 1.3).[7] This classifies patients into separate groups, each having defined

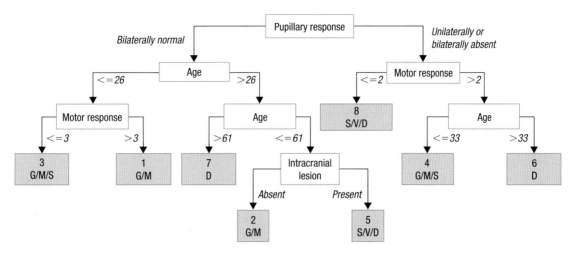

Figure 1.3 Virginia prediction tree. (Republished with kind permission from: Choi SC, Muizelaar JP, Barnes TY, *et al*. Prediction tree for severely head-injured patients. *J Neurosurg* 1991; 75: 251–5. Copyright © 1991 American Association of Neurological Surgeons. All rights reserved.)

Table 1.7 *Revised Trauma Score*

	Value	Coded value	Weighting
Respiratory rate	10–29	4	0.2908
(breaths/min)	>29	3	
	6–9	2	
	1–5	1	
	0	0	
Systolic blood pressure	>88	4	0.7326
(mmHg)	76–89	3	
	50–75	2	
	1–49	1	
	0	0	
Glasgow Coma Scale	13–15	4	0.9368
	9–12	3	
	6–8	2	
	4–5	1	
	3	0	

PROBLEMS WITH SCORING SYSTEMS

Population rather than individual data

Scoring systems are only a model of outcome in intensive care. Using such a model, it is possible to derive the probability of death or survival for an individual patient, but two problems arise: statistical formulae derived from a group are not applicable to individuals, and models derived from logistic statistics fail to provide a probability of 1 (certain to die) or 0 (certain to survive). To give an example: if an individual patient with the high APACHE II score of 30 is admitted to a critical care unit he may survive, against the odds, despite the prediction that he is likely to die. It is only possible to say that out of a group of patients with an APACHE II score of 30 very few are likely to survive. At the extreme, a patient with an APACHE II score of 45 has a predicted mortality of 95.5 per cent. However, it is unlikely that the intensive care unit has ever had a survivor at this level. The APACHE-predicted mortality of 95.5 per cent offers little benefit to the determination of futility of admission for the individual, as it suggests that nearly 1 in 20 such patients will survive. At this probability, admission and prolonged intensive therapy would not be denied. It is therefore impossible to determine whether admission to intensive care is futile for an individual based solely on the score. In the same way, it is also difficult to determine a lower level of risk at which intensive care admission could not possibly benefit a patient with mild illness.

Universal applicability

The original scoring systems were derived from large databases of patients passing through intensive care. These are usually based on large American datasets, and even European databases contain few, if any, UK patients. Furthermore, the databases take years to produce, making many of the data in them historical. ICNARC collects data from intensive care units around the UK, with the government supporting the extension of this programme to more units. Analysis of these data shows that actual observed outcomes with the same APACHE II score vary dramatically between intensive care units in this country (standardized mortality ratio (SMR) between 0.7 and 1.39).

Not only hospitals, but admission diagnoses, also alter the applicability of the score. Patients admitted after neurosurgery or cardiac surgery were more likely to die than were predicted by APACHE II (SMR 1.57 and 1.17, respectively), and patients admitted after surgery with respiratory failure were less likely to die (SMR 0.61).[10] Even comparisons between intensive care units to determine overall quality may be negated by such discrepancies, especially where the units cater for specialist services such as neurosciences or cardiac surgery.

IMPROVING SCORING SYSTEMS

Two recent approaches have attempted to improve the applicability of scoring systems to local intensive care units. The first is calibration of the scoring system, the second is recurrent day-by-day scoring.

Calibration

Local calibration of a system involves reassigning the weightings for the variables of the scoring system to those derived from the local database of patients, or the derivation of a completely new scoring system that is applicable locally. ICNARC uses the UK dataset to provide SMRs to hospitals within its group based on the predicted outcomes for UK intensive care units. Objections about local calibration continue. The size of the underlying database decreases as the data become more local. Relevant recalibration may obscure a high local SMR that is due to poor care, and data remain historical. Recalibration can fail to produce a useful scoring system, as found by Metnitz,[11] in this case due to improvement of mortality since the original scoring system was published.

Daily scoring

Day-to-day scoring offers not only an absolute score, but also a trend that may actually hold more information than the original score. To quote Lemeshow:[12] 'if a patient's clinical profile stays the same, he or she is actually getting worse'. Rue[13] compared MPM II scoring on admission with current-day and previous-day scoring, as well as any combination of the three. He found that the best estimate of hospital

mortality is the probability of death on the current day alone. This may eventually improve our ability to determine when a patient is failing to respond to treatment and move the assessment of likely outcome from the time of admission to a time after resuscitation and the institution of specific therapy. Potential identification of non-responders to therapy may be much more useful for individual outcome analysis.

Doctor assessment

Clinical impression long predates the use of scoring systems in the prediction of outcome from illness, and its use in critical illness is no exception. Scoring systems offer their best prediction in the midrange, where most of the patients in the database from which they are derived are found. Doctors may be better at predicting the extremes, certain survival and certain death. Marks[14] looked at doctors' ability to spot-predict outcome at admission to ITU and compared it with that of nurses and the APACHE II score. Each patient was graded from 1 (expected to die) to 5 (expected to survive). Doctors assessed 77 per cent of outcomes correctly, nurses 72 per cent, and APACHE II 64 per cent. The combination of all three gave 78 per cent correct prediction. Nurses had better specificity than doctors, suggesting that doctors are slightly too pessimistic. Of most interest for the clinician reviewing ward patients with a view to admission were the patients that doctors assigned to group 1 (expected to die). Out of 107 patients in this group 102 (95 per cent) died. The ability of a doctor to predict death may be better than the scoring systems, but doctors remain imperfect to a degree that makes a certain diagnosis of futility for ITU care nearly impossible.

SPECIFIC OUTCOME PREDICTORS

Age

Arguments continue as to whether age is an independent predictor of outcome in critical illness. In the UK ICNARC database age is a significant independent predictor of ITU mortality. In addition, the mean age of survivors is lower than that of non-survivors (54.1 vs 62.4 years). The separate Glasgow follow-up database[5] also found age to be a predictive factor. Outside the UK, patient age has not been found to be as reliable. Chelluri et al.[15] found that elderly patients presented with higher APACHE scores and therefore had a higher mortality, but compared to younger patients with the same APACHE score there was no difference in outcome for the elderly. It is possible that a lower threshold for withdrawal of therapy in the elderly could account for the differences noted.

High-dependency care for the elderly has also been analysed. Ip[16] found that nearly half of patients over 70 were dead 1 month after hospital discharge, but that in the over-85s this figure was 68 per cent. A strong association between the number of organ failures and mortality was demonstrated. Two organ failures gave a mortality of 86 per cent, and there were no survivors with more than two organ failures.

Mortality is not the only important outcome measure, and the potential long-term benefit of critical care in the elderly led to Montuclard's study.[17] He looked at the long-term outcomes of patients aged over 70 who remained in ITU for more than 30 days. Forty-seven per cent survived the hospital admission. He found a significant reduction in independence in activities of daily living as well as a reduction in subjective health and memory, but most survivors felt that their quality of life remained good and most remained independent at home.

CPR

A higher mortality for patients requiring advanced resuscitation before admission to ITU is no surprise. Most scoring systems are weighted for previous CPR, and the ICNARC database found a mortality of 56.8 per cent in patients who had received CPR, against 23.8 per cent for other patients. A recent report in the *New England Journal of Medicine* has set clear criteria to allow identification and the management principles of those patients whose neurological outcome may be improved by admission to a critical care unit following cardiac arrest.[18]

Criteria for patients whose neurological outcome may benefit from critical care management are:

- Witnessed cardiac arrest
- Ventricular fibrillation or non-perfusing ventricular tachycardia as the initial cardiac rhythm
- A presumed cardiac origin of the arrest
- Age 18–75 years
- Interval of 5–15 min from collapse to first attempt at resuscitation
- Interval of less than 60 min from collapse to restoration of spontaneous circulation
- Mean arterial pressure not less than 60 mmHg for more than 30 min after return of spontaneous circulation.

The authors of this report sedated all the patients who met the above criteria and compared the outcome of one group maintained at normothermia with a group cooled to 32–34°C. The cooled group had a significantly better outcome at 6 months than did those maintained at normothermia.

Cancer

Patients admitted to ITU with underlying cancer do not have a greater mortality. In Staudinger's[19] study, 53 per cent survived ITU and 23 per cent were alive at 1 year. APACHE was a poor predictor for these patients' outcomes. Death was associated with respiratory failure, ventilation, septic shock and pre-ITU CPR, all factors associated with mortality in the non-cancer patient. ICNARC also found similar hospital mortality between cancer victims and other patients in intensive care.[4] The presence of cancer does not predict hospital outcome, but obviously the prognosis of the underlying condition guides admission to ITU.

Probable infection

The presence of infection is associated with mortality in ITU. ICNARC found that 42.8 per cent of patients died where the clinician felt that infection was probable, against 21.3 per cent where this was not the case.[4]

SPECIFIC DISEASE OUTCOMES

A small group of illnesses associated with admission to ITU are fully reversible and consequently have a low mortality once the initial phase is passed. Asthma (mortality 12.6 per cent after ITU admission), seizures (12.6 per cent) and drug overdose (11.1 per cent) all fit within this category.

At the other end of the scale, several diagnoses have little reversibility. Cardiogenic shock (mortality 77.5 per cent after ITU admission), septic shock (73 per cent) and respiratory arrest (65 per cent) are not associated with a good outcome. Chronic obstructive airways disease (36.5 per cent) and liver disease (40.6 per cent) do not appear to fit this pattern.

COMMON ITU DIAGNOSES (TABLE 1.8)

The typical ITU patient is a 56-year-old man who has undergone surgery. He has a good chance of having had the operation as an emergency and being admitted with coexisting infection. He has a 1 in 20 chance of requiring readmission to ITU after discharge.

POST-ITU DEATHS

The usual measure of ITU outcome in the UK is survival to hospital discharge. Death between discharge from ITU and

Table 1.8 *Common ITU admission diagnoses in the UK*

Post-operative diagnosis	Percentage	Non-operative diagnosis	Percentage
Peripheral vascular disease	13.3	Cardiac arrest	5.4
Gastrointestinal neoplasm	6.2	Overdose	4.2
Unplanned post-operative respiratory failure	5	Chest infection	4.1
Gastrointestinal perforation or obstruction	4.4	Multiple trauma	2.9
Respiratory obstruction	3.5	Sepsis/septic shock	2.7
Coronary artery disease	3.3	Respiratory arrest	2.2
Multiple trauma	2.8	Asthma	2
Gastrointestinal bleeding	2.1	Head injury	1.8
Renal neoplasm	1.4	Fitting	1
Cancer of the lung	0.9	Gastrointestinal infection	0.7
Cranial haemorrhage	0.7	Gastrointestinal perforation	0.6
		Gastrointestinal bleeding	0.5
		Diabetic ketoacidosis	0.4
		Renal failure	0.3

discharge from the hospital will have a major impact on measured outcomes. A study from Guy's Hospital[20] showed a ward-mortality of 12.4 per cent for ITU patients. A model was produced to predict likely unexpected death after ITU discharge. Significant factors include the acute physiology at discharge, the patient's age, their chronic health and their length of stay on ITU. Patients discharged 'at risk' had a ward mortality of 25 per cent, as opposed to 4 per cent in the 'not at risk' group. It was proposed that a further 48 hours' ITU care could reduce the mortality in the 'at risk' group by 39 per cent.

LONG-TERM SURVIVAL AFTER ITU

Long-term survival may be a better indicator of benefit from intensive therapy than hospital survival, the current standard in measuring success in ITU. The Glasgow study[5] followed 497 patients for 2 years. Of these, 119 died in ITU, 120 died after discharge, and 258 or 52 per cent were still alive 2 years after admission. Age, the severity of the illness and the diagnosis itself were predictors of long-term outcome. Older patients continued dying at a higher rate than expected right to the end of the study period. Seventy-one per cent of trauma victims had survived against 41 per cent of patients with gastrointestinal pathology.

SUMMARY

UK practice has moved to the logical assessment of the requirement for care based on the acute physiological derangement found in an individual patient. Advances in scoring systems for the whole intensive care population do not allow us to assess individual patient outcomes based on a score, but some diseases have guidance for care based on factors associated with poorer outcomes. Assessment of care needs continues to require experienced clinicians and teams from both critical care and the parent specialties, in addition to increased involvement of the patient and their families following recent human rights legislation.

Key points

- Intensive care attempts to focus resources to a group of patients who will have a mortality benefit from higher care.
- Three stepped levels of higher care exist within critical care in the UK.
- Scoring systems quantify risk in groups of patients, and allow comparison of intensive care units.
- Risk of death is associated with the degree of acute physiological disturbance.

REFERENCES

1. Anon. Guidelines for the utilisation of intensive care units. European Society of Intensive Care Medicine. *Intensive Care Med* 1994; **20**: 163–4.
2. Department of Health. Comprehensive critical care. Review of adult critical care services 2002 http://www.doh.gov.uk/compcritcare/compcritcarevw1.htm#compcrit

3. Seneff MG, Zimmerman JE, Knaus WA. Severity of illness indices and outcome prediction: development and evaluation. In: Ayres M. (ed.) *Textbook of Critical Care* (3rd edn). Pennsylvania: WB Saunders, 1995: 1778.

4. Rowan KM, Kerr JH, Major E, *et al*. Intensive Care Society's APACHE II study in Britain and Ireland – I: Variations in case mix of adult admissions to general intensive care units and impact on outcome. *BMJ* 1993; **307**: 972–7.

5. Ridley S, Jackson R, Findlay J, Wallace P. Long term survival after intensive care. *BMJ* 1990; **301**: 1127–30.

6. Bull JP. Revised analysis of mortality due to burns. *Lancet* 1971; **2**: 1133.

7. Choi SC, Muizelaar JP, Barnes TY, *et al*. Prediction tree for severely head-injured patients. *J Neurosurg* 1991; **75**: 251–5.

8. Williams M, Simms HH. Prognostic usefulness of scoring systems in critically ill patients with severe acute pancreatitis. *Crit Care Med* 1999; **27**: 901–7.

9. British Thoracic Society. Community acquired pneumonia in adults in British hospitals in 1982–1983. *Q J Med* 1987; **62**: 195–220.

10. Rowan KM, Kerr JH, Major E. ICS Apache II study in Britain and Ireland II. Outcome comparisons. *BMJ* 1993; **307**: 977–81.

11. Metnitz PG, Valentin A, Vesely H, *et al*. Prognostic performance and customization of the SAPS II: results of a multicenter Austrian study. Simplified Acute Physiology Score. *Intensive Care Med* 1999; **25**: 192–7.

12. Higgins TL. Daily versus admission mortality estimates: is admission severity yesterday's news? *Crit Care Med* 2001; **29**: 208–10.

13. Rue M, Quintana S, Alvarez M, Artigas A. Daily assessment of severity of illness and mortality prediction for individual patients. *Crit Care Med* 2001; **29**: 45–50.

14. Marks RJ, Simons RS, Blizzard RA, Browne DR. Predicting outcome in intensive therapy units – a comparison of Apache II with subjective assessments. *Intensive Care Med* 1991; **17**: 159–63.

15. Chelluri L, Pinsky MR. Long term outcome of critically ill elderly patients requiring intensive care. *JAMA* 1993; **269**: 3119–23.

16. Ip SP, Leung YF, Ip CY, Mak WP. Outcomes of critically ill elderly patients: is high-dependency care for geriatric patients worthwhile? *Crit Care Med* 1999; **27**: 2351–7.

17. Montuclard L, Garrouste-Orgeas M, Timsit JF, *et al*. Outcome, functional autonomy, and quality of life of elderly patients with a long-term intensive care unit stay. *Crit Care Med* 2000; **28**: 3389–95.

18. The Hypothermia after Cardiac Arrest Study Group. Mild therapeutic hypothermia to improve the neurologic outcome after cardiac arrest. *N Engl J Med* 2202; **346**: 549–56.

19. Staudinger T, Stoiser B, Mullner M, *et al*. Outcome and prognostic factors in critically ill cancer patients admitted to the intensive care unit. *Crit Care Med* 2000; **28**: 1322–8.

20. Daly K, Beale R, Chang RW. Reduction in mortality after inappropriate early discharge from intensive care unit: logistic regression triage model. *BMJ* 2001; **322**: 1274–6.

2 Patient assessment

BERNARD RILEY

Viva topics

- How would you recognize a patient with acute airway obstruction and what are the options for treatment?
- How would you examine a patient described to you as being blue and breathless?
- Describe the essential components of formulating a daily management plan.
- How would you decide if a patient was safe to be discharged from High Dependency Care to general ward care?

INTRODUCTION

Critically ill patients may be encountered in all areas of the hospital, from the Accident and Emergency department to medical or surgical wards, operating theatres, recovery wards or critical care units. Patients may be referred by other doctors, ward nurses, physiotherapists or critical care outreach teams. Some may be acutely unwell to the point of requiring immediate resuscitation, whereas others may be relatively stable and require assessment and the formulation of a management plan to ensure continued progress towards full recovery. In either case the aim is to use a systematic approach to assessment to ensure that all immediately life-threatening problems are recognized and the correct treatment is started immediately. Critically ill patients often have multiple problems, and the use of a systematic approach reduces the risk of missed diagnoses and provides a framework for treatment when working under stressful conditions. You are interested in *all* the patient's problems and their responses to the treatments instigated. Documentation is vital, as shift working and frequent handovers provide ample opportunity for failures in communication. Each entry in the notes should be dated and timed, and the person making the entry should sign it legibly.

ASSESSMENT OF THE UNSTABLE PATIENT

Several systems have been recommended for use with particular types of patient, such as the Advanced Trauma Life

Table 2.1 *Immediate assessment*

A – Airway assessment and treatment if needed
B – Breathing assessment and treatment if needed
C – Circulation assessment and treatment if needed
D – Dysfunction of the central nervous system
E – Exposure sufficient to allow complete examination

Support (ATLS) system for trauma patients, or the Care of the Critically Ill Surgical Patient system for non-traumatic problems.[1,2] Both these systems point out that, taken in isolation, certain diseases causing airway obstruction kill more quickly than those causing only pulmonary dysfunction, and in turn these may kill more quickly than certain circulatory problems. This is not an absolute rule, but forms an excellent basis for initial assessment and management, particularly when one is working alone. The system is summarized in Table 2.1.

The process of ABC assessment in an acutely ill patient is predominantly clinical and follows the simple clinical pattern of *LOOK, LISTEN* and *FEEL.*

A – Airway

The first step in assessment is to talk to the patient. A patient who is able to respond appropriately must, at that moment, have control of their airway, and have adequate oxygenation, ventilation and cerebral circulation to be able to reply coherently.

LOOK for the presence of central cyanosis, an obstructed 'seesaw' pattern of respiration or abdominal breathing, the use of accessory muscles of respiration, tracheal tug, alteration in level of consciousness, and any obvious obstruction by foreign body or vomit.

LISTEN for abnormal sounds such as grunting, snoring, gurgling, hoarseness or stridor.

FEEL for air flow on inspiration and expiration.

If an obstruction is present then the immediate goal must be to obtain and secure the airway to allow oxygenation and ventilation. As soon as the airway is patent, high concentrations of oxygen should be administered. Simple methods are used first, such as chin lift, jaw thrust and suction to remove secretions. An oral Guedel airway may be inserted in obtunded patients, or a soft nasopharyngeal airway if the gag reflex is present. If simple methods are not successful then a definitive airway (a cuffed tube secured in the trachea) is required. Such endotracheal tubes may be passed orally or nasally, but the oral route with the larynx visualized by direct laryngoscopy using a laryngoscope is the most usual choice. If the patient is in extremis then this may be accomplished without the use of drugs, but where the patient is responsive and endotracheal intubation is indicated, anaesthetic help is required. **Attempts at intubation without first preoxygenating the patient are futile and dangerous.** Patients can be oxygenated with an airway plus bag and mask ventilation as required while waiting for the anaesthetist – this is often a better option for the non-expert, particularly in hospital, where skilled help is usually rapidly available. If endotracheal intubation is unsuccessful then a surgical airway should be performed, with cricothyroidotomy being the method of choice. If there is a risk of coexisting pathology of the cervical spine than all airway manoeuvres should be performed while maintaining manual inline immobilization of the cervical spine.

B – Breathing

A respiratory rate less than 12 or more than 30 breaths/min, inability to speak in complete sentences because of breathlessness, or breathlessness at rest are all sinister signs of impending respiratory failure.

LOOK for central cyanosis, use of accessory muscles of respiration, high or low respiratory rate, equality and depth of respiration, sweating, raised jugular venous pressure (JVP), patency of any chest drains, and the presence of any paradoxical abdominal or chest wall movement. Note the inspired oxygen concentration (FiO_2) and saturation if pulse oximetry is in use, but remember that pulse oximetry does not detect hypercarbia.

LISTEN for noisy breathing, audible wheeze, clearance of secretions by coughing, ability of the patient to talk in complete sentences (evidence of confusion or decreased level of consciousness may indicate hypoxia or hypercarbia, respectively) and change in percussion note, and auscultate for abnormal breath sounds, heart sounds and rhythm.

FEEL for equality of chest movement, position of the trachea, the presence of surgical emphysema or crepitus,

paradoxical respiration and tactile vocal fremitus if indicated. Percuss the chest superiorly, laterally, and at the lung bases. Abdominal distension may limit diaphragmatic movement and in this respect is part of respiratory assessment.

The best treatment will be determined by the cause and severity of the respiratory failure. During the immediate assessment you should specifically look for signs of the immediately life-threatening conditions of tension pneumothorax, massive haemothorax, open pneumothorax, flail chest and cardiac tamponade, and provide immediate appropriate treatment. Remember that chest drains may become dislodged or blocked, and that their presence does not exclude recurrent pneumothorax. Simple manoeuvres such as sitting the patient up can help, but if the patient is tiring to the point of respiratory arrest then assisted ventilation by bagging may be necessary until help arrives.

C – Circulation

ALL shocked surgical patients should be assumed to be hypovolaemic until proved otherwise.

LOOK for:

- Reduced peripheral perfusion (pallor, coolness, collapsed or under-filled veins) – remember: blood pressure may be *normal* in the shocked patient
- Obvious external haemorrhage from either wounds or drains
- Evidence of concealed haemorrhage into the abdomen, pelvis, soft tissues or thorax. An empty drain does not exclude the presence of concealed bleeding.

LISTEN to the heart sounds: a gallop rhythm, quiet heart sounds or a new murmur may indicate a primary cardiac problem.

FEEL for peripheral and central pulses, assessing volume, equality and rhythm.

Unless there are obvious signs of cardiogenic shock (e.g. raised JVP and gallop rhythm) venous access with a 16 G cannula should be obtained, blood sent for cross-matching and other routine tests, including clotting screen, and appropriate fluid replacement started: a rapid fluid challenge of 10 mL/kg of warmed crystalloid in the normotensive patient or 20 mL/kg if the patient is hypotensive. Patients with known heart failure should receive an initial bolus of 5 mL/kg, and closer monitoring may be needed.

If the patient is actively bleeding from a non-compressible source, then the correct treatment is surgical control. Fluid resuscitation should be maintained at levels to maintain organ perfusion while surgery is being arranged.

Table 2.2 *AVPU mnemonic*

A – Alert and orientated
V – Vocalizing
P – Responding only to pain
U – Unconscious

D – Dysfunction of the central nervous system

A rapid assessment of the CNS may be obtained using the mnemonic AVPU – see Table 2.2.

If time permits, a full Glasgow Coma Score (GCS) should be performed as this is a more repeatable and objective measurement of consciousness. Alteration of conscious level may be due to causes other than a primary brain injury. Hypoxia, hypercarbia, cerebral underperfusion, sedatives or opioid drugs may be responsible. Metabolic or endocrine causes should also be considered, notably hypoglycaemia, uraemia or hypothyroidism. If the diagnosis is not obvious, review the ABCs.

E – Exposure

The patient must be exposed to allow full examination, and the environment should be warm to prevent hypothermia. There should be adequate light, and preserving the patient's privacy by the use of screens is essential. If intimate examinations are planned then a chaperone is required and, where possible, the patient's consent obtained.

At the end of the initial assessment the patient should hopefully have a secure airway, with adequate oxygenation, ventilation and circulation. During the initial assessment the best use should be made of any assistance available. Commence monitoring of vital signs, including pulse, blood pressure, temperature, urine output and pulse oximetry. At this stage consider the need for specialist help and advice, the requirement for additional investigations, and the level of care the patient needs.

ASSESSMENT OF LEVEL OF CARE REQUIRED

Increasingly patients are treated in several distinct areas in the hospital, depending on the severity of their illness. Often these areas are isolated from the specialty wards where stable patients are managed. This has resulted in the development of guidelines for admission and discharge to critical care areas, and the definition of different levels of care (Table 2.3).

Table 2.3 *Levels of care (see www.doh.gov.uk/nhsexec. compcritcare.htm)*

Level	Patients whose needs can be met on a normal acute ward
Level 1	Patients at risk of deterioration, 'step-down' from a higher level of care whose needs can be met on an acute ward with additional advice and support from CCOT
Level 2	Patients requiring more detailed support for single system failure or requiring 'step-down' care
Level 3	Patients requiring advanced respiratory support alone or basic respiratory support together with two other system failures

In general terms the level of care required is determined by the patient's underlying pathology, their medical comorbidity, response to immediate assessment and resuscitation, the likelihood of any deterioration, and the need for preoptimization prior to surgery or for complex postoperative care. In the UK a multidisciplinary working party established criteria for who should be admitted to critical care areas based on the concept of organ systems failure. These were published by the Department of Health in 1996 as *Guidelines on admission to and discharge from intensive care and high dependency units.*[3] The document recommends admission for the following types of patient:

- Patients requiring, or likely to require, advanced respiratory support alone
- Patients requiring support of two or more organ systems
- Patients with comorbidity who require support for an acute reversible failure of another organ system.

Certain types of organ system support (Table 2.4) are only available in specialist centres, e.g. neurosurgery or cardiac surgery, and in this case the patient must be safely transferred to the appropriate unit. The decision to admit or transfer is not one that should be carried out by junior medical staff. The referral should ideally be on a consultant to consultant basis, and no patient should be admitted or refused admission except after discussion with the ICU consultant, one of whom must be available 24 hours a day. The reversibility of the patient's illness must be considered. If it is non-reversible and incompatible with life then the patient should not be admitted. Such decisions are not easily made, and occasionally it is necessary to admit the patient and treat them appropriately for a time and assess any response. Intensive care cannot reverse chronic ill health, and where a patient has significant comorbidity to severely limit their quality and length of life then this may make admission inappropriate. Some patients adapt to comorbidity to the extent that they accept

Table 2.4 *Categories of organ support*

1 Advanced respiratory support

Mechanical ventilatory support (excluding mask continuous positive pressure (CPAP) or non-invasive ventilation)

The possibility of sudden deterioration in respiratory function requires immediate intubation and mechanical ventilation

2 Basic respiratory monitoring and support

The need for more than 40 per cent oxygen

The possibility of progressive deterioration to the point of needing advanced respiratory support

The need for physiotherapy to clear secretions at least 2-hourly

Patients recently extubated after a prolonged period of intubation and ventilation

The need for mask CPAP or non-invasive ventilation

Patients who are intubated to protect their airway but do not need ventilation

3 Circulatory support

The need for vasoactive drugs

Support for circulatory instability due to hypovolaemia from any cause unresponsive to modest volume replacement

Patients resuscitated after cardiac arrest where ICU or HDU care is considered clinically appropriate

4 Neurological monitoring or support

Central nervous system depression sufficient to compromise the airway and protective reflexes

Invasive neurological monitoring

5 Renal support

The need for acute renal replacement therapy

a quality of life that others would regard as unendurable. Denying such patients admission based on the presence of comorbidity alone is difficult to justify, and the patient's views must be respected. The consultant must discuss with them, and their relatives, the range of treatment options and possible outcomes. Where a patient has made an advance directive ('living will') then its contents must be respected.

ASSESSMENT OF THE STABLE PATIENT

Once the patient has been stabilized in a critical care area, they may remain seriously ill but the priorities for daily management are less urgent. A twice-daily visit is necessary to allow thorough examination of the patient and planning to ensure continued progress. The condition of a patient may change dramatically throughout the day, and re-examination and reassessment are the best way to detect early signs of failure to progress. After the clinical examination, the case notes, daily observation charts, fluid charts and X-rays must be reviewed

with the patient's nurse in order to identify any active problems and formulate a plan for the day aimed at ensuring continued progress. Specific patients will have specific problems depending on the nature of the underlying pathology, but all patients have certain potential problem areas, and a systematic review should consider the following points:

- **A – Airway** Is the airway patent or at risk? What do I need to do to secure it? Is the cervical spine at risk? If the patient is intubated, what is the size and length of endotracheal tube? What is the position of the tube? How long has it been in place? Should it be replaced by a tracheostomy? What type of tracheostomy tube? Security of tube? What is coming up the tube? Is the cuff pressure within acceptable limits?
- **B – Breathing** Spontaneous ventilation – rate, depth, character etc? Mechanical ventilation: what is the mode and what are the settings? Inspired oxygen concentration? PEEP (positive end-expiratory pressure) or CPAP (continuous positive airway pressure) level? Position of patient? Clinical examination findings? Arterial blood gas analysis? Chest X-ray or other imaging? Presence and patency of any chest drains? Is drain suction required? Does the patient still need the drain?
- **C – Circulation** ECG, pulse, blood pressure, CVP? Haemodynamic data, e.g. cardiac index, systemic vascular resistance index (SVRI), pulmonary vascular resisitance index (PVRI), wedge pressure etc? Inotropes or other vasoactive agents? Heart sounds? Any new murmurs? Fluid balance, plasma osmolarity? Peripheral circulation/oedema? Any indication for pulmonary artery catheter, oesophageal Doppler or echocardiography?
- **D – Disability/depth of sedation** Sedation score or GCS? What sedation agents should be used, and in what dose? Can the sedation be reduced? Focal neurology? Pupils? Fitting? Cerebral function monitors? Other specialized neurological monitors, e.g. intracranial pressure (ICP), jugular bulb saturation or transcranial Doppler? Any indication for reimaging?
- **E – Equipment** Is it all working, calibrated and accurate? Is there any other monitoring that would safely provide useful information? Is it in the right place, e.g. nasogastric (NG) tubes in the stomach, CVP line tip not below the level of the carina or in the atrium, etc?
- **F – Fluids** How much and what fluid to give? Fluid balance 24 hours/cumulative? Fluid output from where? Fistulae, drains, wounds? What quality and quantity?
- **G – Gut** Is it working? Can I use it to feed the patient? Is there gastric stasis? Are prokinetics required? Dietary supplements/stress ulcer prophylaxis? NG tube

aspirate/drainage? Does the patient require antiemetics, aperients or other drug therapy? Wounds healing or not? Skin sutures or clip removal? Stomas – viable, working or not? Bowel sounds present or bowels working? Distended abdomen – is it gas, fluid or blood? Is there any evidence of abdominal compartment syndrome?

- **H – Haematology** Check *all* blood results, haematology, clotting, biochemistry and serology. Is there any additional blood test that can help? Is transfusion required? What is an appropriate transfusion trigger for this patient?
- **I – Imaging** X-rays? Ultrasound, CT scanning? MRI? Echocardiography (transthoracic or oesophageal)? Doppler? Nuclear medicine?
- **J – Joints and limbs** Fractures, dislocations, other trauma? Deep vein thrombosis (DVT), appropriate prophylaxis, mechanical or low molecular weight heparin? Is DVT prophylaxis contraindicated? Peripheral pulses, perfusion and compartment syndrome? Any evidence of missed orthopaedic injury? Are any splints or immobilization/ elevation devices required?
- **K – Kelvin** Temperature and temperature chart?
- **L – Lines** Examine all lines, intravenous, intra-arterial and others, and ask: When placed? Where placed? Are they necessary? Replacement or removal – send tip to microbiology. Signs of sepsis? Blood cultures from lines?
- **M – Microbiology** Aggressive microbiological surveillance: swabs, blood cultures, sputum – bronchoalveolar lavage or undirected catheter lavage is better than simple sputum sampling – drain fluid, urine, removed line tips. Strict asepsis and cross-infection avoidance – Touch a patient, wash your hands! Always wear gloves and an apron when examining patients. Isolate patients with resistant organisms if possible. Check results daily. Directed antimicrobial therapy only. Antibiotic levels, doses and course duration? Make friends with your microbiologist: joint daily ward rounds
- **N – Nutrition** All patients need feeding. Enteral nutrition is best. NG feeding, oral, percutaneous gastrostomy, jejunal feeding, intravenous feeding? Check trace elements and maintain good control of blood sugar
- **O – Other consultants** Nobody knows everything: arrange appropriate specialist opinions. Let the patient's GP and hospital consultant know one of their patients is on ICU
- **P – Pain relief, psychological support, prescriptions** Prescribe analgesia by appropriate routes, intervals and doses. Talk to your patient always, even if they have a depressed level of consciousness. Explain procedures simply and carefully. Sedation and psychotropic drugs if indicated. Check drug charts to ensure the right dose of any drug in patients with disordered metabolism

- **Q – Question** If you are unsure of what to do, ask your consultant. You should never undertake a task for which you have been inadequately trained. If you decide to perform a new test or investigation, ask yourself whether it will influence the patient's management
- **R – Relatives** Keep relatives fully informed, be honest when discussing prognosis, ask for information on past medical history and daily activity if appropriate. Always hold discussions away from the bedside unless the patient is fully aware/autonomous and can participate. Always hold discussions with the patient's nurse present, and document your comments
- **S – Skin** Examine skin for perfusion, wounds, and signs of systemic disease or infection. Pressure area care, mouth care, etc.
- **T – Trauma and transport** Many trauma patients require multidisciplinary management. Trauma patients may not have had a complete secondary survey; late diagnosis of unrecognized problems may cause significant morbidity and mortality. You must be aware of the potential for missed injury. Trust no-one: look at all the X-rays yourself. Transport of ICU patients within or between hospitals requires the same level of care and monitoring that they receive on the ICU itself
- **U – Universal precautions** The plethora of infectious diseases transmitted by blood and other bodily fluids means that all staff should be aware of the necessity for wearing gloves, aprons, and occasionally faceguards when performing invasive procedures
- **V – Visitors** These may be the patient's relatives or other medical personnel involved in the patient's care. Visiting colleagues should be treated with respect and courtesy, but ultimately all changes to therapy must be discussed with the ICU consultant
- **W – What to do** Once the patient has been fully assessed you must formulate a plan to deal with the patient's problems. This plan must be documented clearly in the notes and discussed with the bedside nurse. Parameters must be agreed within which the nurse is able to vary the components of the therapeutic regimen according to the patient's response, and outside which you need to reassess the patient. Time is an important part of your plan, and regular reassessment is essential
- **Y – Why?** Every time you review the patient ask yourself why they were admitted and what are their active problems are now. Keep on track and forget nothing!

Chart review (Table 2.5)

Critically ill patients can change their physiological status very quickly, and the majority of the parameters measured in ICU are displayed on large-scale paper charts on an hourly basis. Modern electronic data capture allows you to zoom in or out in time to identify more acute changes or longer trends. The doctor must be familiar with the equipment and documentation used in the unit. Accurate chart review is an essential part of patient assessment and treatment planning. Any changes to treatment must be accurately and contemporaneously recorded so that their effects can be observed. The charts should be examined systematically so that all records are scrutinized. If you use the ABCD system of clinical assessment it is logical to use a similar system when analysing the charts. You should remember that *trends* are often more informative than single observations. You may need to look at the previous day's charts in addition to today's, or review the ward charts if this is the patient's first day in a critical care area.

Plan for the day (Table 2.6)

The daily plan should aim to deal with any active problems or, if the patient is stable, to progress to the next stage of treatment. The precise plan should be discussed with the patient's nurse and recorded in the notes. If the nurse is

Table 2.5 *Systematic chart review*

A – Type of tube, cuff pressures, duration of intubation, etc.

B – Mode of ventilation, FiO_2, tidal volumes, PEEP, saturation and blood gases

C – Pulse rate, blood pressure, CVP, PA readings, vasoactive drugs, fluids etc.

D – Sedation or Glasgow Coma Score, pupil size and reactivity, ICP etc.

E – Equipment in use and need for additional investigation

F – Fluid balance and fluid prescriptions, drainage etc.

G – Gastrointestinal losses and nutrition

H – Haematology and biochemistry

I – Imaging results

Table 2.6 *Example of daily management plan*

- Wean from respiratory support – BiPaP/ASB to ASB/CPAP
- Accept $PaCO_2$ between 5.5 and 6.5 kPa
- Accept PaO_2 if $SaO_2 > 90$ per cent
- Reduce epinephrine if MAP > 75 mmHg and CVP > 10
- Repeat chest X-ray
- Stop antibiotics after 1400-hour dose
- Call me (bleep 4691) if chest drainage > 100 mL/h for 2 hours

empowered to titrate therapy against patient response, e.g. rate of infusion of inotropes against mean arterial pressure, then parameters may be set to guide treatment.

The daily assessment and management plan should be clearly written in the notes. Shift changes frequently mean that the results of your plan will often be assessed by a doctor other than yourself. Where the plan looks for a relatively immediate response, e.g. the effect of a fluid challenge on urine output, you must set a time for reassessment and stick to it. Agree success/failure criteria with the nurse and establish recall criteria if you do not intend to routinely return to assess the results of the plan.

ASSESSMENT OF THE PATIENT FOR DISCHARGE (TABLE 2.7)

The decision to reduce the level of care is not always obvious. The patient should be discharged when the condition(s) that necessitated their admission have been successfully treated and they no longer have 1 or 2 types of organ failure. They should be discharged to an appropriate level of care. It is unusual for an ICU patient to be discharged directly to the ward without receiving a period of 'step-down' high-dependency care within the ICU or on a separate high-dependency unit (HDU) to determine that their clinical course is evolving satisfactory. Thereafter they may be discharged to Level 1 care on a suitable ward, as determined by their clinical condition.

It should be remembered that not all ICU patients survive to discharge and that approximately 23 per cent die on the unit. The majority die as a result of withdrawal of life-sustaining treatment in the face of continued deterioration despite maximal appropriate supportive therapy. In such patients palliative, compassionate care should be continued on the ICU if their death is imminent, but where death is

Table 2.7 *Criteria for discharge to Level 1 care*

- No requirement for advanced respiratory support
- Acceptable arterial gases on less than 40 per cent oxygen
- Improving respiratory status with no risk to airway (or tracheostomy *in situ*)
- No requirement for vasoactive drugs
- Haemodynamically normal
- No CNS depression sufficient to compromise airway/gag reflex unless tracheostomy in situ
- No need for renal support
- Analgesia achieved by ward based means
- No requirement for advanced nutritional support

inevitable but likely to be delayed, they should be transferred to a non-ICU/HDU area for terminal care.

ASSESSMENT OF THE PATIENT AFTER DISCHARGE

The discharge criteria listed in Table 2.7 represent the ideal, but in the real world the demand for Level 3 and 2 beds often means that patients are discharged to Level 1 beds before these criteria are met. In such cases the expertise of the critical care area should be exported to follow the patient. In the majority of hospitals this is achieved by some form of Critical Care Outreach Team (CCOT). One of the functions of CCOT is to follow up recently discharged ICU patients and to monitor their condition post discharge to ensure that they continue to make satisfactory progress.

In addition to following up patients after discharge from critical care areas, CCOT allows the early detection of sick patients in Level 1 beds and aims to intervene to provide effective treatment to pre-empt admission to critical care. Goldhill *et al.*[4] investigated physiological parameters for ward patients in the 24 hours prior to admission to ITU. This data was collected over 13 months from 76 patients at the Royal London Hospital. The authors found that respiratory rate, pulse and oxygen saturation were the most important physiological indicators of critical illness; 27 patients (34 per cent) underwent cardiopulmonary resuscitation prior to admission to ITU. Respiratory rate was markedly elevated in the 24 hours prior to admission, but although tachycardia was a useful sign it did not predict the need for intensive care. It is possible to formulate a series of physiological 'tripwires' that mark the limits of abnormality beyond which a response aimed at preventing further deterioration should be triggered. Such systems should be reliable, sensitive, specific and user friendly to ensure they are used consistently and effectively. The initial call-out of the team may be provoked by focus criteria alone, or by a numerical score above a certain level. Focus criteria enable direction of the scoring systems to the patients most likely to benefit from them, thereby increasing the specificity of the system. This prevents the CCOT system from being swamped with unnecessary calls and the ward staff from the pointless task of undertaking scoring on patients who are not in any danger. This should initiate a specific response of calling the patient's own medical team, followed by the outreach team. Focus criteria vary widely from system to system, and often include cardiorespiratory arrest, depressed level of consciousness, post-ICU discharge, pancreatitis, post major surgery, multiple trauma, and the catch-all – any patient causing concern to medical, nursing or physiotherapy staff. The Nottingham CCOT system has specific documentation to aid the calculation of the CCOT score (Appendix 1) and an algorithm to help the ward staff to choose the response most likely to help the patient (Appendix 2). The scoring system enables non-medical staff to identify the objective signs of deterioration from simple clinical assessments.

SUMMARY

The use of a systematic method of assessment aims to minimize the possibility of overlooking serious pathology, particularly where multiple organ systems are involved. When dealing with the acutely ill patient the aim is to identify and treat the greatest threat to life. Once the patient is stabilized a plan is formulated to deal with their active problems after detailed examination and review of all relevant charts and investigations. Repeated reassessment and a rapid response to the early signs of clinical deterioration is aimed at minimizing the effects of the underlying disease processes and promoting recovery. The current system recommended by the Royal College of Surgeons of England (Figure 2.1) was developed primarily for use in Level 1 and 2 areas but forms a sound basis for use in Level 3 areas of critical care.

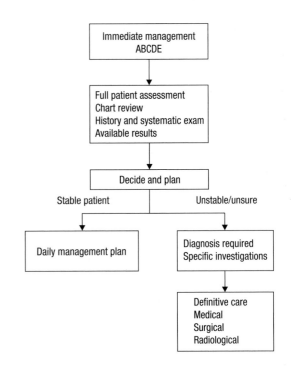

Figure 2.1 Summary of patient assessment

REFERENCES

1. American College of Surgeons. *Advanced trauma life support for doctors*. Chicago: American College of Surgeons, 1997.

2. Anderson ID. (ed.) *Care of the critically ill surgical patient*. London: Arnold, 1999.

3. National Health Service Executive (NHSE). *Guidelines on admission to and discharge from ITU and HDU*. London: Department of Health, 1996.

4. Goldhill DR, White SA, Sumner A. Physiological values and procedures in the 24 hours before ICU admission from the ward. *Anaesthesia* 1999; **54:** 529–34.

APPENDIX 1: CCOT RISK SCORING GUIDELINES

CCOT risk scoring should commence on the following patients:

Any patient:

- Following surgery (all large incisions)
- With peritonitis
- With pancreatitis: If nil by mouth, IVI and urinary catheter
- With obstructive jaundice post percutaneous choliangiography, drainage or instrumentation of the biliary tract
- Following ITU/SHDU discharge
- With chest injury: rib fractures, fractured sternum or lung contusions.

OR

At any time patient condition causes concern.

The following patients should be referred immediately to CCOT/ITU and CCOT risk scoring should be commenced:

Any patient:

- With a compromised airway
- With GCS ≤ 12
- On >60 per cent O_2 **or** With progressive increases in O_2 requirements
- With arterial blood gas analysis showing: pH ≤ 7.2 or ≥ 7.55; $PaO_2 < 8.0\,kPa$; $PaCO_2 > 6.5\,kPa$

OR

At any time that urgent help is needed.

Contact CCOT pager. . . .

APPENDIX 2: CCOT SCORE CHART AND ALGORITHM

Score	3	2	1	0	1	2	3
HR	<40	41–50		51–100	101–110	111–129	≥130
RR	≤ 8			9–14	15–20	21–29	≥30
Temp	<35			35–38.4		38.5–39	>39
Sys. BP	<80	81–90	91–100	101–199			≥200
CNS				Alert	Voice	Pain	Unconscious
Urine	NIL	<20 mL/h					>400 mL/h

Please enter CCOT risk scores below

Date																				
Time																				
HR																				
RR																				
Temp																				
BP CNS																				
Urine																				
Total Score																				
JHO called@																				
CCOT called@																				

If:

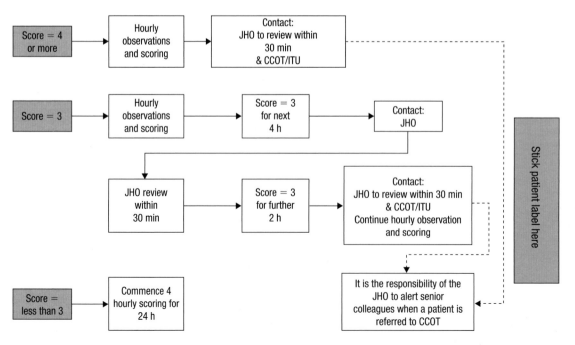

3 Respiratory support

SIMON WHARTON & ROSLYN PURCELL

INTRODUCTION

Respiratory failure remains the principal reason for the vast majority of admissions to intensive care. This chapter will cover a number of important themes. An understanding of the pathophysiology of respiratory failure and objectives of respiratory support is essential in the management of critically ill patients. Because the majority of such patients require respiratory support, the indications for invasive and non-invasive ventilation, the physiological effects and potential complications of mechanical ventilation need to be understood in addition to the different modes of ventilation available and the ventilatory strategies that are used in particular disease states. Weaning a patient following a protracted period of mechanical ventilation may require specific strategies and understanding. The percutaneous tracheostomy

Table 3.1 *Types of respiratory failure*

Ventilatory
Hypoventilation
    Depressed respiratory drive
    Neuromuscular weakness
Ventilation–perfusion mismatch (V/Q mismatch)
    Increased alveolar dead space
    Shunt
Increased impedance to ventilation

Hypoxic
V/Q mismatch
Hypoventilation
Diffusion impairment
Inadequate FiO_2 (only important at altitude)

has become a standard part of critical care management of patients with respiratory failure in recent years, and the indications for and complications of percutaneous tracheostomy will be described.

RESPIRATORY FAILURE – A PHYSIOLOGICAL BACKGROUND

To facilitate the diagnosis of the various causes of acute respiratory failure in ICU and to formulate a treatment plan the relevant physiology will be reviewed briefly (Table 3.1).

HYPOVENTILATION

If hypoventilation is the cause of hypoxia, arterial blood gases (ABG) will *always* reveal an elevated $PaCO_2$; hypoxaemia is generally not severe and can easily be abolished by the administration of supplemental oxygen.

The causes of hypoventilation include:

- Depression of the respiratory centre (e.g. opioid or benzodiazepine overdose)
- High spinal injuries

● Neuromuscular disease (e.g. Guillain–Barré, myasthenia gravis, muscular dystrophy).

The alveolar gas equation may be useful as it allows measurement of the ideal alveolar partial pressure of oxygen (P_AO_2) that the lung would have if there were no V/Q inequality to be calculated. The alveolar–arterial PO_2 gradient (A–a gradient) can then be calculated. The normal value is 2 kPa (15 mmHg). If the A–a gradient is normal, the hypoxia is due to hypoventilation. If the gradient is increased, the hypoxia is due to some form of V/Q mismatch (lung collapse, consolidation).

The alveolar gas equation is as follows:

$$P_AO_2 = P_iO_2 - (P_ACO_2/RQ)$$

When using this equation, a number of assumptions are made. First, RQ stands for the respiratory quotient. This is the ratio of oxygen consumed to carbon dioxide produced and normally has a value of 0.8. However, this value may be altered, classically by a change in diet. Thus, if the diet is changed to being based principally on carbohydrates, the amount of carbon dioxide produced increases to bring the ratio to nearer 1.0. Second, under normal conditions the arterial carbon dioxide tension $PaCO_2$ is very close to the alveolar carbon dioxide tension P_ACO_2. Third, PiO_2 is the inspired partial pressure of oxygen and is affected by both the barometric pressure and the inspired fractional concentration of oxygen, as given by:

$$PiO_2 = P_B \times FiO_2$$

However, this expression also needs to take into account the dilution of oxygen in inspired gas, as the gas is fully saturated in the upper airways.

$$PiO_{2(sat)} = (P_B - P_{H_2O}) \times FiO_2$$

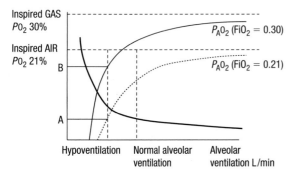

Alveolar PO_2 and PCO_2 (kPa)

Inspired GAS PO_2 30%

P_AO_2 (FiO_2 = 0.30)

Inspired AIR PO_2 21%

B

P_AO_2 (FiO_2 = 0.21)

A

Hypoventilation   Normal alveolar   Alveolar
ventilation   ventilation L/min

Figure 3.1 Relationship between alveolar ventilation and alveolar gases for inspired oxygen concentrations of 21 per cent and 30 per cent during hypoventilation and normal tidal ventilation

Using the alveolar gas equation, the relationship between alveolar ventilation and the alveolar gases can be determined and this is shown in Figure 3.1. It can be seen that hypoventilation will rapidly result in hypoxia, but will be easily corrected by a small increase in the inspired oxygen fraction moving the alveolar PO_2 from point A to point B in the figure.

PULMONARY CAPILLARY PO_2 AND PCO_2

Two factors determine pulmonary capillary PO_2 and PCO_2 in disease states. These are the ventilation–perfusion relationships (V/Q ratio) and impairments to diffusion.

Ventilation–perfusion mismatch

In the normal lung, when standing, from apex to base:

● Ventilation increases ~ 3×
● Perfusion increases ~ 12×.

Therefore, V/Q ratios vary from high values at the apex to low values at the base. The mean value is 0.8.

● Regions with ventilation but no perfusion contribute to *alveolar dead space*
● Regions with no ventilation but perfusion contribute to *shunt*.

The same relationship is true for the lungs in the supine position, but the changes are less marked. V/Q mismatch is an expression that accounts for an increase in either dead space or shunt. This can result in both hypoxia and hypercapnia, and may be caused by a wide variety of disease states.

Dead space is defined as that part of inspired gas that does not take part in gas exchange owing to reduced or absent perfusion of certain areas. Ventilation in these areas is wasted. Dead space is comprised of anatomic dead space (e.g. airways proximal to the respiratory bronchioles) and alveolar dead space (regions of the lung with high V/Q ratios).

The causes of dead space are:

● An abrupt decrease in cardiac output
● Pulmonary embolism, whether due to thrombus, fat, air or amniotic fluid
● ARDS due to intense pulmonary vasoconstriction
● Excessive positive end-expiratory pressure.

An increase in dead space ventilation primarily affects carbon dioxide elimination and will have little effect on arterial oxygenation until the dead space ventilation exceeds 80–90 per cent of the minute ventilation.

Shunt is defined as the blood returning to the arterial circulation that has not passed through ventilated regions of the lungs, and which therefore has not taken part in gas exchange. Physiologic shunt is the term used to describe the effects of both true shunt (anatomical shunt) and regions with low V/Q ratios.

The causes of shunt are:

- Consolidation
- Pulmonary contusion
- Atelectasis
- Pulmonary oedema
- Extrapulmonary shunts (congenital heart disease).

Whereas dead space primarily affects carbon dioxide elimination, shunt primarily inhibits arterial oxygenation and is the predominant cause of hypoxaemia in disease. Blood that is passing through areas of absolute shunt receives no oxygen, and therefore arterial hypoxaemia resulting from absolute shunt is not reversed by the administration of supplemental oxygen. However, rather than absolute shunt the more common clinical phenomenon is that of venous admixture, which occurs where there is deficient alveolar ventilation compared to the degree of perfusion but ventilation is not completely absent. In this situation supplemental oxygen may increase the PaO_2.

Diffusion impairment

This occurs when the blood–gas barrier is so thickened that equilibration between the PO_2 in pulmonary capillary blood and alveolar gas does not occur. Diseases in which diffusion impairment causes hypoxia include cardiac failure, pulmonary fibrosis, interstitial pneumonia, emphysema and connective tissue diseases such as Wegener's granulomatosis and Goodpasture's syndrome. However, although diffusion impairment may be present in patients with these diseases V/Q mismatch still is the most significant contributor to hypoxaemia.

The contribution of diffusion impairment to hypoxaemia in patients is uncertain. Any hypoxaemia caused by diffusion impairment can readily be corrected by oxygen therapy.

INCREASED IMPEDANCE TO VENTILATION

The important impedances to ventilation are:

- Elastic recoil of the lungs and chest wall
- Resistance to gas flow in the airways.

In a normal adult the compliances (the volume change per unit pressure change) of the lungs and chest wall are about the same ($100\,mL/cmH_2O$). In intensive care patients with acute respiratory failure there is frequently a decrease in compliance. This is due mainly to a decrease in the volume of ventilated lung, and not to changes in lung elasticity. The causes of decreased compliance include:

- Decreased lung compliance
  - Pulmonary oedema
  - Consolidation
  - Collapse
- Decreased chest wall compliance
  - Burns
  - Pleural effusions
  - Abdominal distension (which leads to basal atelectasis).

The consequence of a decrease in either chest or lung compliance is a reduction in the functional residual capacity (FRC). The FRC is defined as the volume of gas remaining in the lungs at the end of expiration during normal breathing. The FRC functions essentially as the 'oxygen store'. If oxygen requirements are increased, for example due to sepsis and high basal metabolic rates, this may contribute to both hypoxia, as the lung now has less oxygen storage capacity, and hypercapnia.

The other contributing factor to increased impedance is an increase in airways resistance. The causes of increased airways resistance include:

- Bronchospasm
- Mucosal oedema
- Secretions
- Loss of elastic recoil (as in chronic obstructive pulmonary disease, COPD).

The consequence of high airway resistance is a delay in emptying of the alveoli during the expiratory phase, leading to intrinsic positive end-expiratory pressure (PEEP) (discussed later in the chapter). In addition, there may be extrinsic causes of increased resistance, which include the presence of tracheal or tracheostomy tubes and their connections.[1]

GOALS OF RESPIRATORY SUPPORT

The goals of respiratory support are:

- Treatment of hypoxia (and its cause)
- To decrease the work of breathing.

  Treatment includes:

- Improvement of oxygen delivery
- Removal of secretions
- Ventilatory support.

Pharmacological treatment for respiratory disease is beyond the scope of this chapter.

IMPROVEMENT OF OXYGEN DELIVERY

The PO_2 is only one determinant of oxygen delivery to the tissues. The others are the cardiac output, haemoglobin, and the affinity of haemoglobin for oxygen.

$$O_2 \text{ delivery} = \text{Cardiac output} \times \text{arterial } O_2 \text{ content}$$
$$= 5000 \, \text{mL/min} \times (Hb \times SaO_2 \times 1.34$$
$$+ PO_2 \times 0.023) = 1000 \, \text{mL/min}.$$

Oxygen consumption is $\sim$250 mL/min, so venous blood is $\sim$75 per cent saturated.

where PO_2 is given in kPa. The value 1.34 is the Huffner coefficient for the binding of oxygen to haemoglobin.

Four factors can result in tissue hypoxia:

1 Low cardiac output → stagnant hypoxia
2 Decreased O_2 saturation → hypoxic hypoxia
3 Low Hb → anaemic hypoxia
4 Inability to utilize oxygen → histotoxic hypoxia (CO poisoning).

SO HOW IS OXYGENATION IMPROVED?

1 Administration of supplemental oxygen
2 Application of continuous positive airway pressure (CPAP) and positive end-expiratory pressure (PEEP)
3 Optimization of the cardiac output
4 Ensuring the haemoglobin level is adequate
5 Treatment of the underlying cause (e.g. infection, heart failure).

OXYGEN THERAPY

The response to oxygen therapy is very much dependent on the cause of hypoxia. For example, hypoxaemia due to hypoventilation is easily reversed by relatively low concentrations of oxygen, usually not more than 30 per cent. Hypoxia caused by diffusion impairment is also readily overcome by oxygen administration. The response to oxygen therapy in patients with V/Q mismatch depends upon its pattern. Patients who are hypoxaemic as a result of pure shunts respond poorly to oxygen therapy, as discussed above. Supplemental oxygen may be administered by a number of devices.

Fixed performance systems

These are devices that administer an FiO_2 that is independent of patient factors, principally the inspiratory flow rate.

● **High-flow Venturi masks** These can deliver a set concentration of oxygen, e.g. 28 per cent, 35 per cent, 40 per cent. The flow rate is set according to the FiO_2 chosen, entraining air at a fixed ratio to give a resultant flow rate of 40–60 L/min. At these high flow rates there is negligible rebreathing of expired gas and hence no CO_2 accumulation. In severely dyspnoeic patients who have very high peak inspiratory flow rates these masks may not deliver the intended FiO_2.
● **Low-flow sealed breathing circuits** These include anaesthesia and CPAP circuits. They incorporate a reservoir bag to deliver a set FiO_2 via an endotracheal tube or tight-fitting facemask.

Variable-performance systems

These are devices that deliver an FiO_2 that may vary depending on the patient's inspiratory flow.

● **Nasal cannulae** Usually used at low flow rates (2 L/min), resulting in O_2 concentrations of approximately 25–30 per cent. Because there is insufficient oxygen storage in the nasal passages, the FiO_2 of the next inspiration is dependent on the added oxygen flow and the peak inspiratory flow rate (PIFR).
● **Simple masks (Hudson mask)** The FiO_2 varies with the oxygen flow rate and the patient's ventilation, as for nasal cannulae. However, higher flow rates are tolerated and the maximum FiO_2 delivered is up to 0.6. Once again, as the patient's PIFR increases the FiO_2 decreases.
● **T-piece circuit** This is a simple, non-rebreathing circuit attached directly to an endotracheal or tracheostomy tube. Oxygen is delivered through one limb and expired gas leaves via the other. This can be a fixed-performance device if the fresh gas flow rate and the circuit volume are higher than the patient's PIFR.
● **Plastic masks with reservoir bag (trauma masks)** In this system oxygen is stored in the reservoir bag during expiration and this is made available by the movement of a simple flap valve, during the next inspiration. This allows delivery of a higher FiO_2 than using a simple mask with oxygen flows that can be generated by a standard wall oxygen delivery device.

HAZARDS OF OXYGEN THERAPY

- **CO_2 retention** A small proportion of patients with COPD are dependent on a hypoxic ventilatory drive. These patients have had a chronically raised $PaCO_2$ and the response of the chemoreceptors is obtunded. In this group of patients the administration of high concentrations of oxygen will result in respiratory depression with loss of consciousness. **It should be remembered that it is dangerous to withhold oxygen from patients who are severely hypoxic. The primary cause of death remains hypoxia, NOT hypercapnia.** Also, removal of oxygen from this group of patients may be hazardous. If ventilation is depressed by the administration of supplemental oxygen it will only increase when the blood oxygen tension has decreased again. In the meantime, carbon dioxide tensions will increase and may result in a decreased conscious level. If supplemental oxygen therapy results in decreased ventilation, assistance with mechanical ventilation, preferably non-invasively, should be given until the situation has been reviewed by senior personnel or is resolved.
- **Pulmonary oxygen toxicity** This is dependent on the duration of exposure and the concentration of oxygen. It is extremely difficult to differentiate oxygen toxicity from other causes of lung damage, because all patients requiring high concentrations of oxygen for prolonged periods have severe underlying lung disease. However, it is thought that high concentrations of oxygen deplete the normally protective antioxidants present in the respiratory tract, resulting in pulmonary oedema followed by fibrosis. It is not clear what oxygen concentrations are required for what duration to result in lung damage. However, it is a good principle that inspired oxygen fractions should be decreased as soon as is reasonable to prevent further lung damage.
- **Retrolental fibroplasia** In premature babies oxygen stimulates immature retinal vessels, resulting in proliferation, haemorrhage, retinal detachment and blindness. The absolute safe level of hyperoxia is unknown, but it is recommended that the FiO_2 be restricted to keep the PaO_2 between 8 and 10 kPa.

CONTINUOUS POSITIVE AIRWAY PRESSURE (CPAP) AND POSITIVE END-EXPIRATORY PRESSURE (PEEP)

PEEP is simply positive airway pressure at the end of expiration and is used in combination with mechanical

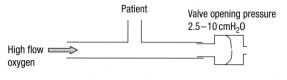

Figure 3.2 A typical CPAP circuit

ventilation. CPAP is a continuous application of pressure throughout the ventilatory cycle during spontaneous breathing (Figure 3.2). There is good evidence to support the use of CPAP in the treatment of patients with cardiogenic pulmonary oedema (CPO). Cardiogenic pulmonary oedema is characterized by interstitial and alveolar oedema, reduced lung compliance and increased work of breathing. This frequently results in hypoxia and, in severe cases, hypercapnia. The potential benefits of CPAP in CPO are correction of hypoxia, alveolar recruitment and a reduction in left ventricular afterload. Several randomized controlled trials support the use of CPAP in the treatment of CPO.[2] CPAP has been shown to significantly reduce the need for intubation and to reduce the length of hospital of stay.

All modes of ventilation may incorporate PEEP, the simplest method being to add a valve to the expiratory end of the breathing circuit that opens at a certain pressure. Commonly, PEEP valves are available that range from 2.5 to 10 cmH$_2$O pressure. PEEP is used both to improve oxygenation and to minimize injury to the lungs. It works by the following mechanisms:

- Recruits collapsed alveoli
- Increases functional residual capacity
- Decreases intrapulmonary shunt.

By reinflating collapsed areas of lung PEEP may improve lung compliance and reduce the work of breathing.

Inadequate amounts of PEEP may contribute to ventilator-induced lung injury (VILI) by permitting tidal opening and closing of alveoli. This creates shearing forces and the release of inflammatory mediators, which contribute to VILI.

Deleterious effects of PEEP

As PEEP increases intrathoracic pressure venous return is reduced, resulting in decreased cardiac output, and oxygen delivery may therefore actually decrease despite an improvement in PaO_2. Therefore, PEEP should be increased carefully, with appropriate monitoring of oxygen delivery and adverse haemodynamic effects.

OPTIMIZATION OF CARDIAC OUTPUT

Cardiac output measurement and optimization are dealt with in another chapter. Suffice to say here, that when oxygenation is the primary deficiency requiring correction, measurement of cardiac output with subsequent manipulation may be the principal intervention required.

OPTIMIZATION OF HAEMOGLOBIN

The optimal haemoglobin for oxygen delivery is contentious. Traditionally, it has been taught that the haemoglobin concentration should be maintained at greater than 10 g/dL. However, in recent years this concept has been examined in critically ill patients. From these studies it appears that there is no additional harm to critically ill patients in maintaining the Hb concentration at 7 g/dL or more (a so-called restrictive transfusion policy) compared to a traditional 10 g/dL transfusion trigger. This has also been shown to hold true in patients with cardiac disease.

VENTILATORY SUPPORT

Non-invasive ventilation

Non-invasive ventilation (NIV) is ventilatory support without endotracheal intubation or tracheostomy. The term incorporates bilevel positive airway pressure (BiPAP), pressure support ventilation (PSV) and non-invasive intermittent positive-pressure ventilation (NIPPV). The rationale behind the use of NIV is to avoid the disadvantages of conventional mechanical ventilation via an endotracheal tube (ETT), which include:

- Trauma to the upper airway
- Laryngeal or tracheal damage
- Patient discomfort
- Loss of verbal communication
- Need for sedation
- Ventilator-associated pneumonia.

NIV cannot be used for all patients with respiratory failure, and the contraindications are listed in Table 3.2.

Table 3.2 Contraindications to NIV

Inability to protect own airway (unconscious patient or those at high risk of aspiration)
Upper airway obstruction
Severe haemodynamic instability
Base of skull fracture (risk of pneumocephalus)

METHODS OF ACTION OF NON-INVASIVE VENTILATION

- Ability to deliver an increased FiO_2 to reverse hypoxia
- Recruitment of collapsed alveoli, improving alveolar ventilation
- Reduction in the work of breathing
- Reduction of left ventricular afterload.

Different modes of NIV

- **BiPAP** Achieves ventilation by cycling the airway pressure between high and low values in synchrony with the patient's own breathing.
- **PSV** In this mode the patient triggers each breath and the ventilator provides positive pressure throughout inspiration, thus reducing the work of breathing by decreasing the elastic and resistive components of respiratory work.
- **NIPPV** A mandatory mode that may be pressure or volume controlled.

The important characteristics of an NIV circuit are:

- An expiratory resistor capable of maintaining positive airway pressure yet offering a low resistance to expiratory flow. This valve should be close to the patient's airway
- Short, wide-bore tubing
- A flow or pressure sensor which detects inspiratory effort, triggering positive inspiratory pressure support (PSV)
- Ability to control FiO_2
- A comfortable and tight-fitting face or nasal mask
- Humidification, monitors and safety features (pressure-relief valves and back-up apnoea ventilation).

The potential complications of NIV are listed in Table 3.3.

The evidence for NIV

Current data support the use of NIV for patients with hypercapnic respiratory failure due to COPD.[3,4] During exacerbations these patients have an elevated resistive work, and all modes of NIV have been shown to be effective in

Table 3.3 Potential complications of NIV

Mask intolerance
Pressure areas (and nasal bridge necrosis)
Oronasal dryness
Gastric distension, reflux and aspiration
Hypotension (especially in the hypovolaemic patient)
Raised intracranial pressure (in patients with traumatic brain injury)

such patients. Those in whom airflow obstruction is the major problem are likely to respond to CPAP. Those with severe hypercapnia and marked respiratory insufficiency are likely to benefit from the addition of inspiratory support (PSV, BiPAP or NIPPV).

One controlled trial of NIV in immunocompromised patients with pneumonia has shown reduced endotracheal intubation rates, reduced serious complications and an improved likelihood of survival to hospital discharge.

In summary, current evidence supports NIV for those patients with hypercapnic respiratory failure, in patients with COPD and in immunocompromised patients with respiratory failure. The role of NIV in other groups of patients remains to be determined.

MECHANICAL VENTILATION

The decision to intubate a patient is made on clinical grounds. It must take into account the likelihood of the patient making a good recovery and their wishes. The factors listed in Table 3.4 are only a guide.

Modes of ventilation

CONTROLLED MECHANICAL VENTILATION (CMV)

This is a mandatory mode of ventilation that provides complete ventilatory support and is typically used for anaesthetized patients intraoperatively. Traditionally, CMV is volume controlled, i.e. a tidal volume is preset. This will depend on the inspiratory time set and the compliance of the lungs. Spontaneous or assisted breaths are not possible during CMV, and so it is only suitable for sedated patients.

VOLUME-CONTROLLED VENTILATION

Synchronized intermittent mandatory ventilation (SIMV) is a form of volume-controlled ventilation which allows spontaneous initiation of breaths. The ventilator will attempt to

Table 3.4 *Indications for mechanical ventilation*

Hypoxia despite supplemental oxygen $\pm$ CPAP

Hypercapnia

To decrease the work of breathing

To allow tight control of CO_2 in patients with raised intracranial pressure

Inability to cough

To stabilize the chest wall in severe chest injury

synchronize the delivery of the mandatory volume with the patient's breaths. If the patient makes no inspiratory effort, the ventilator will continue to deliver the mandatory ventilation as defined by the set tidal volume and respiratory rate. Any spontaneous respiratory effort by the patient between the SIMV breaths can be assisted by pressure support.

PRESSURE SUPPORT VENTILATION (PSV)

In this mode, patients initiate all their own breaths. When triggered, the ventilator applies a preset pressure; the resulting tidal volume depends on inspiratory time and lung compliance. The patient determines the duration of inspiratory time and the respiratory rate. A potential advantage is improved patient comfort, although patients may remain very tachypnoeic. This mode is often used when weaning patients off ventilatory support.

PRESSURE-CONTROLLED VENTILATION

One of the concerns when using volume controlled ventilation is the generation of high intrathoracic pressures resulting in barotrauma, part of the ventilator-induced lung injury spectrum. In pressure controlled ventilation, two pressures are set by the operator: a higher pressure, during which gas will be driven into the lungs, and a lower pressure allowing gas to leave the lungs. The ventilatory rate is set by defining the time spent at each of these pressures. However, should the compliance of the lung change significantly once the pressures are set, the effective tidal volume will either increase or decrease, respectively. This may be responsible for the generation of very large tidal volumes, which in turn may cause volutrauma, another component of VILI.

INVERSE RATIO VENTILATION (IRV)

This form of ventilation inverted the inspiratory:expiratory ratio. Normally 1:2, in IRV this would be changed to 2:1 or greater. The objective was to improve oxygenation by increasing the time spent in inspiration. Unfortunately, no large studies have supported this hypothesis, although interestingly, small studies have shown that IRV does result in a decrease in $PaCO_2$. This is somewhat counterintuitive, and it is suggested that this may occur because of the increased alveolar gas mixing that is allowed to occur during the longer period of inspiration.

Choice of ventilatory mode

With modern ventilators all volume controlled modes of ventilation should be pressure limited to prevent barotrauma and pressure controlled modes volume limited to prevent volutrauma. No controlled studies have shown any significant benefit of volume-controlled over pressure-controlled ventilation. This is true for both gas exchange and complications. Therefore, the choice of mode is entirely dependent on local practice and the ventilator equipment that is available.

VENTILATION FOR SPECIFIC CONDITIONS

ARDS

In acute lung injury (ALI) and acute respiratory distress syndrome (ARDS) the lungs are non-compliant and require high inspiratory pressures if a normal minute ventilation and hence normocapnia is to be achieved.

In 2000, the first multicentre randomized controlled trial demonstrating a mortality benefit comparing different ventilatory strategies for patients with ARDS was published. The trial compared the use of tidal volumes of approximately 12 mL/kg body weight and 6 mL/kg. The theory was that the use of lower tidal volumes would avoid the excessive distension of the alveoli that is accompanied by the release of inflammatory mediators, which could increase lung inflammation and cause injury to other organs. Mortality was decreased by 22 per cent in the group ventilated with lower tidal volumes. Therefore, the use of low tidal volumes is currently considered best practice.[5]

The lung-protective ventilatory strategy used in the aforementioned trial was:

- An initial tidal volume of 6 mL/kg
- Plateau pressure of 30 cmH$_2$O or less
- Permissive hypercapnia.

The term permissive hypercapnia means allowing $PaCO_2$ levels to increase in order to avoid the deleterious effects of ventilating a patient with stiff, non-compliant lungs using a higher minute volume. This will result in a decrease in the pH, which is generally well tolerated to values of 7.1–7.2. If the pH decreases further it is possible to administer bicarbonate to correct it. However, this remains extremely contentious and the pH at which bicarbonate therapy should be commenced, if at all, is yet to be determined.

Further limitation of VILI has been achieved by adopting a practice of permissive hypoxia. This involves allowing the PaO_2 to decrease to approximately 8 kPa rather than 10 kPa or more.

Bronchopulmonary fistulae

These patients can be particularly difficult to ventilate. The aim is to provide adequate oxygenation and ventilation,

while at the same time minimizing the air leak. To achieve this, airway pressures and inspiratory times are decreased as much as possible. However, this is often at the expense of oxygenation. The general principles incorporate the use of:

- Low inspiratory flows
- Short inspiratory times
- Low inspiratory pressures.

Asthma

The patient with severe asthma requiring ventilatory support poses unique problems. All patients with significant airflow obstruction undergo varying degrees of dynamic hyperinflation during mechanical ventilation. This occurs because airflow obstruction slows expiratory gas flow, resulting in incomplete expiration before the next breath is delivered. A proportion of each breath is trapped, causing the lungs to progressively hyperinflate until equilibrium is reached. This equilibrium occurs because at higher lung volumes there is greater lung elastic recoil and larger small airway calibre, both of which improve expiratory flow. The three factors that determine the degree of hyperinflation are:

- Tidal volume
- Time available for expiration
- Severity of airflow obstruction.

Thus when instituting mechanical ventilation for a patient with severe asthma, choose:

- Low tidal volumes 6–8 mL/kg
- Long expiratory time (achieved with a high inspiratory flow rate –80 L/min and short inspiratory time)
- Low respiratory rate (8–10 breaths/min)
- PEEP (none initially).

The use of low tidal volumes in these patients will inevitably result in high $PaCO_2$ levels. Permissive hypercapnia is widely practised, as this is less harmful than increasing minute ventilation to achieve normocarbia. There are no data to support the use of bicarbonate to correct the acidosis caused by the hypercapnia.

The main complication of mechanical ventilation in asthmatic patients is dynamic hyperinflation, which may result in:

- Circulatory compromise, manifested by hypotension and an increased CVP
- Barotrauma, e.g. pneumothorax.

Mechanical ventilation should be regulated by adjusting the respiratory rate to maintain dynamic hyperinflation at a safe level. Many modern ventilators are able to calculate the volume of gas trapped at the end of expiration and the amount of PEEP being generated by the dynamic hyperinflation. This allows measurements to be made following changes in ventilator settings. Thus, in some patients the provision of supplemental PEEP may actually stent the airways, resulting in a decrease in the volume of gas trapped, and therefore be beneficial. Similarly, in spontaneously breathing patients CPAP and NIV have been shown to be helpful. However, the airways resistance in patients with asthma can change dramatically in a short period of time, and facilities for invasive ventilation should always be available if a severely asthmatic patient is requiring non-invasive support.

COMPLICATIONS OF MECHANICAL VENTILATION

Although often life saving, mechanical ventilation has many potential complications: these are listed in Table 3.5.

Ventilator-associated pneumonia

This is nosocomial pneumonia occurring in a ventilated patient and is very common (about 20 per cent). It is due partly to a reduction in the natural defence systems of the respiratory tract that occurs with intubation. Microaspiration from secretions that are regurgitated from the stomach and sit above the tracheal tube cuff has also been implicated, and the supine position may increase its incidence.

Ventilator-induced lung injury

Lung overdistension, due to either excessive pressure or volume, may result in alveolar rupture, causing a pneumothorax

Table 3.5 *Complications of mechanical ventilation*

Complications of intubation
Failure
Dental trauma
Laryngeal trauma

Pulmonary
Ventilator-associated pneumonia
Ventilator-induced lung injury
   Barotrauma
   Volutrauma
   Biotrauma (shearing forces)
Patient–ventilator asynchrony

Cardiovascular
Decreased cardiac output

or a pneumomediastinum. It may also result in diffuse alveolar damage similar to that found in ALI. This is also contributed to by repeated opening and closing of the alveoli (biotrauma), and so the use of adequate PEEP to avoid tidal collapse is advocated.

Patient–ventilator asynchrony

Despite modern ventilators accommodating to the breathing patterns of the patient, in some cases asynchrony between the patient and ventilator remains a difficult clinical problem. In the majority of cases this is resolved by increasing the sedation the patient is receiving. However, further developments in ventilator technology are attempting to address this issue.

Cardiovascular effects of mechanical ventilation

The effects of mechanical ventilation are essentially due to an increase in mean intrathoracic pressure. These include:

- Reduced venous return (VR)
- Reduced left ventricular preload
- Reduced left ventricular afterload
- Increased right ventricular afterload.

The decrease in venous return tends to reduce cardiac output in patients with normal ventricular function, whereas the reduction in left ventricular preload and afterload tends to improve cardiac output in patients with heart failure. This explains the difficulties sometimes encountered when weaning patients with heart failure from mechanical ventilation. In turn, the decreased left ventricular preload results in the release of antidiuretic hormone and aldosterone to increase salt and water retention. Atrial naturetic peptide release is decreased.

WEANING

Once the underlying process that resulted in the institution of mechanical ventilation has started to resolve, withdrawal of ventilatory support should begin. In many critical care patients weaning is not difficult, and return to spontaneous ventilation is achieved within a few days. However, in a relatively small proportion, weaning can be extremely difficult.

In one classic study, patients were assessed as to their suitability for weaning on a daily basis by a respiratory therapist. The assessment comprised five simple weaning criteria, as shown in Table 3.6. Once successful in the screening test, in the intervention group the patient was allowed to breathe through a T-piece circuit as described above for up to 2 hours. If in that time the patient's respiratory rate increased to greater than 35 bpm, or heart rate or BP increased significantly, or the patient became unduly anxious, the trial was abandoned and regarded as not successful. If successful, a message was attached to the patient's chart indicating that they had successfully completed a 2-hour trial of spontaneous breathing and had an 85 per cent chance of staying off mechanical ventilation for 48 hours. The control subjects were screened daily, but no further assessment was made by the respiratory therapist or nursing staff. The study found that patients were weaned on average 1.5 days earlier in the intervention group.

Despite this technique, there may still be difficulty in weaning a patient from mechanical ventilation. In this case a cause for failure should be sought and treated if possible. The more common causes of failure to wean are listed in Table 3.7.

Methods of weaning

Several studies suggest that a weaning protocol, independent of the ventilation mode used, results in faster weaning compared to not having a well-defined protocol.[6]

Table 3.6 *Assessment of a patient's readiness to wean (from Ely EW et al. N Eng J Med 1996; **335**: 1864–9, with permission)*

Respiratory
Oxygen requirements $PaO_2/FiO_2 > 27$ kPa
PEEP ≤ 5 cmH$_2$O
Adequate cough during suctioning
Respiratory frequency:tidal volume ratio < 105 breaths/min/L
Other
No infusions of vasopressors or sedatives

Table 3.7 *Causes of failure to wean*

Respiratory
Infection – ongoing
Pulmonary oedema
Pleural effusions
Chest wall instability (post trauma)
Other
Decreased level of consciousness
Malnutrition
Cardiovascular instability
Critical illness polyneuropathy

The most common methods of weaning are:

- **T-piece weaning** This involves a trial of spontaneous breathing, usually once or twice a day.
- **SIMV** The number of mandatory breaths the patient receives is decreased each day.
- **Pressure support ventilation** The pressure support level is decreased, usually by 2–4 cmH$_2$O each day.

A few studies have attempted to compare these techniques in difficult-to-wean patients. Brochard[7] compared these three methods in a randomized trial and found pressure support to be the most successful with regard to weaning.

Esteban *et al.*[8] compared the above methods and found that daily trials of spontaneous breathing led to extubation more quickly than did SIMV or pressure support ventilation.

This has resulted in much discussion over the optimal weaning method. Most authorities agree that weaning on SIMV is the least efficient method. However, there are few data to support a choice of pressure support ventilation over T-piece weaning or vice versa.

PERCUTANEOUS TRACHEOSTOMY

Critically ill patients frequently require tracheostomy to facilitate their management (Table 3.8). Patients who are intubated for prolonged periods are at risk of laryngeal stenosis; tracheostomy decreases this risk, but is associated with tracheal stenosis which, although still undesirable, is easier to manage than laryngeal stenosis. Tracheostomy also enables patients to speak, to eat, and to have better mouth toilet. It is intuitive that a tracheostomy is rather better tolerated than an oral endotracheal tube, and therefore sedation may be decreased. However, to date this has not been substantiated in clinical trials. The timing of tracheostomy varies depending on many factors, but increasingly there is a tendency for a tracheostomy to be sited if the patient requires intubation at approximately 1 week.

The technique

There are several different percutaneous techniques in use. One of the commonly used is described below.

Table 3.8 *Indications for tracheostomy*

Long-term respiratory support anticipated (>1 week)
To facilitate suctioning if cough remains weak
To prevent aspiration if bulbar reflexes are not intact
Upper airway obstruction, e.g. due to tumour

CIAGLIA'S TECHNIQUE

A small horizontal skin incision is made between the first and second tracheal rings, and blunt dissection is used to separate the underlying strap muscles. A needle is inserted into the trachea and its position confirmed by aspiration of air, and usually also by bronchoscopy. Serial dilators of increasing diameter are then used to dilate the trachea over an intratracheal guidewire. Finally, the tracheostomy tube is inserted mounted on a dilator. A recent modification to this technique is the Ciaglia Blue Rhino, which uses one single tapered dilator in place of multiple dilators.

Contraindication to tracheostomy are listed in Table 3.9.

Like all procedures, percutaneous tracheostomy is not without its complications (Table 3.10). Careful patient selection and good technique will minimize these.

Surgical versus percutaneous tracheostomy

There are few prospective, controlled studies comparing the two techniques, and establishing the absolute superiority of one technique over the other has proved difficult.[9] This particular group of patients has a high mortality, thereby limiting long-term follow-up. Although almost every case scenario previously reserved for surgical tracheostomy has been managed with percutaneous tracheostomy (obesity, previous tracheostomy, emergency tracheostomy, etc.), many

Table 3.9 *Contraindications to percutaneous tracheostomy*

Anatomic
Paediatric airway
Morbid obesity obscuring landmarks
Local mass or tumour (e.g. enlarged thyroid)

Others
Local infection
Emergencies
Coagulopathy

Table 3.10 *Complications of percutaneous tracheostomy*

Immediate	Late
Haemorrhage	Tracheal stenosis
Loss of the airway	Tracheomalacia
Posterior tracheal wall perforation	Granulomas
Paratracheal insertion (pneumothorax)	Tracheocutaneous fistula
Delayed	Tracheoesophageal fistula
Haemorrhage (from tracheoarterial fistulae)	
Infection	
Mucosal ulceration	

institutions still refer these cases for surgical tracheostomy. Conclusions that can be made include:

- The percutaneous technique takes less time to perform
- The percutaneous technique has a lower incidence of infection
- Percutaneous tracheostomy has a lower incidence of early bleeding
- Percutaneous tracheostomy is at least as safe as surgical tracheostomy.

In addition to these advantages the percutaneous technique avoids the need to transport the patient to the operating theatre and is a relatively low-cost technique.

Changing a tracheostomy

Patients who require a tracheostomy for a prolonged period are at risk of airway obstruction due to a build-up of secretions within the tracheostomy itself. For this reason tracheostomies are frequently changed to a type with an inner cannula (e.g. Shiley) that can easily be removed and cleaned at regular intervals. Sufficient time should have elapsed to allow a tract to form prior to any attempt to change the tracheostomy – this usually takes 7–10 days.

When is it safe to decannulate a patient?

The following requirements must be met:

- No requirement for ventilatory assistance
- The patient must have a strong effective cough
- Intact gag reflex.

REFERENCES

1. Sykes K, Young JD. *Respiratory support in ICU*. London: BMJ Books, 1999.
2. Bersten A, Holt A, Vedig A, *et al*. Treatment of severe cardiogenic pulmonary oedema with continuous positive airway pressure delivered by facemask. *N Engl J Med* 1991; **325**: 1825–30.
3. Brochard L, Mancebo J, Wysocki M, *et al*. Noninvasive ventilation for acute exacerbations of chronic obstructive pulmonary disease. *N Engl J Med* 1995; **333**: 817–22.
4. Plant P, Owen J, Elliott M. A multicentre randomised controlled trial of the early use of non-invasive ventilation for acute exacerbations of chronic obstructive pulmonary disease. *Lancet* 2000; **355**: 1931–5.
5. ARDSNET. Ventilation with lower tidal volumes as compared with traditional tidal volumes for acute lung injury and the acute respiratory distress syndrome. *N Engl J Med* 2000; **342**: 1301–8.

6. Vitacca M, Vianello A, Colombo D, *et al.* Comparison of two methods for weaning patients with chronic obstructive pulmonary disease requiring mechanical ventilation for more than 15 days. *Am J Respir Crit Care Med* 2001; **164**: 225–30.

7. Brochard L, Rauss A, Benito S, *et al.* Comparison of three methods of gradual withdrawal from ventilatory support during weaning from mechanical ventilation. *Am J Respir Crit Care Med* 1994; **150**: 896–903.

8. Esteban A, Frutos F, Tobin MJ, *et al.* A comparison of four methods of weaning patients from mechanical ventilation. *N Engl J Med* 1995; **332**: 345–50.

9. Freeman B, Isabella K, Lin N, Buchman T. A meta-analysis of prospective trials comparing percutaneous and surgical tracheostomy in critically ill patients. *Chest* 2000; **118**: 1412–19.

4 The acute respiratory distress syndrome

MARK EHLERS

Viva topics

- How is the diagnosis of acute respiratory distress syndrome made? What difficulties are associated with making this diagnosis?
- Describe the pathogenesis of ARDS.
- What is the place of inhaled nitric oxide in the management of ARDS?
- What information would you wish to convey to the family of a young patient on an intensive care unit with the diagnosis of ARDS?

INTRODUCTION

The acute respiratory distress syndrome (ARDS) and acute lung injury (ALI) are syndromes that commonly affect intensive care patients. Initially termed the *adult* respiratory distress syndrome, because it was thought to only occur in adults, it has now been renamed the *acute* respiratory distress syndrome, as it does also occur in children. Despite recent important advances in management and our understanding of its pathophysiology, ARDS still carries a high mortality. This chapter outlines the definition, epidemiology, pathophysiology and clinical presentation of this disease complex as well as discussing current treatment modalities, both conventional and alternative.

DEFINITION

The original description of the acute respiratory distress syndrome (ARDS) in 1967 was by Ashbaugh and colleagues.[1] They described 12 patients presenting with a combination of acute respiratory distress, hypoxaemia refractory to oxygen therapy, decreased lung compliance and the appearance of diffuse infiltrates on chest X-ray. Although this description summarized the clinical presentation well, it was not specific enough to exclude other conditions. This made it difficult to determine the true incidence and mortality of the disease. It could also not be used to predict outcome.

In 1988, Murray and colleagues[2] proposed a more specific definition that was based on a 4-point lung injury scoring system, namely, the level of positive end-expiratory pressure (PEEP), the ratio of partial pressure of arterial oxygen (PaO_2) to fraction of inspired oxygen (FiO_2), static lung compliance, and chest X-ray changes. The cause of lung injury and the presence or absence of non-pulmonary organ dysfunction were also included. This new definition was not only more specific, but also allowed the severity of the lung injury to be graded. However, it was only able to predict outcome partially. A score of >2.5 between days 4 and 7 predicted a need for prolonged ventilation, but the score in the first 72 hours did not correlate at all with outcome. This definition was also not specific enough to make the important exclusion of cardiogenic pulmonary oedema.

It had become increasingly apparent that ARDS was not a syndrome on its own, but rather the more severe form of a disease complex that affected the lungs of critically ill patients. There was also a 'less severe' form of ARDS, which is more common and has a similar pathogenesis but a lower mortality than true ARDS. This was termed acute lung injury (ALI). Not all patients with ALI go on to develop ARDS. A new definition was proposed by the American–European Consensus Conference Committee in 1994 that would encompass both extremes of the disease complex, but at the same time distinguish between them.[3]

ALI/ARDS may be diagnosed if the onset is acute; bilateral pulmonary infiltrates are present on chest X-ray (Figure 4.1); and the pulmonary artery wedge pressure is ≤18 mmHg. In addition to these, if the ratio of $PaO_2:FiO_2$ is ≤300 this is termed ALI, and if the $PaO_2:FiO_2$ ≤ 200 it is ARDS (where PaO_2 is measured in mmHg and FiO_2 is measured as a fraction of 1).

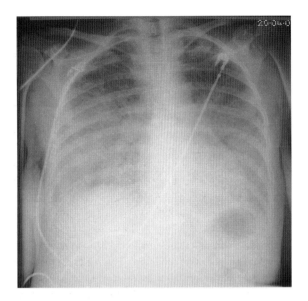

Figure 4.1 Chest X-ray of ARDS

Table 4.1 *Clinical disorders associated with ALI/ARDS*

Direct lung injury	Indirect lung injury
Pneumonia	Sepsis – most common
Aspiration of gastric contents	Severe trauma
Near-drowning	Shock
Pulmonary contusion	Acute pancreatitis
Inhalational injury – smoke, corrosive gases	Massive transfusion of blood products (Transfusion-related acute lung injury)
Fat embolism	Disseminated intravascular coagulation
Amniotic fluid embolism	Eclampsia
Post lung transplantation or pulmonary embolectomy	Cardiopulmonary bypass
High altitude	Drug overdose – heroin, barbiturates

For example, a patient meeting the other criteria, with a PaO_2 of 80 mmHg on an FiO_2 of 0.50 (50 per cent inspired oxygen), would have a PaO_2:FiO_2 of 160, and therefore, by definition, would have ARDS. This definition is simple, easy to use, recognizes the spectrum of the clinical disorder (ALI vs ARDS), and excludes a diagnosis of cardiogenic pulmonary oedema. The disadvantages are that it does not recognize non-pulmonary factors that may influence outcome, and the chest X-ray appearance of bilateral infiltrates is not specific enough to exclude diseases such as Wegner's granulomatosis, Goodpasture's syndrome and acute lupus pneumonitis (for which the treatment would be different). In addition, it may still be difficult to exclude a patient with acute cardiogenic pulmonary oedema in whom the pulmonary artery wedge pressure may have been normalized prior to measurement.

EPIDEMIOLOGY

Incidence

Because of problems with the definition, the incidence of ALI/ARDS has previously been difficult to determine. In 1977 the incidence in the USA was reported to be 75 per 100 000 population. The first epidemiologic study to use the 1994 consensus definition, conducted in Scandinavia, reported an incidence of 17.9 per 100 000 population for ALI and 13.5 per 100 000 for ARDS. The first prospective epidemiologic study based on the 1994 consensus definition is currently under way.

Risk factors

Certain clinical disorders are risk factors for the development of ALI/ARDS. These can be divided into those causing direct and those causing indirect lung injury (Table 4.1). Sepsis is the most common disorder associated with ALI/ARDS, with approximately 40 per cent of patients having sepsis developing ALI/ARDS. Secondary risk factors for the development of ALI/ARDS include chronic alcohol abuse, chronic lung disease and a low serum pH.

There may be a difference between ARDS due to direct lung injury and ARDS due to indirect lung injury, in terms of both pathophysiology and response to therapy. Computed tomography (CT) scanning of the chest demonstrates a difference between ARDS due to direct lung injury (ARDSd) and ARDS due to indirect lung injury (ARDSind). In the ARDSd group, the CT scan shows a picture of patchy consolidation, whereas in the ARDSind group the scan has a more symmetrical ground-glass appearance (owing to the presence of more alveolar collapse and interstitial oedema).

There may also be a difference in response to therapy between the two groups. Gattinoni and colleagues[4] showed a difference in pulmonary mechanical changes in response to varying levels of positive end-expiratory pressure. The lungs appear to be stiffer in ARDSd, less responsive to sigh manoeuvres, and less amenable to a recruitment strategy than in ARDSind. There may also be a difference in the response to pulmonary vasodilators: one study showed that oxygenation improved more in ARDSind in response to prostacyclin, although mortality was unchanged. It is unclear whether there is a difference in the response to nitric oxide. It may be that eventually treatment will vary according to the underlying clinical disorder.

Outcome

The quoted mortality rate is between 40 and 60 per cent, although most deaths are due to sepsis or multiple organ dysfunction rather than to the ALI/ARDS itself. The recent success of low tidal volume ventilation in reducing mortality indicates that in some patients, death may be related directly to lung injury.

It is possible that the mortality rate from ALI/ARDS is decreasing. One study from the USA and another from the UK showed a decrease in the mortality rates over the last 10 years in the same centres. This could be explained by improved general supportive care, better treatment of patients with sepsis, and improved ventilation strategies. However, interestingly, the initial PaO_2:FiO_2 ratio does not correlate with the risk of death.

Recently, a number of publications have examined the 1-year outcome of patients with ARDS. These have demonstrated that at 1 year survivors have significantly impaired respiratory function, as evidenced by decreased tidal volume and carbon monoxide diffusing capacity. These factors are in turn associated with a decreased health-related quality of life that is due to physical limitations. One paper has suggested that the avoidance of steroids, the lack of hospital-acquired illness and a rapid resolution of the lung injury and multiorgan dysfunction were associated with an improved 12-month outcome.

ARDS network

In 1994 the National Heart, Lung, and Blood Institute and the National Institutes of Health in the USA established the ARDS Network group. The group consists of a clinical network of 10 centres with a total of 75 intensive care units in 24 hospitals. This has had a significant impact on ALI/ARDS research, as it allows the collection of controlled epidemiological data and well designed, multicentre randomized clinical trials for the assessment of new therapies to be conducted. The first trial completed by the ARDS Network was on the use of ketoconazole in patients with acute lung injury.

PATHOPHYSIOLOGY

The pathophysiology of ALI/ARDS can be divided into the acute phase and the resolution phase (or fibrosing alveolitis if resolution does not occur).

Acute phase

The acute phase of ALI/ARDS is characterized by alveolar flooding with protein-rich fluid as a result of loss of the integrity of the normal alveolar–capillary barrier (Figure 4.2). This is a complex process and there are several mechanisms by which it occurs.

The normal alveolar epithelium consists of two types of cell. Flat type I cells make up 90 per cent of the epithelium and their function is essentially to provide a lining for the alveoli. Cuboidal type II cells make up the remaining 10 per cent, and their functions are to replace damaged type I cells by differentiation; and to produce surfactant and transport ions and fluid. Damage to type I cells disrupts the integrity of the alveoli and allows any interstitial fluid in the lungs to leak into the alveoli. Damage to type II cells results in a decreased surfactant production, inability to pump ions and fluid back out of the alveoli, and impaired replacement of damaged type I cells. The decreased surfactant production contributes to atelectasis. The surfactant that is produced is of low quality and is inactivated by the fluid in the alveoli. In addition, if the type II cells have been severely damaged, then repair occurs by fibrosis. Endothelial damage and increased permeability occur either due to direct lung microvascular injury or as part of the generalized inflammatory process seen in patients with the systemic inflammatory response syndrome or sepsis. The disruption of the alveolar–capillary barrier allows not only fluid to leak into the alveoli, but also protein, neutrophils, red blood cells and fibroblasts.

Alveolar epithelial damage is probably neutrophil mediated. Alveolar macrophages secrete proinflammatory cytokines. These include interleukins (IL)-1, 6 and 8 and tumour necrosis factor-α (TNF-α). TNF-α is responsible for neutrophil chemotaxis and activation in the alveoli. The activated neutrophils secrete oxidants, proteases, leukotrienes and platelet-activating factor, all of which cause lung injury. In addition, proinflammatory cytokines are also produced by alveolar epithelial cells, and systemically as part of the systemic inflammatory response syndrome. IL-1 stimulates fibroblasts to lay down fibrin (after 5–10 days), and the fibroblasts in turn secrete IL-8. The anterior pituitary gland secretes macrophage inhibitory factor. This cytokine acts on the alveolar macrophages to increase their secretion of IL-8 and TNF-α.

In addition to the proinflammatory cytokines, anti-inflammatory cytokines are also found in the alveoli of patients with ALI/ARDS. These include IL-1 receptor antagonist, soluble TNF-α receptor, IL-8 autoantibody, IL-10 and IL-11. Under normal circumstances these anti-inflammatory cytokines would inhibit the proinflammatory cytokines and thus modulate the inflammatory response. In patients with

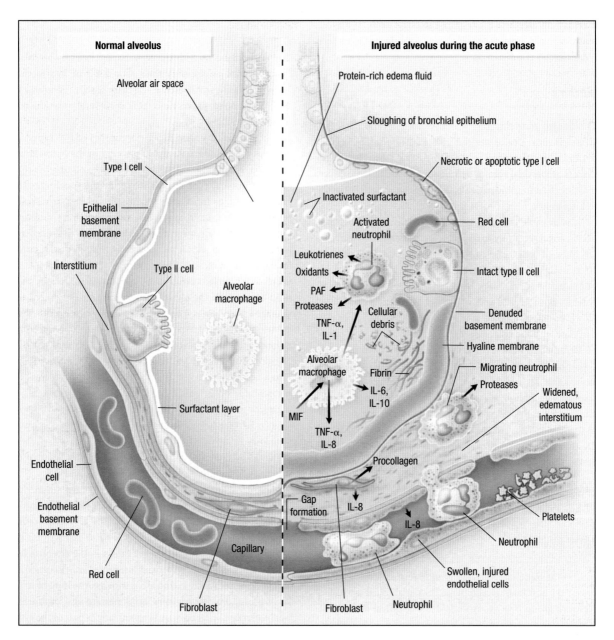

Figure 4.2 The normal alveolus (left-hand side) and the injured alveolus in the acute phase of acute lung injury and the acute respiratory distress syndrome (right-hand side). In the acute phase of the syndrome (right) there is sloughing of both the bronchial and the alveolar epithelial cells, with the formation of protein-rich hyaline membranes on the denuded basement membrane. Neutrophils are shown adhering to the injured capillary endothelium and marginating through the interstitium into the air space, which is filled with protein-rich oedema fluid. In the air space an alveolar macrophage is secreting cytokines, interleukins (IL)-1, 6, 8 and 10, and tumour necrosis factor-α, which act locally to stimulate chemotaxis and activate neutrophils. Macrophages also secrete other cytokines, including IL-1, IL-6 and IL-10. IL-1 can also stimulate the production of extracellular matrix by fibroblasts. Neutrophils can release oxidants, proteases, leukotrienes and other proinflammatory molecules, such as platelet-activating factor (PAF). A number of anti-inflammatory mediators are also present in the alveolar milieu, including IL-1 receptor antagonist, soluble tumour necrosis factor receptor, autoantibodies against IL-8, and cytokines such as IL-10 and IL-11 (not shown). The influx of protein-rich fluid into the alveolus has led to the inactivation of surfactant. MIF, macrophage inhibitory factor. (Republished with kind permission from: Ware LB, Matthay MA. The acute respiratory distress syndrome. *N Engl J Med* 2000; **342**: 1334–49. Figure 3. Copyright © 2000 Massachusetts Medical Society. All rights reserved.)

ALI/ARDS, this natural balance is disturbed and the proinflammatory effects predominate.

Although cytokines and neutrophils are central to the inflammatory process that occurs, there are other mechanisms of injury at work in the lungs that also occur throughout the body as part of the systemic inflammatory response syndrome. Of particular interest are the coagulation abnormalities that result in microvascular occlusion within the lung as a result of the presence of platelet- and fibrin-rich thrombi and abnormal fibrinolysis.

The characteristic hypoxaemia in ALI/ARDS is due to increased intrapulmonary shunting and a ventilation–perfusion (V_A/Q) mismatch. The increased intrapulmonary shunting is due to loss of the alveolar microvascular bed caused by direct damage and thrombi. The ventilation–perfusion mismatch is due to alveolar collapse and a decrease in the number of alveoli that are ventilated. Alveolar flooding and decreased surfactant increases the surface tension within the alveoli, whereupon they collapse and are unable to re-expand. Alveolar dead space increases and hypercapnia ensues, causing respiratory acidosis. Pulmonary compliance is decreased and patients hyperventilate in an attempt to compensate.

Ventilator-induced lung injury

Mechanical ventilation per se may cause lung injury by several mechanisms. Although the lungs of patients with ALI/ARDS are diffusely injured, the damage is not homogeneous. There may be one area of lung with normal compliance and gas exchange. In a second area there may be alveolar flooding and atelectasis present, but alveoli can be recruited for gas exchange by safely raising airway pressures. There may also be a third area with severe alveolar flooding and inflammation, in which the alveoli cannot be recruited without using 'unsafe' high airway pressures. The first area of apparently healthy lung may only represent 30 per cent of the total lung volume. This small area has been referred to as the 'baby lung' and is easily overventilated, thereby exposing it to potential damage. The alveolar overdistension associated with ventilation at high volumes (volutrauma) and pressures (barotrauma) can damage the pulmonary capillaries and cause pulmonary oedema in both normal and abnormal lung tissue. In addition, the repeated opening and closing of collapsed alveoli causes shearing stresses in the alveoli (biotrauma). These mechanisms can in turn initiate proinflammatory cytokine release. In an attempt to minimize the injury associated with mechanical ventilation, a number of lung-protective strategies have been developed.

Resolution

Resolution depends on the repair of the alveolar epithelium, clearance of the pulmonary oedema fluid and the removal of proteins from the alveolar space (Figure 4.3). Type II cells proliferate across the alveolar basement membrane and then differentiate into type I cells. The proliferation of type II cells is controlled by epithelial growth factors, such as keratinocyte growth factor and hepatocyte growth factor. The removal of alveolar fluid is dependent on the active transport of sodium and perhaps chloride. Sodium passes through sodium channels on the alveolar surface of the type II cells and then is pumped out of the cells through their basal membrane by the Na^+/K^+-ATPase pump. Water then follows passively down the resultant osmotic gradient via transcellular water channels (aquasporins) on type I cells. Soluble proteins are removed by diffusion between alveolar epithelial cells, and insoluble proteins are removed by endocytosis and transcytosis by alveolar type I cells, and by phagocytosis by macrophages. The mechanism for the removal of the inflammatory-cell infiltrate is unclear, although apoptosis (programmed cell death) may be important in the clearance of neutrophils.

Fibrosing alveolitis

For reasons that are unclear, some patients do not undergo resolution but progress to fibrosing alveolitis instead. This may begin as early as 5–7 days after the onset of ALI/ARDS, and may be promoted by IL-1. The alveolar spaces become filled with acute and chronic inflammatory cells, mesenchymal cells, fibrin, collagen, fibronectin and blood vessels, eventually leading to fibrosis and only partial resolution of the pulmonary oedema. The hypoxaemia, decreased compliance and increased alveolar dead space persist. Patients who develop fibrosing alveolitis are at increased risk of dying.

CLINICAL FEATURES

Acute phase

The diagnosis of ALI/ARDS should always be considered in patients with respiratory failure who have risk factors for developing the syndrome. Onset is usually gradual, within 12–72 hours of the precipitating event, although it may be within 6 hours in patients with sepsis. Patients have symptoms and signs of acute respiratory failure, with hypoxaemia that is characteristically resistant to oxygen therapy alone. On chest auscultation diffuse, fine crepitations can be heard

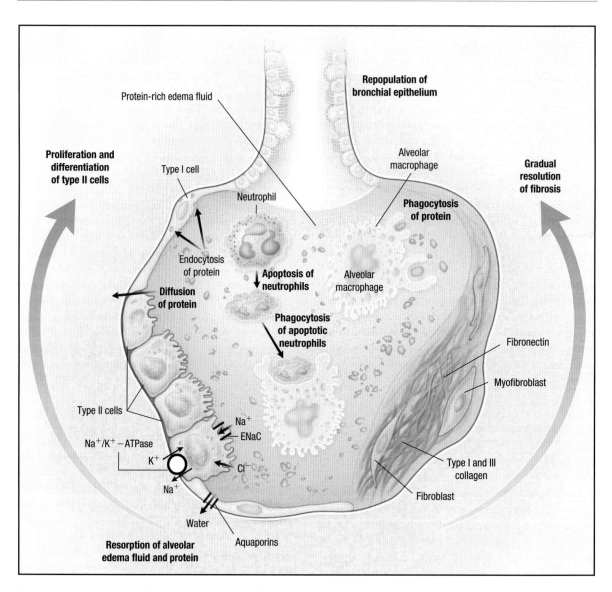

Figure 4.3 Mechanisms important in the resolution of acute lung injury (Republished with kind permission from: Ware LB, Matthay MA. The acute respiratory distress syndrome. *N Engl J Med* 2000; **342**: 1334–49. Figure 4. Copyright © 2000 Massachusetts Medical Society. All rights reserved.)

that are indistinguishable from those found in pulmonary oedema. The diagnosis is established when patients fulfil the criteria outlined in the 1994 consensus definition. As mentioned above, the chest X-ray findings are non-specific and show bilateral patchy infiltrates, which may or may not be symmetrical. In addition, pleural effusions and pneumothoraces may also be seen. The incidence of pneumothoraces is 10–13 per cent and does not appear to be related to levels of inspiratory airway pressure or positive end-expiratory pressure.

The CT scan typically shows patchy areas of alveolar consolidation and atelectasis in the dependent zones (Figure 4.4).

Resolution

Resolution usually starts after about 7 days. As the alveoli clear the fluid and cells and the alveolar epithelium is rebuilt, the hypoxaemia resolves and lung compliance gradually returns to normal. Pulmonary function can be expected to

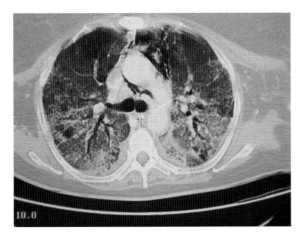

Figure 4.4 A CT scan of ARDS

return to normal within 6–12 months in survivors. The chest X-ray features also resolve and return to normal.

Fibrosing alveolitis

In patients who develop fibrosing alveolitis, the hypoxaemia, increased alveolar dead space and decreased compliance persist. Failure of respiratory function to improve after the first week may imply the onset of fibrosing alveolitis. The survival rate is lower in this group of patients. Survivors can be expected to have persistent impairment of gas exchange and abnormal lung compliance, and thus may remain short of breath. In severe cases, pulmonary hypertension, as a result of permanent damage to the pulmonary capillaries, may occur and, if severe, may cause right ventricular failure. The chest X-ray does not return to normal and linear opacities are seen. The CT scan shows diffuse ground-glass opacities throughout both lung fields, and bullae may also be seen.

TREATMENT

The treatment of ALI/ARDS should be aimed at the underlying cause, managing any infection that may be present, comprehensive supportive therapy, and an appropriate ventilation strategy. In addition, there are a large number of alternative therapies (ventilation strategies and pharmacological agents) that are available which have not proved beneficial (Figure 4.5).

Treatment of the underlying cause

Where possible, the underlying cause should be identified and the appropriate treatment started. This is particularly important when the underlying cause is sepsis or pneumonia.

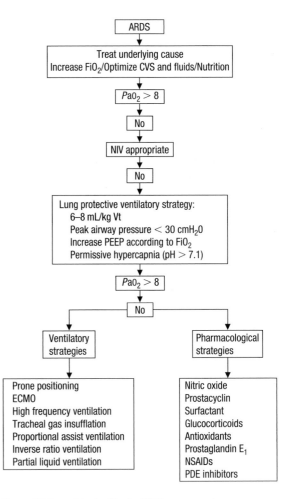

Figure 4.5 A possible algorithm for ARDS management

Management of infection

The treatment of infections is important, as it is associated with a better outcome. This includes infections of any origin – sepsis, pneumonia, intra-abdominal infections, nosocomial infections and catheter-related infections. Treatment should be by appropriate surgical drainage and/or antimicrobial therapy. Patients with ALI/ARDS frequently die as a result of uncontrolled infection, rather than from primary respiratory failure.

Ventilator-associated pneumonia is common in patients with ALI/ARDS, and the incidence may be as high as 60 per cent. The diagnosis of pneumonia in patients with ALI/ARDS is often difficult, because fever and a raised white cell count are often present as a result of concomitant systemic inflammatory response syndrome, and the chest X-ray findings associated with ALI/ARDS can mask any new changes as a result of pneumonia. In addition, patients who have been ventilated for prolonged periods often have colonized airways, which makes the interpretation of endotracheal aspirates difficult. Specimens obtained by bronchoalveolar lavage may assist in the diagnosis of pneumonia.

Supportive care

The reduction in mortality due to ALI/ARDS over the last 10 years may be due in part to improvements in general supportive care. Attention to detail regarding adequate nutrition, appropriate fluid and haemodynamic management, stress ulcer prophylaxis and thromboembolic prophylaxis is as important as the ventilation strategy.

Nutrition

Although there is no randomized controlled trial that shows conclusively any benefit to nutritional support in critically ill patients, it has become part of standard practice, including in patients with ALI/ARDS. The goal of adequate nutrition should be to provide the correct nutrients, vitamins and trace elements to meet the needs of each individual patient. It is not yet clear whether patients with ALI/ARDS have any specific nutritional requirements. Overfeeding may result in a high respiratory quotient and increased production of carbon dioxide, which may increase the work of breathing and delay weaning. It has been suggested that a high-fat low-carbohydrate diet may reduce the respiratory quotient and hence the duration of ventilation. Adding immunomodulatory nutrients such as arginine, glutamine, ribonucleotides and ω-3 fatty acids has been shown to decrease nosocomial infections and hospital stay, but not to improve mortality. The addition of fish oil, γ-linolenic acid and antioxidants has been shown to shorten the duration of ventilation but had no effect on mortality. In general, the enteral route of administration is preferable to the parenteral route.

HAEMODYNAMIC MANAGEMENT

Haemodynamic management includes the administration of fluids, vasopressors, and occasionally vasodilators.

Whether or not to restrict fluids in patients with ALI/ARDS is controversial. Because of the increased pulmonary vascular permeability in ALI/ARDS, it is difficult to control the movement of fluid from the pulmonary capillaries into the pulmonary extravascular space. It may seem logical that by restricting fluids it would be possible to decrease total lung water, and several animal studies have shown this to be true. Clinical studies have shown that oxygenation and pulmonary compliance can be improved by restricting fluids. A reduced mortality has been demonstrated in patients with ALI having a low cumulative net fluid gain. However, this may be because fluid accumulation is a marker of disease severity. The disadvantage of fluid restriction is that it may decrease cardiac output and tissue perfusion, which may worsen non-pulmonary organ failure.

It has been suggested that outcomes may be improved by aiming for levels of supranormal oxygen delivery using aggressive volume replacement, increased haemoglobin levels and inotropes. A trend towards decreased mortality has been shown in postoperative or post-trauma patients using this approach, but no advantage has been shown in ALI/ARDS patients.

There remains no clear evidence to suggest whether colloids or crystalloids are the optimal fluid for resuscitation in ALI/ARDS. The ARDS Network group will soon be conducting a randomized trial to compare fluid restriction with liberal fluid use, based on monitoring with either a pulmonary artery flotation catheter or central venous pressure measurement in patients with ALI/ARDS. Until then a reasonable compromise would be to maintain the intravascular volume at the lowest level that will maintain adequate systemic perfusion. If necessary, vasopressors should be used to improve systemic perfusion, rather than liberal fluid administration. Provided an adequate cardiac output is obtained, there is no mortality benefit to a particular vasopressor or combination of vasopressors being used.

Most ALI/ARDS patients have some degree of pulmonary hypertension. This may be due to hypoxic vasoconstriction, destruction of the pulmonary bed, or high levels of PEEP. The pulmonary hypertension is usually mild and does not require treatment, but occasionally it can be severe enough to cause right heart failure. Intravenous agents can be used to counteract the increase in pulmonary vascular resistance. An ideal agent would be one that vasodilates the pulmonary vessels that supply only the ventilated lung areas, as dilating lung areas that are not being ventilated would increase the shunt fraction and worsen V_A/Q mismatching. However, the available intravenous agents are relatively non-selective in this respect. Sodium nitroprusside decreases right heart afterload (thus increasing cardiac output) but increases the shunt fraction. Hydralazine and prostaglandin E_1 (alprostadil) both decrease right heart afterload but do not increase the shunt fraction. Hydralazine has not been evaluated in randomized controlled trials, and the results from a double-blind randomized multicentre study using prostaglandin E_1 were disappointing. Inhaled vasodilators, such as nitric oxide, will be discussed later.

Ventilation

The ventilation strategy remains central to the treatment of ALI/ARDS. The aim should be to optimize oxygenation while at the same time avoiding ventilator-induced lung injury. Many ventilation strategies have been proposed over the years; these can be divided into lung-protective strategies that have been shown to be effective by good evidence, and alternative therapies that have not.

NON-INVASIVE VENTILATION

Non-invasive ventilation in general has several advantages. It is well tolerated by non-sedated patients and it allows them to talk and eat. There is also a lower incidence of nosocomial pneumonia, and the duration of ventilation is shorter. It is not suitable for patients who are confused or obtunded, and ventilation requiring high airway pressures may produce an unacceptable leak. There are few studies of its use in patients with ALI/ARDS, but its use is limited to patients with less severe disease who are likely to require ventilation for a short period only, and with lower airway pressures.

LUNG-PROTECTIVE VENTILATION STRATEGIES

Most authors currently recommend a ventilation strategy that includes an increased fraction of inspired oxygen, PEEP and lung protection. This has evolved into a low tidal volume with permissive hypercapnia method of ventilation, the best example of which is the ARDS Network low tidal volume study.

FRACTION OF INSPIRED OXYGEN

The primary aim of ventilation in patients with ALI/ARDS is to provide adequate oxygenation, usually regarded as a $PaO_2 > 8\,kPa$. Initially, this can be achieved by simply increasing the fraction of inspired oxygen (FiO_2). However, prolonged high FiO_2 (>60 per cent) may contribute to lung injury due to oxygen toxicity.

PEEP AND FiO_2

Since the first description of ARDS, PEEP has been shown to improve oxygenation and allow the FiO_2 to be reduced, thereby avoiding lung injury due to oxygen toxicity.

PEEP improves oxygenation by the following mechanisms:

- Increased functional residual capacity by recruiting collapsed alveoli
- Reduced intrapulmonary shunting
- Improved ventilation/perfusion ratio (V_A/Q).

Table 4.2 *Suggested PEEP at increasing levels of FiO_2*

FiO_2	PEEP (cmH_2O)
0.3	5
0.4	5–8
0.5	8–10
0.6	10
0.7	10–14
0.8	14
0.9	16–18
1.0	18–24

In addition, PEEP has the following advantages:

- Avoid lung damage from repeated opening and closing of small bronchioles and alveoli
- Decreased inflammatory cytokines in alveolar fluid
- Decreased extravascular lung water in animal models.

PEEP now forms a standard part of the treatment of ARDS. However, the evidence is currently unclear as to what level of PEEP should be applied, and whether PEEP should be adjusted according to the FiO_2 or according to the lower inflection point of the compliance curve for the lung (see below). The ARDS Network low tidal volume study varied the amount of PEEP according to the FiO_2 (Table 4.2). Although the prophylactic use of PEEP has been shown to prevent lung injury in animal models this has not been substantiated in clinical trials.

PEEP also has several physiological disadvantages:

- Decreased cardiac output
- Increased pulmonary oedema formation
- Increased dead space
- Increased resistance of the bronchial circulation
- Increased lung volume and stretch during inspiration.

The ARDS Clinical Trials Network has published a prospective randomized controlled trial comparing low PEEP and high PEEP in patients ventilated with tidal volume goals of 6 mL/kg. The study did not demonstrate a survival difference between the regimes or significant difference in important clinical outcomes.[5]

LUNG-PROTECTIVE STRATEGY

The optimal method for ventilating the lungs of patients with ARDS has always been controversial. Historically, a tidal volume of 12–15 mL/kg body mass has been used. This is double the normal physiological tidal volume of 6–7 mL/kg and results in high airway pressures and overdistension of relatively unaffected lung areas, leading to ventilator-associated lung injury. Large-scale alveolar collapse and repeated lung reopening and overdistension with mechanical ventilation may further worsen lung injury. The obvious question that arises is whether such injury can be avoided by ventilating patients with more physiological tidal volumes, thereby improving outcome.

In a small study of 53 patients, Amato and colleagues[6] compared conventional ventilation (tidal volume 12 mL/kg and normocapnia) to a lung-protective ventilation strategy (target tidal volume 6 mL/kg). The aim of the lung-protective strategy was to avoid alveolar collapse and repeated reopening by keeping the alveoli open with PEEP that was set at the lower inflection point of the static lung pressure–volume curve, to prevent ongoing collapse by repeated recruitment manoeuvres (Lachmann's 'open lung approach' – 30–40 cm H_2O continuous positive airway pressure for 40 s), and to prevent overdistension by limiting peak airway pressure below the upper inflection point of the pressure–volume curve (taken to be <20 cmH_2O above the PEEP level). Limiting peak airway pressure in preference to delivering an adequate tidal volume often resulted in a rise in the partial pressure of arterial carbon dioxide ($PaCO_2$) – so-called 'permissive hypercapnia'. Sodium bicarbonate was administered if the arterial pH was <7.2. The 28-day mortality in the lung-protective group was 38 per cent, compared to 71 per cent in the conventional group. The patients in the lung-protective group also weaned faster from the ventilator and had a lower incidence of barotrauma. Although the results of this study are impressive, several criticisms must be borne in mind:

- Small study group (the study was stopped after 53 patients were enrolled because the difference in mortality between the two groups at that point was statistically significant)
- The mortality in the conventional group was higher than would be expected (71 per cent)
- The lower inflection point can be difficult to measure accurately, and may vary with time
- The set tidal volume of 12 mL/kg used in the conventional group may be considered as being the high end of 'conventional'
- The study was not blinded.

A number of other studies have shown no benefit in terms of outcome when using low tidal volumes. However, a recent study conducted by the ARDS Network group showed a 22 per cent reduction in mortality in patients ventilated with low tidal volumes.[7] This multicentre randomized controlled trial compared traditional ventilation (12 mL/kg predicted body weight) with low tidal volume (6 mL/kg) in 861 patients. In the low tidal volume group, peak airway pressure was limited to 30 cmH_2O and PEEP was adjusted according to the FiO_2. Acidosis due to hypercapnia in the low tidal

volume group was treated by increasing the respiratory rate to 35 breaths per minute (bpm) and, if the pH was still less than 7.3, by the administration of sodium bicarbonate. In-hospital mortality rate was lower in the group receiving low tidal volumes (31.0 per cent vs 39.8 per cent, $p = 0.007$). Morbidity was also reduced in the low tidal volume group, as evidenced by a shorter duration of both ventilation and organ failure. The results of this study need to be viewed with the following considerations in mind:

- The study does not tell us whether 6 mL/kg is the optimal tidal volume, simply that it is better than 12 mL/kg
- The mean tidal volume of patients enrolled in the ARDS Network study *prior to randomization* was 10.3 mL/kg predicted body weight, and so the patients assigned to the conventional group were receiving a higher tidal volume than was actual 'conventional' practice at the time
- In practice, many physicians have been reluctant to implement the ARDS Network low tidal volume recommendations
- The study included only 10 per cent of patients with ARDS at the participating centres
- Sodium bicarbonate was used to correct acidosis: previous studies have tolerated a lower pH because of the hypercapnia.

Subsequent studies have suggested that the higher respiratory rate used in the low tidal volume group may have led to an increase in intrinsic PEEP, and that the beneficial effects were due to high total or intrinsic PEEP rather than to low tidal volumes.[8] The ARDS Network group is currently studying the effects of high levels of PEEP.

Both volume-controlled (e.g. Synchronized Intermittent Mandatory Ventilation, SIMV) and pressure-controlled modes (e.g. Biphasic Positive Airway Pressure, BiPAP) can be used in the treatment of ALI/ARDS. The risk of volutrauma and barotrauma is the same for both modes, provided a lung protective strategy is used.

Alternative ventilation strategies

A number of alternative ventilation strategies have been proposed. They have been shown either to improve oxygenation but not mortality (e.g. prone positioning), or to be of no clear benefit. Prone positioning or extracorporeal membrane oxygenation may be considered in patients with severe refractory hypoxaemia.

PRONE POSITIONING

Mechanical ventilation of patients in the prone position may improve oxygenation by allowing recruitment of the dorsal lung segments. Thus more even distribution of the tidal volume and improved V_A/Q matching occurs. There is good evidence that prone positioning improves oxygenation by 60–70 per cent, but it does not appear to reduce mortality. A recent multicentre trial in 304 ALI/ARDS patients randomized to prone or supine positioning for an average of 7 ± 1.8 hours per day for 10 days improved oxygenation in 70 per cent of patients.[9] There was no improvement in survival at the end of the 10 days, at the time of discharge from intensive care, or at 6 months. The post hoc analysis of subgroups suggested that in the patients at highest risk, the 10-day survival might have been greater in the prone group. This may suggest that a longer period of prone positioning might have been more beneficial.

There are a number of disadvantages to prone positioning. It is technically difficult to position patients and care for them once they are prone. Common complications include the need for increased sedation and muscle relaxants, airway obstruction (due to secretions), facial oedema and pressure sores. Fortunately, accidental extubation is uncommon. There are also no clear guidelines as to which particular patients will respond to prone positioning, at which stage prone positioning should be considered, how long patients should be prone in a 24-hour period (periods used vary from 6 to 20 hours/day), nor for how many days the therapy should be continued.

Continuous rotation of patients has also been used as an alternative to prone positioning in a number of prospective uncontrolled trials.

Based on current evidence, prone positioning should be considered as rescue therapy in patients with refractory hypoxaemia.

Extracorporeal membrane oxygenation (ECMO)

Extracorporeal membrane oxygenation (ECMO) is a modified form of cardiopulmonary bypass. It aims to provide gaseous exchange across an artificial membrane external to the body, allowing the lungs time to recover. It has been used with varying degrees of success for the treatment of ARDS since the 1970s. Because it has generally been used in patients with severe disease with a high expected mortality, it is difficult to demonstrate any advantage. Indeed, at least two randomized trials have shown no benefit, and one multicentre prospective randomized trial comparing ECMO to conventional ventilation showed a high mortality of 90 per cent in both groups. Recent technical advances in the ECMO circuit may make this treatment more effective. ECMO does improve oxygenation, and so at present it may have a place in the treatment of severe refractory hypoxaemia. The Conventional ventilation or ECMO for Severe Adult Respiratory Failure (CESAR) study is ongoing and the results are awaited with interest.

High-frequency ventilation

High-frequency ventilation uses respiratory rates of more than 60 bpm and very small tidal volumes. In theory this should prove advantageous in the treatment of ALI/ARDS, as it would prevent atelectasis and avoid overdistension. However, results from randomized controlled trials have shown conflicting results. Although it is safe and may improve oxygenation, it does not appear to affect outcome.

Tracheal gas insufflation

In patients with ALI/ARDS physiological dead space is increased, particularly if small-volume ventilation is applied. This increase in dead space causes a rise in $PaCO_2$. Tracheal gas insufflation is used as an adjunct to conventional ventilation to wash out the carbon dioxide in this dead space using a constant stream of fresh gas into the distal trachea via a small catheter or a channel in the endotracheal tube. This flushes out the CO-rich gas during expiration. The catheter may accumulate secretions, damage the mucosa, and the constant stream of gas may desiccate the airways and increase auto-PEEP.

Proportional-assist ventilation

This is a form of positive-pressure ventilation in which the inspiratory airway pressure can be varied breath-to-breath according to the patient's effort. This is more comfortable for patients than conventional pressure support ventilation, and may therefore be used in non-sedated patients being supported with non-invasive ventilation.

Inverse ratio ventilation and airway pressure release ventilation

The aim of these modes of ventilation is to limit peak inspired pressure and to improve recruitment. Reversing the ratio of inspiration to expiration prolongs inspiration. This allows the desired tidal volume to be delivered over a longer period and hence at a lower peak airway pressure. It also holds the lungs in an inflated position for longer and thus improves recruitment. However, not allowing normal time for expiration results in hypercapnia and increased auto-PEEP. Patients also need to be paralysed to tolerate inverse ratio ventilation. The benefits that have been shown may only be due to the increased auto-PEEP.

Airway pressure release ventilation is a more extreme form of inverse ratio ventilation where the lungs are held open in prolonged inspiration and exhalation is limited to brief periods where the inspired airway pressure is released. Patients do not need to be paralysed, and can breathe on top of the inspired pressure. There are no controlled trials looking at these modes of ventilation.

Partial liquid ventilation

Reduced surfactant in ALI/ARDS results in alveolar collapse owing to increased surface tension. Organic fluorocarbon liquids reduce surface tension, have a high oxygen-carrying capacity, are non-toxic, not absorbed, and are excreted by evaporation from the lungs. Organic fluorocarbon can thus increase lung compliance, reduce atelectasis and improve gas exchange. *Partial* liquid ventilation (PLV) means that the lungs are only filled to functional residual capacity (FRC) with the fluorocarbon liquid.

Gas exchange is improved in animal models with PLV, especially if combined with higher PEEP, inverse ratio ventilation or prone positioning. Studies in humans have shown that PLV is safe. A randomized controlled pilot study in 90 patients showed no improvement in oxygenation or 28-day mortality. Subgroup analysis showed a trend towards a shorter period of ventilation in patients under 55 years of age. Until further studies have been done, this intriguing treatment modality remains experimental.

PHARMACOLOGICAL

No pharmacological agents have shown to be of benefit in patients with ALI/ARDS, with the possible exception of glucocorticoids when given to patients with fibrosing alveolitis. Nitric oxide could be considered in patients with severe refractory hypoxaemia. A number of these agents warrant further review.

Inhaled vasodilators

In a model of patients with ALI/ARDS the lungs can be divided into four ventilation–perfusion regions: region 1, which is well ventilated and well perfused; región 2, which is well ventilated but poorly perfused; region 3, which is poorly ventilated but well perfused; and region 4, which is both poorly ventilated and poorly perfused. Regions 2 and 3 are responsible for the V_A/Q mismatch, increased shunt fraction and resultant hypoxaemia that are seen. Ventilation strategies are aimed at improving the mismatch in region 3. It would seem logical that a pulmonary vasodilator would improve the mismatch in region 2. If this vasodilator were to

be delivered intravenously, it would indiscriminately increase the perfusion in all regions, including those that are not ventilated, and would thus worsen the V_A/Q mismatch and further increase the shunt fraction. However, if the vasodilator were to be delivered by inhalation and only had a local effect, it would only vasodilate region 2, and thus would have the desired effect of improving V_A/Q matching, increasing the shunt fraction and improving oxygenation. Nitric oxide and prostacyclin are two such agents that can be delivered by inhalation.

NITRIC OXIDE

Nitric oxide (NO) is a potent vasodilator delivered by inhalation and has the advantage that it is not systemically absorbed and is rapidly inactivated, so that its effect is limited to the site of action. In theory, NO would seem an ideal agent for treating hypoxaemia due to V_A/Q mismatching, and for reducing the pulmonary hypertension in ALI/ARDS.[10] Prospective randomized controlled trials have shown that inhaled NO does indeed significantly reduce hypoxaemia in ALI/ARDS patients. However, it has not been shown to make a significant difference to outcome in terms of mortality or duration of ventilation. This may be because the improvement in oxygenation is not sustained beyond 24 hours. It also has the disadvantages that it is expensive, requires specialized equipment and training to deliver, and produces toxic degradation products. Some success in the use of NO in neonates (leading to a reduced need for ECMO) cannot be translated to its use in adult patients with ALI/ARDS. At present NO only has a place as a rescue therapy in the treatment of refractory hypoxaemia or pulmonary hypertension.

PROSTACYCLIN

Inhaled nebulized prostacyclin has effects similar to inhaled NO. However, it has the advantages that it is cheaper, easier to administer, and has no toxic byproducts. Case-controlled studies have shown that it improves oxygenation to the same degree as inhaled NO. One study has suggested that patients with ALI/ARDS due to indirect lung injury may respond better. No prospective randomized controlled trials have been performed, and thus there is insufficient evidence to recommend its use.

Surfactant

Surfactant is normally produced by type II cells in the lungs. Its primary function is to reduce surface tension in the alveoli and thus prevent alveolar collapse during normal respiration. It also protects against pulmonary infection. In patients with ALI/ARDS surfactant production and quality are reduced, resulting in alveolar collapse and an increased susceptibility to infection.

In experimental models, pulmonary compliance and oxygenation are improved by surfactant. There is good evidence to support the use of surfactant in premature infants with immature lungs who have a deficiency in surfactant. This is not the case in adults with ALI/ARDS. In a multicentre randomized placebo-controlled trial, continuous surfactant was given by aerosol to 725 patients with ARDS.[11] There was no difference in mortality, duration of ventilation or oxygenation between the two groups. The type of surfactant used in this study was an artificial protein-free version (Exosurf). Studies using a natural bovine surfactant instilled directly into the tracheobronchial tree have shown an improvement in oxygenation and a possible reduction in mortality in certain patient subgroups. However, until further studies are undertaken, the use of surfactant in adults with ALI/ARDS is not recommended.

Inflammatory modulators

The ability to modulate the inflammatory process and all its proinflammatory and anti-inflammatory components is the Holy Grail of intensive care. One pharmacological agent after another has come and gone without any proven benefit. The reason for this is twofold. First, the inflammatory process is complex, involving a number of pathways. Successful modulation would require the simultaneous manipulation of several pathways. Second, once the inflammatory process has been started, it is difficult to stop. It may be that some agents would only be beneficial if given early, or even before the event.

GLUCOCORTICOIDS

Glucocorticoids act at several points of the inflammatory cascade, which may seem an advantage. Numerous randomized double-blind controlled trials have shown no benefit to high-dose glucocorticoids (120 mg/kg methylprednisolone per day) when given in an attempt to prevent the development of ALI/ARDS (in patients with sepsis), nor when given early in the course of the disease. However, several smaller trials have shown that there may be some benefit to giving lower doses of glucocorticoids (2–3 mg/kg methylprednisolone per day) to patients in the later, fibroproliferative phase. Any advantage has to be weighed against the increased risk of nosocomial infection that occurs with the administration of glucocorticoids. The ARDS Network group is currently conducting a large prospective randomized double-blind trial looking at the late use (after 7 days) of glucocorticoids in patients with ALI/ARDS.

ANTIOXIDANTS

Sepsis, endotoxins and hyperoxia all increase reactive oxygen species (free radicals) in the lungs of patients with ALI/ARDS. In addition, these patients have reduced levels of natural antioxidants. These free radicals increase damage to the lung endothelium. To determine whether the administration of exogenous antioxidants would counteract this, a number of antioxidants have been tried, including *N*-acetylcysteine, procysteine, glutathione precursors and enteral antioxidant vitamins. Earlier studies showed a trend towards improved oxygenation and faster recovery, but a large placebo-controlled trial with procysteine did not show any benefit.

PROSTAGLANDIN E_1

Prostaglandin E_1 exerts its anti-inflammatory action by decreasing neutrophil activation and preventing platelet aggregation. Early clinical studies were encouraging, but the results of a multicentre study with intravenous prostaglandin E_1 and a phase II study with inhaled liposomal prostaglandin E_1 in patients with ALI/ARDS failed to demonstrate any benefit.

IBUPROFEN

Ibuprofen, a non-steroidal anti-inflammatory agent, inhibits the cyclooxygenase inflammatory pathway. A prospective double-blind randomized trial in 455 patients with sepsis showed no difference in mortality or in organ failure-free days despite successfully inhibiting the cyclooxygenase pathway (as measured by an 89 per cent reduction in prostanoid levels).

KETOCONAZOLE

Ketoconazole, a synthetic imidazole, inhibits the production of thromboxane and leukotrienes. A multicentre phase III trial in 234 patients showed no difference in mortality or duration of ventilation.

LISOFYLLINE

Lisofylline is a phosphodiesterase inhibitor that inhibits the release of free fatty acids from cell membranes, and in animal models has been shown to inhibit the release of various cytokines (TNF, IL-1, IL-6) in lung injury. A phase III trial conducted by the ARDS Network was stopped for lack of efficacy.

PENTOXIFYLLINE

Pentoxifylline is also a phosphodiesterase inhibitor that inhibits neutrophil chemotaxis and activation in animal lung injury models. It requires further study in humans.

OTHER INFLAMMATORY MODULATORS

Antiendotoxin monoclonal antibody, anti-TNF-α and anti-IL-1 have all been tried and failed. Recently, activated protein C has been shown to significantly reduce mortality in patients with sepsis. It may follow that this therapy could reduce the mortality of patients with ALI/ARDS due to sepsis, although there is as yet no evidence to support this theory. Other anti-inflammatory therapies that probably warrant testing in patients with ALI/ARDS are monoclonal antibodies against IL-8 (to mitigate neutrophil chemotaxis), platelet-activating factor inhibitors, antiproteases and coagulation cascade inhibitors.

β-Agonists

Alveolar fluid reabsorption by the alveolar epithelium is an important part of the resolution process in patients with ALI/ARDS. This alveolar fluid clearance depends on active sodium transport across the epithelium. β-Agonists have been shown experimentally to increase sodium and fluid clearance both in normal animal lung and in animal lung injury models. This response is noted with β-agonists delivered either by aerosol or intravenously. This therapy may prove useful in the resolution phase of ALI/ARDS, but needs to be evaluated by clinical studies.

Hepatocyte growth factor and keratinocyte growth factor

In ALI/ARDS the alveolar epithelium begins the repair process by a provisional proliferation of type II cells. However, gaps in this repair can allow myofibroblasts to migrate into the alveoli, which can then proliferate and cause fibrosing alveolitis. Therefore, anything that may enhance the initial proliferation of type II cells may prevent this fibroproliferative response. Hepatocyte growth factor and keratinocyte growth factor have both been shown to enhance proliferation of type II cells in experimental animal lung injury models.

Muscle relaxants

Muscle relaxants may occasionally be necessary to facilitate ventilation in patients with severe ARDS. The use of these drugs may be associated with a polymyopathy in the critically ill, and the train-of-four ratio should always be monitored while these agents are being administered. Use should be limited to the amount and duration required to maintain acceptable oxygenation.

CONCLUSION

Mortality due to ALI/ARDS has decreased in the last decade. This is due to improvements in general supportive care, management of infections and ventilation management, rather than to any one specific therapy. Based on the current evidence, patients should be ventilated with a protective lung strategy, along the lines of the ARDS Network low tidal volume study. This strategy will no doubt continue to evolve and be refined. In addition, there are a number of alternative ventilation strategies and pharmacological interventions that warrant further study.

REFERENCES

1. Ashbaugh DG, Bigelow DB, Petty TL, Levine BE. Acute respiratory distress in adults. *Lancet* 1967; **2**: 319–23.
2. Murray JF, Matthay MA, Luce JM, Flick MR. An expanded definition of the adult respiratory distress syndrome. *Am Rev Respir Dis* 1988; **138**: 720–3.
3. Bernard GR, Artigas A, Brigham KL, *et al.* The American–European Consensus Conference on ARDS: definitions, mechanisms, relevant outcomes, and clinical trial coordination. *Am J Respir Crit Care Med* 1994; **149**: 818–24.
4. Gattinoni L, Pelosi P, Suter PM, *et al.* Acute respiratory distress syndrome caused by pulmonary and extrapulmonary disease. Different syndromes? *Am J Respir Crit Care Med* 1998; **158**: 3–11.
5. The National Heart, Lung and Blood Institute, ARDS Clinical Trials Network. Higher versus lower positive end-expiratory pressures in patients with the acute respiratory distress syndrome. *N Engl J Med* 2004; **351**: 327–35.
6. Amato M, Barbas C, Medeiros D, *et al.* Effect of a protective-ventilation strategy on mortality in the acute respiratory distress syndrome. *N Engl J Med* 1998; **338**: 347–54.
7. The Acute Respiratory Distress Syndrome Network. Ventilation with low tidal volumes as compared with traditional tidal volumes for acute lung injury and the acute respiratory distress syndrome. *N Engl J Med* 2000; **342**: 1301–8.
8. Richard J-C, Brochard L, Breton L, *et al.* Influence of respiratory rate on gas trapping during low volume ventilation of patients with acute lung injury. *Intensive Care Med* 2002; **28**: 1078–83.
9. Gattinoni L, Tognoni G, Pesenti I, *et al.* The Prone–Supine Study Group. Effect of prone positioning on the survival of patients with acute respiratory failure. *N Engl J Med* 2001; **345**: 568–73.
10. Rossaint R, Falke KJ, Lopez F, *et al.* Inhaled nitric oxide for the adult respiratory distress syndrome. *N Engl J Med* 1993; **328**: 399–405.
11. Anzueto A, Baughman RP, Guntupalli KK, *et al.* Aerosolised surfactant in adults with sepsis-induced acute respiratory distress syndrome. *N Engl J Med* 1996; **334**: 1417–21.

5 Cardiovascular support in critical care

RAVI MAHAJAN & IAIN MOPPETT

Viva topics

- Describe the arterial pressure waveform. What information may be obtained from this?
- Describe three clinical methods for the measurement of cardiac output and the advantages and disadvantages of each.
- What assumptions are being made in the interpretation of central venous pressure (CVP) as an estimate of preload?
- Describe a simple algorithm for the management of hypotension in a postoperative patient.
- What is the place of dopamine in the critical care management of hypotension?

INTRODUCTION

The aim of cardiovascular support is to perfuse vital organs with sufficient blood to meet their oxygen and metabolic requirements and waste elimination needs without initiating or maintaining pathological effects. A large proportion of patients admitted to critical care units have a compromised cardiovascular system, and cardiovascular support is a vital aspect of their management.

The objectives of this chapter are to review the anatomical and physiological basis of cardiovascular support, review the current monitoring options, and discuss the management of the common cardiovascular pathologies encountered in critical care.

PHYSIOLOGICAL BASIS OF CARDIOVASCULAR SUPPORT

The purpose of the cardiovascular system is to provide an efficient mechanism for the transport of oxygen and other nutrients to the tissues and the removal of waste products. To achieve this blood is pumped around two circuits – the pulmonary and systemic circulations. Deoxygenated blood

from systemic veins enters the right side of the heart, which pumps it into the pulmonary circulation, a low-pressure system. The left side of the heart receives oxygenated blood from the pulmonary veins, from where it is pumped into the aorta for systemic circulation, a high-pressure system.

Electrophysiology

The electrical impulse originates spontaneously from the sinoatrial (SA) node at a rate of 70–80 beats/min (bpm). The impulse travels to the atrioventricular (AV) node, and then to the bundle of His. The bundle of His is divided into right and left bundle branches, which in turn divide into a network of Purkinje fibres. Normally, the SA node assumes the role of cardiac pacemaker because of its higher intrinsic discharge rate compared with the AV node (40–60 bpm) or Purkinje fibres (15–40 bpm). The pacemaker cells contain calcium, sodium and potassium channels and β receptors.

- The pacemaker activity of the heart can be influenced by the level of sympathetic/parasympathetic activity, temperature, oxygenation, serum potassium and other electrolyte imbalances
- The atria are innervated by both sympathetic and parasympathetic fibres, whereas the ventricles are innervated predominantly by sympathetic fibres
- Stimulation of the vagus nerves causes bradycardia, and stimulation of the sympathetic nervous system causes tachycardia.

The heart as a pump

The ventricles are filled during diastole with approximately 130 mL of blood (end-diastolic volume). During systole, a portion of the blood in the ventricle is ejected (ejection fraction) into the aorta. The ejection fraction is normally >60 per cent of end-diastolic volume, which equates to a stroke volume of about 70–80 mL. Atrial contraction contributes up to 25 per cent of ventricular filling. This component is lost during atrial fibrillation, leading to reduced ventricular filling and reduced stroke volume. Other factors that may reduce ventricular filling due to failure of the atrial pump are increased heart rate (reduced diastolic time), mitral stenosis and hypertrophic myopathies (Table 5.1). Significant dysfunction of left ventricular contractility is indicated if the ejection fraction is <40 per cent (as determined by echocardiography or angiography). The causes of decreased myocardial contractility are discussed below.

Venous return

Systemic veins are capacitance vessels. About 60 per cent of the total blood volume is contained in small veins and venules. The venous return is regulated by changes in vascular tone, which in turn is mediated by the sympathetic and parasympathetic nervous systems. Increased sympathetic activity causes constriction of the veins that can add up to 1 L of blood into the circulation, whereas dilatation of the veins can accommodate as much as 70–75 per cent of the systemic blood volume. Venous return is the major determinant of cardiac preload and cardiac output. Therefore, factors that decrease venous return also decrease cardiac output (Table 5.1).

During changes in posture, positive-pressure ventilation and hypovolaemia, compensatory mechanisms increase the tone of the vessels, leading to an increase in venous return. These mechanisms may be impaired in critically ill patients.

Cardiac output

Cardiac output can be defined as the amount of blood leaving the left ventricle per minute.

Thus:

Cardiac output = heart rate × stroke volume.

Therefore, the factors that affect heart rate, stroke volume, or both will also affect cardiac output. The stroke volume is determined by:

- Preload (ventricular filling)
- Force of contraction of the myocardium
- Afterload (systemic vascular resistance).

The typical Starling curve (Figure 5.1) determines the relationship between the initial length of cardiac muscle fibre and the force of contraction. According to this relationship, an increased initial length of muscle (i.e. if the cardiac muscle is stretched) would result in a greater force of contraction. Thus, an increase in venous return (or preload) would result in an increase in the force of contraction of the myocardium and hence an increase in cardiac output.

Table 5.1 *Causes of decreased venous return*

Causes of reduced ventricular filling

Reduced venous return
Loss of atrial pump
   Atrial fibrillation
   Ischaemia
Mitral stenosis
Poor ventricular relaxation
   Ischaemic heart disease
   Sepsis

Causes of decreased venous return

Hypovolaemia – fluid or blood loss
Venous dilatation – sepsis
Autonomic neuropathy
Vasodilator therapy
Positive-pressure ventilation of the lungs
Loss of compensatory increase in venous tone in response to
   changes in posture

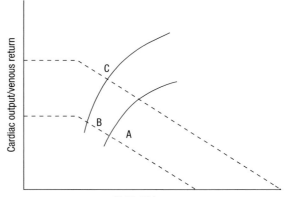

Figure 5.1 Starling curve – the effect of venous return and contractility on cardiac output. The response to changes in venous return and cardiac contractility. Stroke volume (and therefore cardiac output) is determined by Starling's law. Thus as end-diastolic volume increases (approximated by right atrial pressure) so does stroke volume. Increased contractility moves the curve up and to the left. Venous return (equal to cardiac output at steady state) is also a function of right atrial pressure: as right atrial pressure decreases, venous return will increase until the point at which venous collapse is reached when a plateau occurs (dashed lines). Addition of volume to the venous circulation causes this curve to move up and to the right. At equilibrium, the two lines must intersect (A). If contractility alone is increased then cardiac output rises a modest amount (B). If venous compliance reduces (higher pressures for the same venous return) along with increased contractility, then there is a marked increase in cardiac output (C)

However, the right atrial pressure will also govern venous return, and at steady state venous return must be equal to cardiac output. As right atrial pressure decreases venous return will increase until the right atrial pressure is less than intrathoracic pressure, when the great veins will collapse and limit further venous return (Figure 5.1).

Afterload is usually determined by the systemic vascular resistance.

Blood pressure

Traditionally, the systemic circulation has been thought of as analogous to an electric circuit where voltage is equal to resistance times current (Ohm's Law), thus:

Mean arterial pressure − mean central venous pressure
= systemic vascular resistance × cardiac output.

This is an oversimplification, but it provides an essential guide to what is happening clinically.

Given that the mean central venous pressure is usually relatively small (compared to the mean arterial pressure) and constant, the equation can be simplified to:

Mean arterial pressure = systemic vascular resistance
× cardiac output.

Therefore:

- If the mean arterial pressure increases there must be an increase in peripheral resistance or cardiac output, or both
- If mean blood pressure decreases there must be a decrease in peripheral resistance or cardiac output, or both
- Blood pressure alone cannot give any indication about cardiac output.

The factors that decrease or increase systemic vascular resistance are given in Table 5.2.

Myocardial function

In critical care, a number of indices can be used to assess myocardial function. These are given in Table 5.3. The advantage of using indexed measurements is that allowance is made for the size of the patient. Measurements of work incorporate values for pressure and flow. Myocardial contractility is a function of the preload in addition to adrenergic receptor stimulation and effects of disease states. Factors that can affect myocardial contractility are given in Table 5.4.

Myocardial oxygen balance

The oxygen consumption of the myocardium is among the highest of all organs. A balance must exist between oxygen

Table 5.2 *Factors affecting systemic vascular resistance*

Factors decreasing systemic vascular resistance
Anaemia
Exercise
Hyperthermia
Hyperthyroidism
Arteriovenous shunts
Vasodilators
Sepsis
SIRS (burns, multiple trauma), etc.

Factors increasing systemic vascular resistance
Polycythaemia
Hypothermia
Vasoconstriction
Application of tourniquets
Sympathetic stimulation

Table 5.3 *Commonly used indices of cardiac function*

	Normal values
Cardiac output = Stroke volume × heart rate	4–6 L/min
Cardiac index = Cardiac output/body surface area	2.5–4 L/min/m^2
Stroke index = Stroke volume/body surface area	40–60 mL/beat/m^2
Stroke work index = (MAP − PAOP) × stroke index	>3000 mL/ mmHg/m^2

Table 5.4 *Factors affecting myocardial contractility*

Factors increasing myocardial contractility
Increased ventricular filling (preload)
Decreased systemic vascular resistance (afterload)
Sympathetic stimulation
Inotropes
   β_1 agonists
   Phosphodiesterase inhibitors
   Glucagon
   Calcium

Factors decreasing myocardial contractility
Decreased preload
β blockade
Calcium channel blockade
Electrolyte imbalance
Myocardial ischaemia
Uraemia
Sepsis, particularly meningococcal
Cardiomyopathy
Acidosis

Table 5.5 *Factors affecting myocardial oxygen supply and demand*

Factors decreasing myocardial oxygen supply
Decreased coronary perfusion pressure
    Decreased aortic diastolic pressure
    Increased left ventricular end-diastolic pressure
Increased coronary arterial resistance
    Failure of diastolic relaxation
    Coronary artery disease
Decreased arterial oxygen content
Increased heart rate (decreased time for diastole)

Factors increasing myocardial oxygen demand
Increased heart rate
Increased force of contractility
Increased ventricular wall tension (increased LVEDP)

consumption and oxygen supply to avoid myocardial ischaemia. The blood supply to the myocardium occurs during diastole, because the tension in the myocardial wall is lowest at this time, reducing coronary arterial resistance. Therefore:

Coronary perfusion pressure = diastolic arterial pressure − left ventricular end-diastolic pressure.

Thus, myocardial blood supply is decreased if diastolic arterial pressure is decreased or left ventricular end-diastolic pressure (LVEDP) is increased (e.g. stiff ventricular wall due to ischaemia, sepsis or hypertrophy).

The length of diastole also affects coronary blood flow: if the heart rate is increased the diastolic time is shortened more than systolic, and this can impair coronary perfusion.

Factors affecting the supply and demand of myocardial oxygen are summarized in Table 5.5.

Physiological responses to changes in blood pressure

Blood pressure is the lateral pressure exerted by the blood on the vessels. As previously stated:

Mean arterial pressure = cardiac output × systemic vascular resistance.

Physiologically, changes in blood pressure normally activate a number of compensatory mechanisms; these may be impaired in critical care patients, because of either pre-existing disease or the precipitating illness. The most important of these mechanisms are:

- **Baroreceptor reflexes** Receptors in the carotid body respond to acute changes in systemic blood pressure by changing their firing rate, in turn altering the degree of activation of the vasomotor centre. An increase in blood pressure thus results in arterial and venous dilatation, bradycardia, and a reduction in cardiac output.

- **Atrial reflexes** Receptors in the atria respond to the degree of stretch in the low-pressure venous system, giving feedback on volume status. Increased stimulation occurs with increased venous pressure and results in vasodilation and usually a decrease in blood pressure. This also causes tachycardia. A reduction in stimulation due to reduced extracellular fluid (ECF) volume or positive-pressure ventilation results in increased sympathetic activity and increased vasopressin (ADH) release.

- **Central nervous system ischaemic reflex (Cushing reflex)** This is activated during ischaemia of the central vasomotor centre. This results in intense activity of the sympathetic nervous system and a classic picture of hypertension and bradycardia.

- **Catecholamines** These may be released as mediators of the above reflexes. Norepinephrine (noradrenaline) is the most important α-receptor agonist: it constricts arteries and veins independently of their neural supply. Epinephrine (adrenaline) is an important β-agonist that increases myocardial contractility.

- **Renin–angiotensin system** Renin release from the kidneys is provoked by a reduction in renal perfusion. It initiates the formation of angiotensin I, which is converted to angiotensin II in the lungs (angiotensin-converting enzyme). Angiotensin II is a vasoconstrictor and also stimulates the secretion of aldosterone, which conserves sodium and retains water.

- **Vasopressin** This posterior pituitary hormone is released in response to reduced extracellular fluid volume, positive-pressure ventilation and physiological stress. It results in vasoconstriction and fluid retention by the kidney.

- **Atrial natriuretic peptide (ANP)** This is stored principally in atrial myocytes and is released in response to increased vascular volume (atrial distension). ANP decreases blood pressure by peripheral dilatation, natriuresis and diuresis.

Pulmonary circulation

The pulmonary circulation is a low-pressure high-flow system. Its principal function is the transport of blood through the lungs for gas exchange. A hypoxic gas mixture in alveoli causes pulmonary vasoconstriction (hypoxic pulmonary vasoconstriction). This is a protective response that diverts the blood from less ventilated (atelectatic) areas to the ventilated ones, thus minimizing the V/Q mismatch. Persistent hypoxic pulmonary vasoconstriction in critical care patients can lead to increased pulmonary artery pressure and subsequent right heart failure.

Table 5.6 *Advantages and disadvantages of various methods of monitoring cardiac output*

	Fundamental technique	Cannulae required	Continuous, real time	Degree of invasiveness	Confidence in absolute value	Confidence in trends	Usefulness in predicting response to fluid
PAFC	Indicator dilution	PA	Yes	High	High	High	Moderate
LiDCO	Indicator dilution + pulse contour analysis	Any venous, arterial	Yes	Moderate	High for LiDCO Moderate for pulse wave analysis	High	High
PiCCO	Indicator dilution + pulse contour analysis	CV, Art	Yes	Moderate	Moderate	High	Moderate
TOD	Doppler derived blood flow velocity	None	Yes	Low	Poor	High	High
TOE	Doppler-derived blood flow velocity + estimation of flow conduit size	None	No	Moderate	Moderate	High	High
NICO	Fick principle with partial rebreathing of CO_2	None	Yes	Low	Moderate	High	Moderate

TOE = transoesophageal echocardiography

MONITORING

Monitoring of the cardiovascular system ranges from clinical assessment to the use of invasive, complex technical equipment. There is little evidence to suggest that more complex methods of investigation confer survival benefit, or that any one device is preferable to another. The decision as to which monitor to use and when is a balance of factors such as diagnostic uncertainty, the familiarity with and risks of using the monitor, and the secondary benefits (such as blood sampling) that are present (Table 5.6).

Clinical assessment

In critical care much dependence is placed on available mechanical monitoring. However, clinical examination may be neglected, and values obtained from technical equipment may be accepted inappropriately. Examination of the patient may indicate the presence of hypovolaemia, poor cardiac output or peripheral vasodilatation.

Technical assessment

Equipment is now commonly available to measure blood pressure, central venous pressure/right atrial pressure and cardiac output. The range of techniques used varies in the requirement for invasive access and the methods of calibration. The limitations and potential benefits of each monitoring device need to be appreciated before data obtained can be interpreted appropriately.

Invasive blood pressure measurement

ARTERIAL CANNULATION

Invasive blood pressure measurement allows beat-to-beat assessment of blood pressure and the ability to take repeated arterial blood samples. However, a number of common errors result in inaccurate blood pressure recording:

- The pressure transducer should be at the level of the heart; if lower than this the recorded pressure will be inappropriately high, and vice versa
- The equipment should be calibrated correctly. Commonly this involves zeroing the transducer at the level of the heart. If readings continue to be unexpected and significantly different from non-invasive measurements, further calibration at pressures of 100 and 200 mmHg should be performed using a manometer
- If the arterial pressure trace is flattened in amplitude this is termed a damped trace. Common causes are air in the arterial cannula and obstruction of the cannula by clot. The simplest way to assess damping is using a flush test, as shown in Figure 5.2
- Resonance is said to occur if the resonant frequency of the monitoring system is close to the measured frequency, as shown in Figure 5.2A. This can usually be overcome by

using short, stiff tubing to connect the arterial cannula to the transducer.

The arterial pulse can be analysed to measure or estimate a number of variables (Figure 5.3).

The change in systolic pressure, pulse pressure, or stroke volume with cyclical changes in intrathoracic pressure may

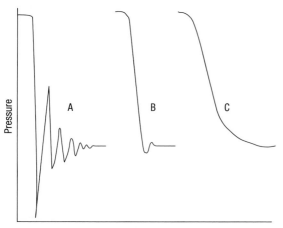

Figure 5.2 Examples of arterial waveforms. Flush test. The pressure is raised to a high level using the flush on the pressure system and then released. If the system is resonant or underdamped (A), then significant overshoot and oscillation occurs. In an optimally damped system the pressure just overshoots the baseline (B), but still reflects the timecourse of pressure change. In the overdamped system there is no overshoot (C), but the timecourse of pressure change is too slow

be used as a measure of preload (see below). LiDCO (lithium indicator dilution), PiCCO and Finometer technologies use analysis of the arterial waveform to give information about peripheral vascular resistance and cardiac output.

SYSTOLIC PRESSURE VARIATION

During positive-pressure ventilation, inspiration is associated with an increase in intrathoracic pressure. As this occurs, venous return is decreased and so cardiac output and blood pressure also decrease, with a phase length equal to the respiratory rate. This may be manifest by a 'swing' on the arterial pressure trace. It is possible to examine the variation in systolic pressure during the respiratory cycle mathematically and use this measure (the systolic pressure variation) to estimate the extent of right heart filling. Similar effects are seen with pulse pressure and stroke volume. In clinical practice observation of the 'swing' on the arterial pressure trace is more commonly used (Figure 5.4).

CENTRAL VENOUS PRESSURE MEASUREMENT

Central venous pressure is measured traditionally to allow an estimate of right atrial preload. The relationship between right atrial volume and right atrial pressure is shown in Figure 5.5. It is immediately apparent that there is no direct relationship between these two variables, although between the points marked VV' and PP' the relationship is approximately linear. The absolute measurement of central venous pressure is not a helpful measure of right atrial filling. However, the change in central venous pressure due to a

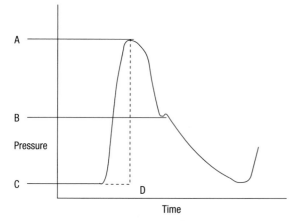

Figure 5.3 Information obtained from arterial waveform. A, systolic blood pressure; B, approximation of aortic valve closure and end of systole; C, diastole; D, the rate of change of pressure with time gives an indication of contractility

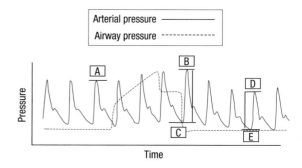

Figure 5.4 Pulse wave variation. A, baseline systolic pressure – SBP bl; B, maximum systolic pressure – SBPmax; C, maximum pulse pressure – PPmax; D, minimum systolic pressure – SBPmin; E, minimum pulse pressure – PPmin. Systolic pressure variation is defined as deltaUp + deltaDown. Normal < 10 mmHg. DeltaUp is SBPmax − SBPbl, deltaDown is SBPbl − SBPmin. Pulse pressure variation is defined as PPmax − PPmin/((PPmax + PPmin)/2). Normal < 10 per cent

rapid fluid bolus may allow estimation of whether the circulation is underfilled, overfilled or appropriate (Figure 5.5b). An underfilled system will respond with an immediate rise in right atrial pressure, but this will quickly fall as venous compliance increases. An overfilled system will respond with a marked and prolonged increase in right atrial pressure, as not only is venous compliance low already, but also the cardiac output will not increase. However, this is only of value at the time of assessment. Changes in cardiac contractility and myocardial ischaemia may require this to be repeated frequently.

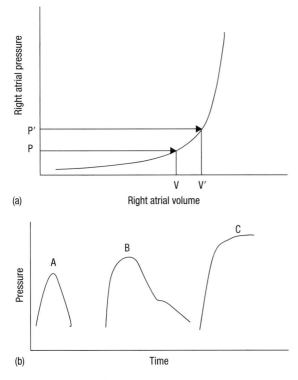

Figure 5.5 (a) The relationship between atrial volume and pressure is non-linear, and so measuring pressure alone gives little indication of absolute atrial volume. The relationship will appear linear between relatively small changes in volume. For instance, between V and V′ the pressure increases approximately linearly from P to P′. (b) Response of right atrial (or left atrial) pressure to a fluid bolus. A: The underfilled system has a brief rise in pressure, which then returns to its previous value as venous compliance increases. B: The well-filled system has a brief rise, followed by a fall back to a higher value than before. This will then gradually return to the initial value as fluid is redistributed/excreted. C: The overfilled system has a large rise in pressure, which is sustained. Note, the initial pressures in this diagram are all the same, emphasizing that static values of atrial pressure are poor predictors of fluid responsiveness

CARDIAC OUTPUT MEASUREMENT

Since the introduction into clinical practice of the pulmonary artery flow catheter in the 1970s the place of this tool in the assessment of the critically ill patient has been contested. The debate intensified following the publication of a paper by Connors *et al.* in 1996,[1] in which the mortality of a cohort of critically ill patients managed with a pulmonary artery catheter was shown to be greater than that of a similar cohort managed without, even when allowance was made for the patients' level of sickness. Despite much criticism of this study pulmonary artery catheter use declined following its publication. In recent years, alternative, less invasive methods of cardiac output monitoring have been made available, and interest in cardiac output monitoring appears to be increasing again.

PULMONARY ARTERY FLOTATION CATHETER (PAFC)

Right heart (Swann–Ganz) catheterization allows measurement of:

- Right atrial (RAP), right ventricular (RVP), pulmonary artery (PAP) and pulmonary artery occlusion pressures (PAOP) (Figure 5.6)
- Cardiac output using intermittent or continuous thermodilution techniques
- Mixed venous oxygen tension
- Central blood temperature.

Using these measured variables a whole range of additional parameters can be calculated, including systemic vascular resistance, pulmonary vascular resistance, stroke volume index, cardiac index, and left and right ventricular stroke work indices.

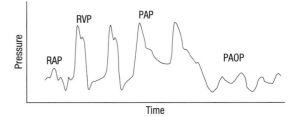

Figure 5.6 PAFC waveforms. Typical waveforms seen on passage of a pulmonary artery flotation catheter. On passing from the right atrium to the ventricle systolic pressures are markedly higher, but diastolic pressures fall to atrial values. When the pulmonary valve is crossed systolic pressures remain the same, but there is now a significant diastolic pressure. When the balloon is inflated, there is (in theory) a complete column of blood between the catheter tip and the left atrium. Hence, PAOP represents left atrial pressure

In clinical practice, pulmonary artery measurement of the cardiac output is still considered the gold standard against which other techniques are compared. However, it is an extremely invasive technique that carries real risks of pulmonary embolism/infarction, infection, arrhythmias, pulmonary artery rupture, valve rupture, and catheter knotting requiring surgical removal.

The pulmonary artery occlusion pressure (PAOP) is in many ways analogous to the central venous pressure discussed above. However, although in theory the PAOP gives a guide to left ventricular volume and hence cardiac function, more assumptions are required than for the central venous pressure assessment of right ventricular volume. This relationship only holds true if:

- The relationship between LVEDP and LVEDV is known – essentially similar to Figure 5.5
- There is no significant gradient across the mitral valve
- There is a continuous column of blood between the catheter and the left atrium (i.e. PV > PA)
- The relationship between intrathoracic pressure and left atrial pressure is known
- There is no overdistension of the right heart resulting in paradoxical septal movement.

Very rarely will these assumptions hold true in the critically ill. PAOP therefore suffers from similar limitations as CVP, but with rather more assumptions.

If the patient's lungs are ventilated mechanically and positive end-expiratory pressure (PEEP) is applied, this will affect intrathoracic pressure and the measurement of both CVP and PAOP. Again, this relationship is not linear. Disconnecting the ventilator circuit for a short period at end expiration and taking the nadir PAOP value will allow a measurement independent of PEEP. However, this will result in changes in oxygenation and fluid shifts owing to the change in PEEP that may, therefore, render the measurement meaningless. At least one author has suggested that the practice of giving volume to a patient based on targeting the PAOP may actually result in right heart failure.

THERMODILUTION TECHNIQUES

The traditional, clinical approach to cardiac output measurement using the pulmonary artery catheter involves the administration of a bolus of ice-cold water into the right side of the heart. A thermistor placed at the tip of the catheter in the pulmonary artery records the temperature change as the cold water, mixed with blood, is ejected from the right ventricle through the pulmonary artery. If the cardiac output is low the curve showing temperature change over time will be quite different from that in a high-output situation (Figure 5.7).

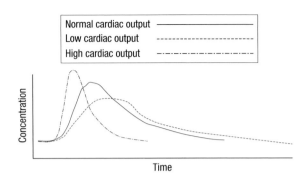

Figure 5.7 Indicator dilution curves. The cardiac output is calculated as mass of indicator/area under time concentration curve. A lower cardiac output results in a lower peak and a longer time to reach baseline, hence a larger area under the curve. The converse is true for high cardiac output

The stroke volume can be calculated by measuring the area under the temperature curve. This value is then multiplied by the heart rate to give cardiac output.

The limitations of this technique are that it is operator dependent: the injectate has to be at a significantly different temperature from blood to allow accurate determination, and the timing and speed of injection in the respiratory cycle will alter the measurement.

The current gold standard cardiac output measurement technique is semicontinuous monitoring using a pulmonary artery catheter. In this situation a copper coil is wrapped around the catheter to heat blood in the right side of the heart. The decrease in temperature as blood is ejected into the pulmonary artery is then detected by the distal thermistor. Although this is thought of as being a continuous cardiac output measurement, this is not true. The system takes some time to stabilize after insertion, the cardiac output recorded is an average of several measurements, and if cold fluid such as homologous blood is added to the system the temperature change may result in erroneous measurements for a period.

Alternative methods of cardiac output estimation

PULSE CONTOUR ANALYSIS

As indicated already, the peripheral arterial pulse waveform is a function of the input pressure, the cardiac output, and the peripheral vascular compliance and resistance. As such, the peripheral arterial waveform can be used to estimate cardiac output. If the cardiac output is then measured for a given peripheral pulse waveform, the relationship between the two can be defined. Once calibrated, changes in the peripheral pulse waveform can then be used to derive changes in the cardiac output. Both the LiDCO and PiCCO systems use intermittent cardiac output determination to calibrate continuous pulse wave analysis.

- **Lithium indicator dilution (LiDCO)** A small bolus (0.15 mL) of lithium chloride is given into a vein. The Li^+ level is measured by a lithium-sensitive electrode in a flow-through cell connected to an arterial line. The cardiac output calculated from this can then be used to calibrate the cardiac output determined by pulse wave contour analysis.
- **Cold technique/PiCCO** This is similar to the lithium technique except that the indicator is a cold fluid which is sensed by a thermistor in a centrally placed (femoral) arterial catheter. Using this equipment, the catheter can also be used to measure indocyanine green, which is cleared almost entirely by the liver. The elimination curve for indocyanine green therefore gives an indication of hepatic function.

DOPPLER TECHNIQUES

The velocity of blood flow in the aorta can be measured using Doppler ultrasound. Suprasternal approaches allow access to the ascending aorta and transoesophageal (TOD) approaches to the descending aorta. Because of difficulty in fixing the suprasternal probe, the transoesophageal route is usually used. Characteristically, a triangular time/velocity waveform is seen (Figure 5.8). A number of measurements can be made from this waveform.

The peak velocity (PV) is the height of the apex of the waveform and is an index of left ventricular contractility, which varies with age. In a 20-year-old the normal peak velocity would be of the order of 90–120 cm/s, whereas in those aged 70 it would be approximately 60–80 cm/s. The flow time is reflected by the base of the waveform and is corrected for heart rate to give an index of left ventricular filling. The area under the curve – the stroke distance – is proportional to the stroke volume (SV) passing the probe.

The area of the aorta is not measured but is estimated using nomograms based on height, weight, age and gender. This allows the velocity measurements to be converted to estimated flow, and hence cardiac output can be assessed. However, because the oesophageal probe only examines the descending aorta, assumptions also have to be made on the proportion of total cardiac output flowing through the descending aorta. Therefore, the absolute value of cardiac output may be significantly different from that obtained from a pulmonary artery catheter. However, because any errors due to incorrect assumptions tend to be constant, the trends obtained should remain reliable. Some transoesophageal Doppler manufacturers have included an M-mode ultrasound facility to measure aortic area directly, but there is little

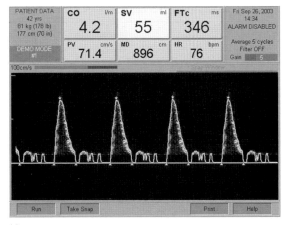

(a)

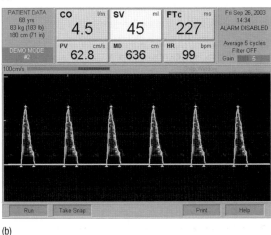

(b)

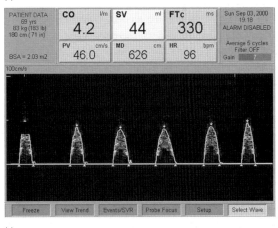

(c)

Figure 5.8 (a) A normal transoesophageal Doppler waveform. (b) A transoesophageal Doppler waveform typical of that seen in hypovolaemia. Note the decreased corrected flow time (FTc) and stroke volume (SV). (c) A transoesophageal waveform typical of that seen during left ventricular failure. Note the decreased peak velocity and 'blunted' waveforms

Table 5.7 *Causes of cardiovascular failure*

	Indicators of preload	Cardiac output	Peripheral resistance	Precipitants/ risks
Cardiac pump failure	High	Low	High	Acute coronary syndromes, hypertension
Hypovolaemia	Low	Low	High	Trauma, surgery, coagulopathy
Sepsis	Low	Low → High	Low	Infection, trauma, surgery
Anaphylaxis	Low	High	Low	Drug/plant/animal allergy

evidence to suggest that this makes the absolute values more reliable.

Limitations of this technique include the following. The probe is positioned by a combination of the sound and the waveform that the monitor generates. If the probe position changes between measurements it is possible that the reflected Doppler signal will have altered, resulting in inaccurate readings. It is possible to detect both intracardiac, pulmonary vessels and venous waveforms, and these need to be excluded.

The advantages of transoesophageal monitoring are that it is inserted very quickly and that waveforms can be analysed within a few minutes of a decision to monitor the cardiac output. The probe can be manipulated by nursing as well as medical staff with relatively little training. Despite many hundreds of probes being sited there are no life-threatening complications associated with this technology.

Figure 5.8 shows a typical Doppler waveform and how this will be changed in various disease and treatment states.

NICO (NON-INVASIVE CARDIAC OUTPUT MONITOR)

This technique relies on the accurate estimation of carbon dioxide elimination and is therefore only suitable for patients who are intubated and receiving positive-pressure ventilation. The mass of carbon dioxide eliminated in a unit of time is equal to the cardiac output multiplied by the arterial/mixed venous CO_2 content difference. By measuring CO_2 elimination at baseline and during partial rebreathing of CO_2 an estimate of cardiac output can be made without the need to measure either arterial or mixed venous CO_2 content. Various assumptions have to be made about the slope of the CO_2 dissociation curve and the constancy of ventilation dead space, cardiac output and shunt during the measurement period. However, the technique shows good correlation with thermodilution.

MANAGEMENT OF CARDIOVASCULAR SYSTEM FAILURE

Cardiovascular system failure (shock) occurs when there is inadequate tissue perfusion of the vital organs to meet metabolic demands. Table 5.7 summarizes the different causes of shock and the likely changes that will be seen in preload, cardiac output and peripheral resistance.

The cardiovascular system may also be 'failing' as a result of uncontrolled hypertension, and although this is not as common as hypotension in the critically ill, strategies for management need to be based on the same physiological principles as described above.

Endpoints for assessment of management

The objective of cardiovascular management is to provide adequate tissue perfusion. There are no specific monitors of tissue oxygenation in current everyday use. Therefore, the prime objectives are:

- To maintain the blood pressure in the normal range for the patient
- To maintain tissue perfusion as evidenced by:
  - An adequate urine output
  - A normal lactate concentration, i.e. <2 mmol/L (a marker of anaerobic respiration and inadequate perfusion)
  - A base excess that is either in or returning to the normal range (0–2 mEq).

Management of hypotension

The possible causes of hypotension are listed in Tables 5.1, 5.2 and 5.4. Management options for hypotension can be divided into fluids to increase preload, inotropes to increase myocardial contractility, and vasopressors to increase peripheral vascular resistance. Figure 5.9 illustrates the effect of administering fluids on the venous return curve and the effect of inotropes on the cardiac output curve. Both modalities may increase the cardiac output. Notice, though, in Figure 5.9 the situation in the failing heart. The cardiac output curve has been flattened as in myocardial failure, and the addition of fluid now results in a rise in the position of the venous return curve but the cardiac output remains unchanged. However, in this situation inotropes increase the cardiac output, and after this the addition of fluid may further increase the cardiac output.

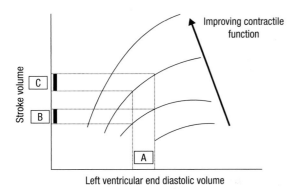

Figure 5.9 Starling curve. The 'normal' response curve results in increased stroke volume (B) (and hence cardiac output) in response to increased preload (A) (e.g. a fluid challenge). In the presence of positive inotropes the curve is shifted to the left and upward – thus for the same degree of preload there is an increased stroke volume, and the same increase in preload has a proportionally greater effect (C). In the presence of impaired cardiac contractility – such as ischaemia, heart failure and sepsis – the curve is shifted downward and to the right. It is also flatter. For a given preload cardiac output is reduced, and increased preload may have little or no effect

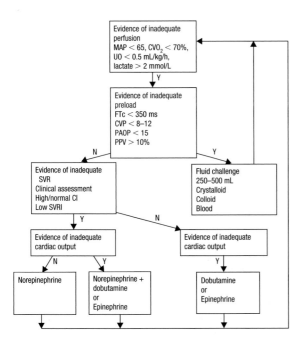

Figure 5.10 Approach to hypotension/underperfusion

A typical management plan for hypotension in the critically ill is shown in Figure 5.10. While monitoring the arterial pressure and the central venous pressure, a fluid bolus is given (e.g. 250 mL colloid as fast as possible). If the CVP

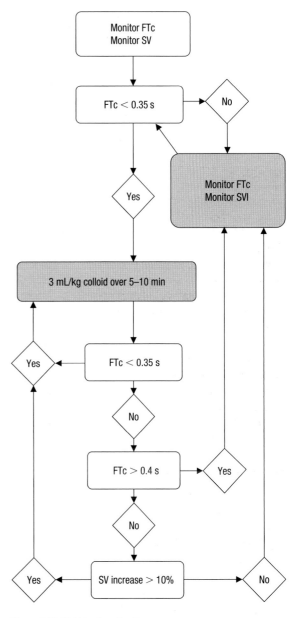

Figure 5.11 Fluid loading algorithm

increases marginally or rapidly returns to the previous value, this may be repeated. If the CVP rises and stays within a 'normal' range but the blood pressure remains low, a further fluid bolus may be given. If the CVP rises dramatically and stays high no further fluid should be given, but consideration given to the addition of a vasoactive agent. An algorithm for fluid loading based on the transoesophageal Doppler is shown in Figure 5.11. Further information on management of sepsis as a whole can be found in recently published guidelines from the Surviving Sepsis campaign.[2] These guidelines are discussed in more detail in Chapter 6.

Table 5.8 *Considerations in unresolving hypotension*

Cardiac	Drugs
Arrhythmia	Sedation
Acute coronary syndromes	Propofol
Pulmonary embolism	Benzodiazepines
Acute/chronic valvular disease	Opioids
Pericardial tamponade	Clonidine
Pulmonary	**Allergy**
Excessive intrathoracic pressures	**Maladminstration/blocked lines for vasoactive drugs**
Pneumothorax	**Metabolic**
PEEP/inspiratory ventilator pressures	pH < 7.2
	Hyper/hypo – K, Ca, Mg
Visceral	Marked hyper/hypocapnia
Bleeding	Temperature > 39.5

Table 5.9 *Alternative strategies for unresolving hypotension*

Vasopressin analogues
  Terlipressin 1–2 mg bolus 12-hourly

Methylene blue
  0.5 mg/kg/h for 6 hours
  2 mg/kg bolus

Steroids
  50 mg qds hydrocortisone $\pm$ fludrocortisone

Active cooling
  Cooling blankets
  Cardiopulmonary bypass (CPB)/Continuous veno-venous haemofiltration (CVVH)

Metabolic correction
  CVVH

The commonest cause of hypotension in the critically ill patient, when hypovolaemia is excluded, is peripheral vasodilatation. Therefore, the first-line vasoactive agent used tends to be a vasopressor. The drug of choice depends to some extent on local practice, but will often be norepinephrine. Norepinephrine is normally administered in a range between 0 and 1 µg/kg/min, and would normally be commenced at approximately 0.05 µg/kg/min and titrated to response. There is no absolute/correct dose. If the patient remains hypotensive despite fluid filling and vasopressor therapy, or if there is a history of myocardial disease, cardiac output monitoring will be essential to balance the need for inotropy and vasoconstriction. Details of the fluids and vasoactive agents available are given below. Unresolving hypotension despite these treatments may occur. Table 5.8 details factors that may be overlooked in the treatment of such patients. Table 5.9 provides some alternative strategies for managing unresolving hypotension, based largely on anecdote and clinical experience. There is no good evidence to support their use. There is some evidence that early aggressive therapy in the critically ill improves outcome.[3]

FLUIDS

The debate over whether colloid or crystalloid solutions are the 'best' has been ongoing for over 30 years without an unequivocal answer.

Crystalloids

These can be divided into salt-containing solutions (e.g. 0.9 per cent saline, compound sodium lactate) and dextrose solutions. The latter are distributed throughout the total body water and

should never be used as resuscitation fluids, whereas approximately 25 per cent of infused salt-containing solutions will remain in the intravascular compartment. Inevitably, the majority of the sodium (and with it water) remains in the extracellular, extravascular compartment. There is now a substantial amount of evidence to support the use of 'physiological' salt solutions rather than normal (0.9 per cent) saline for resuscitation. This is based on the relatively high concentration of chloride (150 mmol/L) in normal saline, which results in a hyperchloraemia and is manifested as metabolic acidosis. This is due to the strong ion difference (SID) created by large volume saline resuscitation, which is beyond the scope of this chapter. Although there is no evidence to date that a hyperchloraemic acidosis is essentially harmful, correction of base excess to normal levels by resuscitation is one well-defined endpoint. It is counterintuitive, therefore, to use a resuscitation fluid which itself will contribute to a change in this endpoint.

Hyperosmolar electrolyte solutions have some experimental evidence to support their use, particularly in the resuscitative phase of burns and head trauma. They act as intravascular volume expanders by virtue of their high osmolality, which reduces tissue oedema. The most commonly used hyperosmolar solution is 8.4 per cent sodium bicarbonate, and some authors attribute much of the benefit of this fluid to its osmolality rather than the pH changes. At present there is insufficient evidence to support the routine use of these solutions in resuscitation.

Colloids

Colloids can further be divided into gelatins and starch-containing solutions. Gelatins are solutions of molecules with higher molecular weight (30 000 Da) than crystalloids, and these might be expected to remain in the intravascular compartment for longer. However, the capillary leak that occurs in critical illness means that the intravascular half-life of these molecules is also short. Starches have been promoted for prolonged intravascular expansion in critically ill patients. However, these solutions contain a range of molecules of varying molecular size (mean 200 kDa). There is some evidence that a proportion of these molecules in fact stay in the extracellular compartment, where they promote further oedema formation owing to their colloidal properties. These fluids also cause deposition of starch in the reticulo-endothelial system, which may contribute to the long-term itching that is also associated with their use.

All synthetic colloids in the UK are currently marketed in a saline-based solution, and the same strong ion difference problems discussed with saline are true of these solutions. One starch is now available in the USA in compound sodium lactate. Some studies have already shown a marked improvement in acid–base changes using this solution. Synthetic colloids also dilute coagulation factors and affect platelet function, resulting in a coagulopathy. This needs to be monitored and corrected appropriately. Again, studies of starch in Ringer's lactate indicate that this problem is reduced with this solution compared to other starches. However, there remains no evidence that one colloid is particularly better than any other in terms of clinical outcome.

Human albumin solution has been the subject of much debate, with a Cochrane meta-analysis indicating an increased mortality associated with its use. However the SAFE (Saline versus Albumin Fluid Evaluation) study, a multicentre, randomized, double-blind trial that recruited nearly 7000 patients, demonstrated no significant difference in outcomes at 28 days, including mortality, between patients in the ICU resuscitated with 4 per cent albumin or crystalloid.[4] As a natural substance albumin has some theoretical advantages over the synthetic colloids: low risk of anaphylaxis, physiological metabolism and excretion, free radical scavenging, and negligible effect on the coagulation pathway.

VASOACTIVE AGENTS

The ideal vasoactive agent would provide a predictable, titratable increase in tissue perfusion without worsening the oxygen supply:demand ratio for any of the vital organs. No such agent exists. Those currently available are largely sympathomimetics, though a few non-adrenergic drugs are being used (Tables 5.10 and 5.11). Numerous studies have failed to identify which are the best agents in which situation. A logical approach based on the pathophysiology of the patient is the best solution.

Sympathomimetics

These drugs all act via a combination of α, β and dopaminergic stimulation. Although classified largely according to their central cardiovascular effects, they also have important effects on local blood supply and organ perfusion. In addition, these drugs may have significant immunomodulatory effects, altering cytokine release.

The effect of pharmacological stimulation of the adrenergic system in both the healthy and the critically ill is becoming clearer. A summary is given in Table 5.12.

NOREPINEPHRINE

Norepinephrine is a naturally occurring catecholamine which stimulates both α and β adrenoceptors at pharmacological doses, though its α effects predominate. Administration therefore results in peripheral vasoconstriction and an increase in blood pressure. There may be a reflex reduction in heart rate, though this is less than seen with pure α agonists such as phenylephrine. Cardiac output may also decrease owing to an increase in afterload. If administered to a patient with a failing heart this may result in worsening hypotension.

There are concerns regarding splanchnic vasoconstriction during the administration of norepinephrine. However, studies have shown that renal and gut perfusion is pressure dependent and, provided doses are not causing excessive vasoconstriction, the beneficial increase in mean arterial pressure (MAP) outweighs the potential disadvantage.

EPINEPHRINE

Epinephrine is a naturally occurring catecholamine. It stimulates both α and β adrenoceptors at pharmacological doses. This results in both positive inotropy and peripheral vasoconstriction. This makes it an extremely useful agent when it is not clear whether the primary cause of hypotension is myocardial depression or vasodilatation, and may increase the blood pressure while additional monitoring is used to assess the cardiovascular system more fully. However, in contrast to norepinephrine, epinephrine has been shown to cause a reversible lactic acidosis, due in part to intestinal ischaemia. This has been associated with a poorer outcome and gives rise to concerns that the duration of its use should be limited. Epinephrine has various metabolic effects, including stimulation of both glycogenolysis and insulin secretion.

DOBUTAMINE

Dobutamine is a synthetic catecholamine. It stimulates predominantly β_1 and β_2 adrenoceptors at pharmacological doses, though there is also some α activity. It therefore acts

Table 5.10 *Drugs used for cardiovascular support*

Drug	Effect	Mode of action	Dose range	Method of administration
Epinephrine	Inotrope			Central venous infusion
	Peripheral vasoconstriction	α and β agonist	0.01–0.1 μg/kg/min 0.1–1 mg bolus	
Norepinephrine	Peripheral vasoconstriction	α agonist	0.01–1 μg/kg/min	Central venous infusion
Dobutamine	Inotrope			Central venous infusion
	Peripheral vasodilation	β agonist	0.5–40 μg/kg/min	
Dopamine	Inotrope			Central or peripheral venous infusion
	Variable effects on peripheral vasculature	β, α and dopa agonist	1–20 μg/kg/min	
Dopexamine	Peripheral vasodilator			Central or peripheral venous infusion
	Mild inotrope	β and dopa agonist	0.5–6 μg/kg/min	
Vasopressin	Peripheral vasoconstriction	Vasopressin agonist	4 units/h	Central or peripheral venous infusion
Terlipressin	Peripheral vasoconstriction	Vasopressin agonist	1–2 mg bolus 6–12-hourly	Central or peripheral venous infusion
Methylene blue	Peripheral vasoconstriction	Guanylate cyclase inhibitor	2–4 mg/kg	Central venous infusion
Levosimendan	Positive inotrope	Calcium sensitiser	24 μg/kg bolus over 10 min 0.1 μg/kg/min	Central or peripheral venous infusion

Table 5.11 *Hypotensive and negatively inotropic agents*

Sodium nitroprusside	Veno- and arteriodilator	NO donor	2.5–10 μg/kg/min 0.25–1 mg/kg bolus	Central or peripheral venous infusion
GTN	Veno- and arteriodilator	NO donor	0.3 mg s/l 0.4–0.8 mg buccal spray 0.1–8 μg/kg/min	Central or peripheral venous infusion, sublingual, buccal
Hydralazine	Arteriodilator	Smooth muscle relaxation	20–40 mg bolus	Central or peripheral venous infusion
Methyldopa	Arteriodilator	Inhibition of sympathetic transmitter release	0.5–3 g/day (oral) 0.25–1 g over 4 h (iv)	Oral Peripheral venous
Nifedipine	Arteriodilator	Calcium channel blocker	10–20 mg	Sublingual or enteral
Clonidine	Peripheral vasodilator	Central inhibition of sympathetic drive	Up to 4 μg/kg/h 25–50 μg/h	Central or peripheral venous infusion
Enalaprilat	Peripheral vasodilator	Inhibition of ACE	1.25–5 mg/bolus	Central or peripheral venous infusion
Esmolol	Negative inotrope	β blockade	50–150 μg/kg/min 1 μg/kg bolus	Peripheral venous infusion
Labetalol	Negative inotrope, peripheral vasodilator	β and α blockade	2 mg/min 20–50 mg bolus	Peripheral venous infusion

Table 5.12 *Effects of stimulation of adrenergic and dopaminergic receptors*

	Heart	Peripheral vessels	Splanchnic vessels	Metabolic
α_1	Nil	Constriction	Constriction	
α_2	Centrally mediated bradycardia	Vasodilation		Platelet aggregation
β_1	Inotrope and chronotrope	Nil	Nil	
β_2	(Inotrope and chronotrope)	Vasodilation	Vasodilation	Increased glycogenolysis and insulin release
DA1			Vasodilation	
DA2				Anterior pituitary inhibition

as an inodilator, with an increase in cardiac output and a decrease in systemic vascular resistance. This makes it an ideal agent for use in pure cardiogenic shock, where the myocardium is failing and the systemic vascular resistance is increased to maintain the blood pressure. However, in the critically ill patient the peripheral vasodilatation will often be associated with hypotension. Tachycardia can also occur, limiting atrial filling and decreasing cardiac output. Clinically, it may be used in combination with norepinephrine when both cardiac output and peripheral resistance are low. The normal dose range is 0–20 µg/kg/min.

DOPEXAMINE

Dopexamine is a synthetic catecholamine. It has most activity at β_2 and dopaminergic receptors, with some small β_1 effect. Initially it was thought to have particularly beneficial effects on splanchnic perfusion, but this has not been borne out by later studies.

DOPAMINE

Dopamine is a naturally occurring catecholamine. It is metabolized to norepinephrine and at pharmacological doses it stimulates α and β adrenoceptors and dopaminergic receptors. Several studies have shown that the traditional view of selective dopaminergic effects, followed by β followed by α effects at increasing doses does not occur in the critically ill. 'Low-dose' (renal) dopamine (quoted as 1–4 µg/ kg/min) does not have selective renal vasodilatory effects and has been shown to raise cardiac output in sepsis at these doses. Stimulation of central DA2 receptors leads to inhibition of anterior pituitary hormone release. Because of the unpredictable receptor effects and the hormonal side effects many authors have suggested that this agent should no longer be used in critical care.

Vasopressin analogues

Vasopressin is a naturally occurring peptide that is part of the cardiovascular regulatory system. Subjects with sepsis have inappropriately low levels in the face of systemic hypotension. This may in part be due to altered baroreceptor responsiveness in sepsis and depletion of vasopressin stores in the posterior pituitary. This has led to the use of vasopressin as a vasoconstrictor in septic shock. Initial reports suggest that vasopressin infusion (4 units/h) allows the reduction/discontinuation of high-dose catecholamines. Infusion at 2–4 units/h restores blood vasopressin concentrations to those seen in other forms of hypotension. Vasopressin appears to act mainly as a pure vasoconstrictor, with constriction of resistance arterioles. There is also some improvement in indices of cardiac function. This may be due to suppression of cardiotoxic mediator release, and also to a reduction in catecholamine dosage, thereby reducing tachyarrhythmias. Also, vasopressin may increase intracellular calcium concentrations, with direct inotropic effects. The improvement in blood pressure would also be expected to improve coronary perfusion. High doses of vasopressin are associated with gastrointestinal ischaemia, but this does not appear to occur at 4 units/h, though an increase in bilirubin concentrations has been described. The synthetic analogue terlipressin may also be used, as it is longer acting and can be given as intermittent boluses rather than an infusion. A recent study has compared the use of vasopressin (40 units) with epinephrine (1 mg) as the first-line drug in out-of-hospital resuscitation from cardiac arrest.[5] No difference was found in rates of hospital admission or hospital discharge, though a post-hoc subgroup analysis suggested that survival may be improved when it is used in asystole. The UK Resuscitation Council does not recommend its use in resuscitation, though it is an option in the USA.

Methylene blue

Methylene blue acts as a guanylate cyclase inhibitor, thereby reducing the production of cyclic guanosine monophosphate (cGMP). Cyclic GMP is one of the mediators produced by the action of nitric oxide, and is responsible for vascular smooth muscle relaxation. In theory, methylene blue is therefore more selective than direct nitric oxide synthase inhibitors, which block the beneficial as well as the harmful effects of nitric oxide.

Anecdotal evidence and small uncontrolled trials suggest that infusions or bolus administration of methylene blue (2–4 mg/kg) can reverse refractory hypotension. The effects are mainly due to a rise in systemic vascular resistance and an improvement in systolic left ventricular function. There is no trial evidence of improvement in mortality.

Levosimendan

Levosimendan is a new drug that sensitizes cardiac myocytes to calcium and is said to improve contractility without increasing oxygen demand. Preliminary evidence suggests that it is better than dobutamine in improving cardiac function in low-output cardiac failure, with a reduction in mortality. There have been no randomized controlled trials in the critically ill, and at present there is no UK distributor for this drug.

MECHANICAL SUPPORT

For patients with primary cardiac pump failure, mechanical support of the circulation using intra-aortic balloon pumping may be of benefit. This is most commonly used after cardiac surgery and myocardial infarction, but may sometimes be of benefit in the general critical care area. A balloon is placed under fluoroscopic guidance so that the tip lies just distal to the origin of the left subclavian artery. The balloon is inflated in time with diastole to augment diastolic pressure, and hence coronary perfusion. The balloon is deflated at the start of systole to provide a dynamic reduction in afterload. Complications include leg ischaemia, infection, haemolysis and coagulopathy.

MANAGEMENT OF ARRHYTHMIAS

If an arrhythmia develops in a critically ill patient this needs the following assessment:

- If the rhythm is life threatening or contributing to resistant hypotension, ensure that it is not being stimulated by a central venous catheter/pulmonary artery catheter irritating the endocardium. If this is a possibility, pull back the catheter and see if it resolves. If not, treat according to standard ALS algorithms (Figure 5.12)
- If the rhythm is judged not to be life threatening the following may be considered:
  - Check recent electrolytes, including serum potassium and magnesium levels, and correct if necessary.

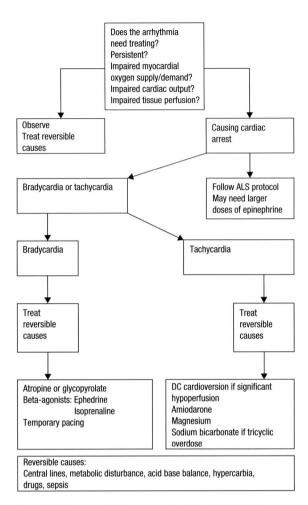

Figure 5.12 Flow chart for the management of arrhythmia in the critically ill

- Is this a self-limiting run of atrial/nodal/ventricular ectopic beats that requires no treatment?
- Is this worsening myocardial oxygen supply:demand ratios or reducing cardiac output?
- Reversible causes of a new-onset arrhythmia should be sought and treated if possible before using potentially harmful drugs or cardioversion (Table 5.13).

Bradycardia

- This is most commonly an appropriate physiological response to sudden hypertension (e.g Cushing's reflex, or an inadvertent bolus of vasoactive drug), in which case it should not be treated.
- Symptomatic bradycardia following myocardial infarction may need temporary pacing.

Table 5.13 *Reversible causes of arrhythmia*

Cause	Treatment
Intracardiac lines	Pull catheter back to beyond pericardial reflection
Intrathoracic infection	Look for and treat pneumonia/mediastinitis
New onset sepsis	Look for and treat extrathoracic sepsis
Drugs	Review charts
Sympathomimetics	
Tricyclic antidepressants	
H_2 antagonists	
Digoxin	
Electrolyte imbalance	Replace missing ions
Particularly K^+ and Mg^+	
Acid–base balance	Correct severe acidosis or alkalosis
Uraemia	Consider renal replacement therapy

- Excessive β-blockade can be overcome by:
  - Stopping the drug
  - Glucagon adminstration
  - Large doses of β-agonists
  - Atropine/glycopyrrolate (may be ineffective)
  - Temporary pacing.

Tachycardias

Usually narrow complex tachycardias will be supraventricular (atrial or nodal) in origin, and broad complex tachycardias will be ventricular. Occasionally, patients will have 'rate-dependent' conduction defects so that supraventricular tachycardias (SVT) become broad complex. Adenosine given as a rapid intravenous bolus (6–12 mg) may help to differentiate between supraventricular and ventricular tachycardias (VT). Awake patients must always be warned of its unpleasant effects. It may cause severe, but almost always self-limiting, bradycardia.

The distinction between SVT and VT in the critically ill is often academic, as the three most commonly used treatments will treat both.

Amiodarone

Amiodarone has been shown to be effective for both cardioversion back to sinus rhythm and rate control. It can be used for both SVT and VT. It should be given as a loading dose (300 mg over 20 min) followed by continuous infusion (900 mg over 24 hours for up to 7 days). It has a panoply of side effects, but fortunately for the intensive care physician most of these are reversible and relate largely to long-term use. It may cause peripheral vasodilation and hypotension if given too quickly. Because of its very large volume of distribution amiodarone levels decrease very slowly after discontinuation.

Magnesium

There is some evidence that magnesium (8 mmol) is more effective than amiodarone for cardioversion in the critically ill. Hypomagnesaemia should be treated in all critically ill patients as it predisposes to arrhythmia. Magnesium is effective as an antiarrhythmic even when serum Mg^+ levels are in the normal range. It is specifically indicated for arrhythmia secondary to long QT syndromes (e.g. *Torsades de pointes*). It may cause peripheral vasodilation, flushing and nausea.

Cardioversion

Cardioversion is an effective treatment for the current arrhythmia but will not stop the next event. If it is used, then the clinician must consider whether there is a reversible cause that needs treating, and whether prophylaxis with amiodarone or magnesium may be beneficial.

β-blockade

For patients with paroxysmal arrhythmias (e.g. Guillain–Barré syndrome) a β-antagonist may be appropriate. Short-acting drugs such as esmolol have the obvious advantage of titration to effect in the critically ill, but otherwise there is little evidence that one drug is any better than another.

Digoxin

Digoxin is used for rate control of atrial fibrillation and flutter. Its therapeutic index is relatively narrow and blood levels do not correlate well with effect or toxicity. Toxic effects include brady- and tachydysrhythmias. It is not removed by haemofiltration, and toxic effects may require reversal with specific antibodies (Digibind).

MANAGEMENT OF UNCONTROLLED HYPERTENSION

In critically ill patients uncontrolled hypertension is less common than hypotension. However, the effects of uncontrolled hypertension may be life threatening, particularly in terms of neurological and cardiac function. As discussed above, blood pressure may be decreased either by reducing the stroke volume, heart rate or systemic vascular resistance, or by a combination of these. Table 5.11 (page 62) classifies these agents according to their predominant site of action.

SUMMARY

The management of cardiovascular system failure is based firmly on physiology. The different causes of hypotension have been discussed, along with modes of monitoring and the management of critically ill patients with cardiovascular failure.

REFERENCES

1. Connors AF Jr, Speroff T, Dawson NV, *et al*. The effectiveness of right heart catheterization in the initial care of critically ill patients. SUPPORT Investigators. *JAMA* 1996; **276**: 889–97.

2. Dellinger RP, Carlet JM, Masur H, *et al*. Surviving Sepsis Campaign Management Guidelines Committee. *Crit Care Med* 2004; **32**: 858–73.

3. Rivers E, Nguyen B, Havstad S, *et al*. Early goal directed therapy in the treatment of severe sepsis and septic shock. *N Engl J Med* 2001; **345**: 1368–77.

4. The SAFE study investigators. A comparison of albumin and saline for fluid resuscitation in the intensive care unit. *N Engl J Med* 2004; **350**: 2247–55.

5. Wenzel V, Krismer AC, Arntz HR, *et al*. European Resuscitation Council Vasopressor during Cardiopulmonary Resuscitation Study Group. A comparison of vasopressin and epinephrine for out-of-hospital cardiopulmonary resuscitation. *N Engl J Med* 2004; **350**: 105–113.

6 Sepsis and disseminated intravascular coagulation

KEITH GIRLING

Viva topics

- What do you understand by the term 'source control'? What may this involve in the management of a septic patient?
- Explain how the release of cytokines is initiated following infection with a Gram-negative organism.
- The gut has been termed the 'motor of critical illness'. What is the basis for this assertion?
- What is DIC and how does it relate to sepsis?
- What information would you need to be able to give the family of a patient with septic shock an estimate of the patient's likely outcome?

INTRODUCTION

Sepsis remains an important and life-threatening problem and continues to be the principal cause of death in patients admitted to an intensive care unit. Approximately 150 000 people die annually in Europe from severe sepsis, and more than 200 000 in the USA.[1] In recent years there have been a number of changes in our understanding and management of sepsis, although the mortality remains high.

The objectives of this chapter are to review the pathological processes that take place in sepsis and then to discuss the clinical presentation, differential diagnosis and specific medical and surgical treatment pathways that are available.

DEFINITIONS

Many terms are used within the all-embracing term 'sepsis', leading to confusion between clinicians and misunderstanding of published material. The definitions of the following

terms have been taken from the 2001 International Sepsis Definitions Conference that was reported in both *Critical Care Medicine* and *Intensive Care Medicine* in 2003.[2]

- **Infection** is a microbial phenomenon characterized by an inflammatory response to the presence of microorganisms or the invasion of the normally sterile host tissue by those organisms.
- **Bacteraemia** is the presence of viable bacteria in the blood as determined by culture. The presence of viruses, fungi, parasites and other pathogens in the blood can be described in a similar manner (i.e. fungaemia).
- **Septicaemia** is a term that the Consensus Conference in 1992 suggested should no longer be used because of the confusion its use causes.
- **Systemic inflammatory response syndrome (SIRS)** is a term that may be used to describe the manifestations of systemic inflammation that are seen but are not necessarily attributable to infection. The common non-infective causes of SIRS are shown in Table 6.1. SIRS is considered to be present when a patient has more than one of the following clinical findings:
  - Temperature $>38°C$ or $<36°C$
  - White cell count <4000 or $>12\,000$ cells/mm^3, or the presence of >10 per cent immature neutrophils ('bands')
  - Tachycardia HR >90 bpm
  - Tachypnoea or supranormal minute ventilation, i.e. respiratory rate (RR) >20 or P_aCO_2 <4.3 kPa, or the need for mechanical ventilation for a non-respiratory cause.

It is immediately apparent that although this definition enables the diagnosis to be agreed on, it is not particularly discriminatory, and therefore neither specific nor sensitive. The most recent conference sought to extend the list of possible signs of systemic inflammation in response to infection and produced lists of general parameters, inflammatory parameters, haemodynamic parameters and tissue perfusion parameters.

- **Sepsis** has been defined as SIRS plus infection.
- **Severe sepsis** occurs if an organ system begins to fail because of the effects of sepsis, e.g. renal function deteriorates as evidenced by poor urine output, or cerebral function is affected, resulting in confusion.

    Organ system failure may be defined by either the Multiple Organ Dysfunction score[3] or the Sequential Organ Failure Assessment score.[4] The Multiple Organ Dysfunction score takes six physiological parameters that indicate the extent of organ failure (Table 6.2). Each of

these is then given a score depending on the variation from normal, and the scores for the six systems are combined. In the original description of this scoring system the authors showed that a total score of 13–16 equated to an ICU mortality of approximately 50 per cent, and a score greater than 21 equated to an ICU mortality of 100 per cent.

- **Septic shock** is defined as sepsis with documented hypotension, i.e. a systolic BP <90 mmHg or a decrease in MAP (mean arterial pressure) of >40 mmHg from baseline persisting despite 'adequate' fluid resuscitation. Septic shock is further considered to be *refractory* if the state of shock lasts more than 1 hour, with no response to intervention with intravenous fluids or pharmacological agents.

Clearly, this plethora of terms and definitions may lead to significant diagnostic confusion. Care needs to be taken to compare relevant research findings with the appropriate condition.

Recent published surveys from the USA and Europe have suggested that between 2 and 11 per cent of all admissions to hospitals or intensive care units are attributed to severe sepsis. The mortality associated with sepsis depends on both the series being examined and the exact diagnostic criteria being applied. It is true to say that the majority of patients on the intensive care unit at one time or another fulfil the criteria for SIRS, and the mortality in this group is of the order of 15–20 per cent (i.e. that associated with general intensive care). However, series that describe the mortality of patients with septic shock indicate that this may rise to 50 per cent. If septic shock then incorporates multiple organ failure (MOF) the mortality may be in excess of 90 per cent, depending on the number of organ systems affected and the extent of the deviation from normal parameters.

Table 6.1 *Non-infective causes of SIRS*

Category	Details
Tissue injury	Surgery/trauma
	Haematoma/venous thrombosis
	Myocardial/pulmonary infarction
	Transplant rejection
	Pancreatitis
	Erythroderma
Metabolic	Acute adrenal insufficiency
	Thyroid storm
Treatment related	Transfusion of blood products
	Cytokines
	Malignant hyperpyrexia
	Neuroleptic malignant syndrome
Malignancy	Tumour lysis syndrome
	Hypernephroma/lymphoma
Neurological	Subarachnoid haemorrhage

Table 6.2 *Multiple Organ Dysfunction score*

Organ system	Score				
	0	1	2	3	4
Respiratory					
PO_2/FiO_2 (mmHg)	>300	226–300	151–225	76–150	<75
Renal					
Serum creatinine (μmol/L)	<100	101–200	201–350	351–500	>500
Hepatic					
Serum bilirubin (μmol/L)	<20	21–60	61–120	121–240	>240
Cardiovascular					
HR $\times$ CVP/MAP	<10.0	10.1–15.0	15.1–20.0	20.1–30.0	>30.0
Haematologic					
Platelet count/mL/10^{-3}	>120	81–120	51–80	21–50	<20
Glasgow Coma Score	15	13–14	10–12	7–9	<6

Delegates at the International Symposium on Intensive Care and Emergency Medicine (ISICEM) in 2003 on definitions in sepsis attempted to go a stage further than previously and proposed a staging system to stratify patients with sepsis. This classified patients according to the following parameters:

- **Predisposition**, such as premorbid health status and the reversibility of concomitant diseases
- **Infection**: the site, type and extent of the infection have a significant impact on prognosis
- **Response**: markers that may give some estimation of the host response to sepsis include procalcitonin and interleukin-6, among others
- **Organ dysfunction**, either as the number of failing organs or the composite score.

This PIRO (*Predisposition*, *Infection*, *Response*, *Organ dysfunction*) system was proposed as a template for future investigation and further studies are still awaited.

PATHOLOGICAL PROCESSES ASSOCIATED WITH SEPSIS

Our understanding of the pathways involved in the sepsis 'cascade' has advanced tremendously in recent years and the process is known to be incredibly complex. In this section only a basic overview will be given. Figure 6.1 is intended to provide an outline of some of the pathways involved in the septic process. In recent years a number of key observations have been made regarding the pathology of sepsis. First, the endothelium, once regarded as a relatively inert blood vessel barrier, is now known to be a highly active organ in its own right and is responsible for mediating the immune response and the production of nitric oxide. Second, the relationship between thrombin and inflammation has been defined, such that the interaction between sepsis and disseminated intravascular coagulation (DIC) is now much more fully understood. The essential steps of the 'sepsis cascade' are discussed below.

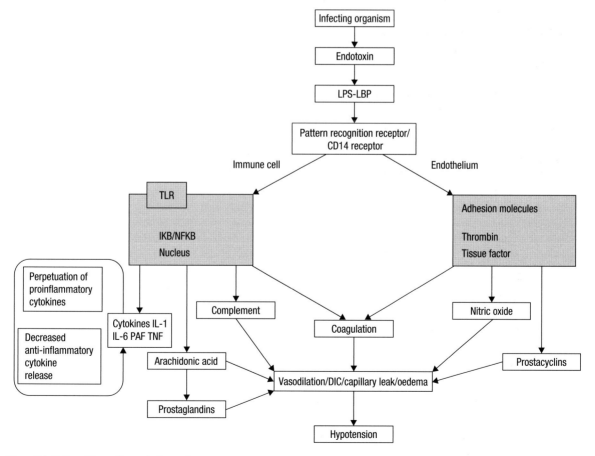

Figure 6.1 Outline of key pathways in the septic process

Initiation

The initiating event in sepsis is most commonly bacterial, and traditionally this has been attributed to Gram-negative organisms, but recent studies suggest that the ratio of Gram-positive to Gram-negative infections is now approaching one to one. This is principally because of the vast increase in staphylococcal infections and the appreciation that even non-coagulase staphylococci, such as *Staphylococcus epidermidis*, may result in the clinical picture of sepsis. Candida is the third most common cause of systemic sepsis, with other fungi and viral infections making up the rest. It is worthy of note that one of the essential differences between Gram-negative and Gram-positive organisms is the toxin produced: Gram-negative organisms are responsible for the production of endotoxin, compared to exotoxin production by Gram-positive organisms. Endotoxin is extruded from the bacterium with an outer layer of lipopolysaccharide, whereas exotoxin has no such outer lining.

A wide range of patients are predisposed to life-threatening infections. These include immunocompromised patients, diabetic patients, those with indwelling metalwork, and patients who have had large bowel surgery etc.

Detection

The detection of invading microorganisms is mediated by pattern recognition receptors expressed on the surface of immune cells. These receptors recognize structures common to many microbial pathogens, including lipopolysaccharide associated with Gram-negative organisms. However, peptidoglycan, lipoteichoic acid, lipopeptides and viral RNA allow recognition of many other substances as being part of microbial pathogens. These recognizable structures are called pathogen-associated molecular patterns and are essential for the survival of the microorganism and do not undergo major mutations.

Macrophage activation

Endotoxin, when produced, is comprised of three essential constituents: a lipopolysaccharide membrane, core substance, and lipid A. Each of these parts is antigenic and may result in the generation of an inflammatory response.

Endotoxin (lipopolysaccharide, LPS) binds to a specific LPS-binding protein (LBP) in the plasma. The LPS–LBP complex binds to a macrophage membrane receptor, CD14. These receptors are not transmembrane and have to be linked to a Toll-like receptor (TLR, in this case TLR4) in order to stimulate intracellular effects. Other pathogen-associated molecular patterns bind to other Toll-like receptors, e.g. lipoteichoic acid produced by Gram-positive organisms binds to TLR2 receptors. Soluble CD14 receptors exist in the bloodstream which promote LPS binding to endothelial (CD14-negative) cells. Once the CD14–TLR complex is activated inhibitory κB kinase allows NFκB to be activated, such that cytokine, thrombin and nitric oxide production is initiated. This results in stimulation of the cytokine cascade and production of the proinflammatory cytokines, which include interleukins (IL)-1, 6 and 8 and tumour necrosis factor (TNF)-α. These cytokines result in the widespread activation of molecular pathways, including arachidonic acid, complement and the coagulation cascade. In addition, inflammatory cytokine production has the immediate effect of decreasing anti-inflammatory cytokine (IL-10, soluble TNF receptors and IL-1ra, a competitive inhibitor of the IL-1 receptor) production and perpetuating the release of further proinflammatory cytokines.

Arachidonic acid metabolism leads to the formation of prostaglandins, thromboxane and leukotrienes. These locally acting metabolites are potent agents with widespread functions. For example, prostaglandin E_2 (PGE$_2$) is a vasodilator which also inhibits platelet aggregation.

Complement activation results in increased release of IL-1 and TNF, perpetuating the sepsis response. Complement factor C5a also stimulates the adhesion and degranulation of leukocytes, resulting in the release of reactive oxygen species and proteases, causing endothelial damage.

ENDOTHELIUM

In normal conditions endothelial cells have a number of mechanisms that prevent coagulation occurring. These include the expression of thrombomodulin, which both binds thrombin and is integral to the activation of protein C; proteoglycans such as heparan sulphate on the surface bind and potentiate antithrombin III; tissue factor pathway inhibitor prevents the formation of the tissue factor–factor VII complex; and small amounts of tissue-type plasminogen activator (tPA) are continually released. Once activated by the presence of various cytokines and inflammatory mediators, the endothelial functions are grossly altered. The endothelium becomes procoagulant in an attempt to wall off infection. Thrombomodulin and heparan sulphate are no longer expressed by the endothelial cells, and tissue factor is synthesized. Protein C activation is diminished and tissue factor–FVII complexes are formed. The latter results in the production of factors VIIa and Xa and thrombin, all of which will further activate endothelial cells, which then start to express adhesion molecules such as P-selectin and E-selectin. These molecules interact with leukocytes in the blood, causing them to marginalize and initially roll over the endothelium before becoming strongly adhered to it and finally transmigrating into the tissues. This causes extravascular inflammation and coagulation.

In addition to the changes in coagulant properties a number of vasoactive molecules are produced by the endothelium, including nitric oxide and prostacyclins.

Nitric oxide

This molecule, formerly known as endothelium-derived relaxing factor, is produced by the enzyme nitric oxide synthase acting on L-arginine (the most abundant amino acid in the body). The enzyme has two isoforms – inducible nitric oxide synthase (iNOS) and constitutive nitric oxide synthase (cNOS). cNOS can further be divided into endothelial NOS (eNOS) and neuronal NOS (nNOS). Nitric oxide is released in smooth muscle, and by activating the soluble guanylate cyclase of smooth muscle cells causes the production of cyclic guanosine monophosphate (cGMP) to be increased. This results in smooth muscle relaxation. In physiological concentrations NO plays an essential role in modulation of basal vascular tone. Excessive formation of NO and cGMP, as occurs in sepsis, is associated with profound vasodilatation, decreased reactivity to catecholamines and myocardial depression. Large concentrations of NO also result in the modification of gene expression, mediation of oxidative stress, and have cytotoxic actions. These effects contribute to multiple organ failure and increased mortality.

At the present time nitric oxide effects may be inhibited in one of two ways. The production of nitric oxide may be decreased by inhibiting NOS using false substrates (L-NAME and L-NMMA), or the effects of nitric oxide may be inhibited by blocking the guanylate cyclase enzyme using methylene blue. There are limited data available using these agents in humans. However, they are both non-selective NOS inhibitors blocking both inducible and constitutive isoforms. Using a false substrate appears to result in an increase in mortality and selective inhibition of the inducible isoform is still awaited. Methylene Blue has been used to some beneficial effect in small clinical trials in patients with severe sepsis and septic shock but the benefits have not been confirmed by any large prospective blinded studies.

DISSEMINATED INTRAVASCULAR COAGULATION (DIC)

Although the association between sepsis and DIC has been well documented, the extent of the interaction between these two pathological processes has only been detailed relatively recently. It is now established that DIC is an integral part of sepsis, and the two processes should be considered together.

Definition

Disseminated intravascular coagulation is an acquired syndrome characterized by systemic activation of the blood coagulation system, resulting in the generation and deposition of fibrin and the formation of microvascular thrombi, which contribute to the development of multiorgan failure.

Coagulation, anticoagulants and fibrinolysis

Thrombin is now recognized to be a molecule that is central to both the coagulation pathway and the sepsis cascade. The traditional coagulation pathway is shown in Figure 6.2 and comprises the intrinsic and the extrinsic components. These pathways come together at the activation of factor X to form the common pathway, which results in the formation of thrombin and then fibrin.

Naturally occurring anticoagulants prevent the perpetuation of clot whenever the coagulation cascade is stimulated, and include tissue factor pathway inhibitor, antithrombin III and activated protein C, as indicated in Figure 6.3. As described above, the endothelium under normal conditions is a source of all these anticoagulants, but this process becomes altered significantly in sepsis. Fibrinolytic enzymes are shown in Figure 6.3. These are present to break down clot and prevent intravascular coagulation.

DIC occurs in situations in which the balance between procoagulant compounds, anticoagulants and fibrinolytic compounds is altered, as shown in Figure 6.4.

DIC results in the deposition of clot, particularly in small and medium-sized vessels, and it is this that may contribute to the development of multiorgan failure (Figure 6.5).

Although it has been recognized for many years that coagulation disorders form a part of sepsis, more recently it has been appreciated that thrombin is also a significant inflammatory mediator in the sepsis cascade.

Within the understanding of coagulation, it is now clear that the extrinsic pathway and the generation of tissue factor are the principal initiators of coagulation, and the intrinsic pathway acts as an accelerator for the extrinsic pathway and is possibly only very rarely, if ever, the initiator of coagulation. As noted above, tissue factor may be exposed by stimulated endothelium as well as synthesized by monocytes challenged with endotoxin. In DIC the naturally occurring anticoagulants antithrombin III and tissue factor pathway inhibitor are decreased.

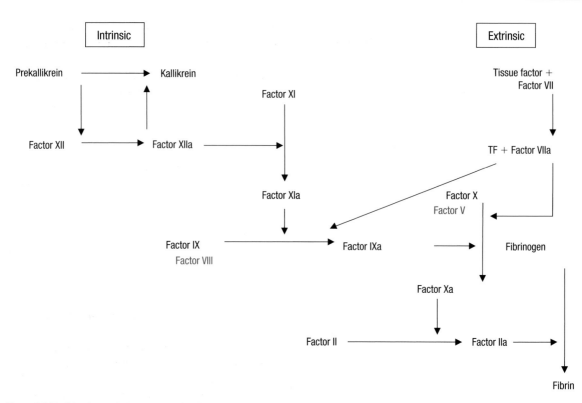

Figure 6.2 Traditional coagulation cascades showing intrinsic and extrinsic pathways

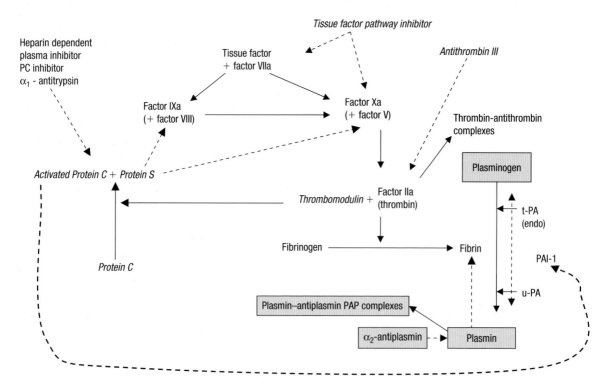

Figure 6.3 Simplified coagulation pathway to show essential parts of the extrinsic pathway. Naturally occurring anticoagulants are shown in italics and fibrinolytic pathway in tinted boxes. Solid lines indicate positive effect and dashed lines indicate antagonistic effect

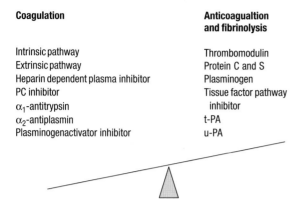

Coagulation	Anticoagualtion and fibrinolysis
Intrinsic pathway	Thrombomodulin
Extrinsic pathway	Protein C and S
Heparin dependent plasma inhibitor	Plasminogen
PC inhibitor	Tissue factor pathway inhibitor
α_1-antitrypsin	t-PA
α_2-antiplasmin	u-PA
Plasminogenactivator inhibitor	

Figure 6.4 The imbalance between factors tending to result in coagulation and those tending to anticoagulate or cause fibrinolysis

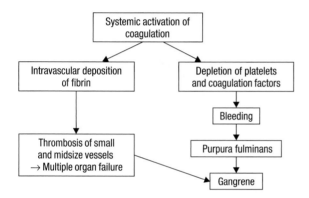

Figure 6.5 Mechanism of DIC

THROMBIN

Thrombin has very complex actions and is now regarded as central to the coagulation pathway but it is also a very potent proinflammatory mediator. Thrombin acts as a procoagulant and generates the fibrin plug, however it also activates protein C via the expression of thrombomodulin and also promotes prostacyclin formation. In inflammation, thrombin binds to specific receptors found on platelets, endothelial cells and white blood cells known as protease-activated receptors (PARs). Thrombin and other coagulation factor-mediated activation of cells increases proinflammatory cytokine synthesis and calcium flux, alters intracellular signaling cascades such as the mitogen activated protein (MAP) kinase pathway, and induces nitric oxide synthesis. Thrombin also stimulates platelet activating factor production. Platelet activating factor is a potent neutrophil and platelet activating substance, and thrombin promotes the surface expression of P-selectin on endothelial cells and platelets. P-selectin is a major adhesin facilitating the initial interaction of circulating granulocytes, monocytes and lymphocytes with endothelial cells at sites of tissue injury. By these mechanisms, thrombin generation is a potent inducer of inflammation.

The importance of the understanding of the relationship between sepsis and DIC is manifest by the development of activated protein C in the management of sepsis, as discussed below.

SPECIFIC ORGAN SYSTEMS AND SEPSIS

Gut

Since the 1960s it has been proposed that the gut is the 'motor of critical illness' and the source of the mediators of sepsis. This proposal suggests that initially, gut mucosal perfusion, and hence tissue oxygenation, is compromised by hypotension or altered distribution of blood flow away from the splanchnic circulation. This results in disruption of the mucosal barrier, and toxic entities normally contained within the bowel lumen are allowed to pass into the systemic circulation. These toxins may include bacteria or bacterial components, e.g. endotoxin and other chemicals. Many studies are available to support this theory, and in the majority of these in humans gut perfusion is assessed using gastric tonometry. This consists of a semipermeable balloon that is placed into the stomach lumen. Carbon dioxide from the gastric mucosa diffuses into the balloon, and this can then be sampled. The original technique involved placing saline in the balloon. This has been replaced by an automated semicontinuous air tonometry that uses infrared spectrophotometry to measure CO_2. This allows more rapid equilibration of the CO_2 and reduces the manual aspects of the measurement. It also allows the derivation of the CO_2 gap, defined as the gastric PCO_2 – either the arterial or the end-tidal CO_2. The assumption is that when local perfusion is compromised, oxygen delivery is reduced and anaerobic metabolism increases, with a consequent increase in local lactic acidosis and the generation of CO_2. Alternatively, the decrease in splanchnic blood flow may result in an inadequate washout of carbon dioxide due to low blood flow.

In sepsis the total hepatosplanchnic blood flow is increased, with higher splanchnic oxygen extraction and consumption. This increase in blood flow is attributed to cytopathic hypoxia, and many possible cellular mechanisms have been postulated. Endothelial functions are altered due to a panendothelial injury that may be generated by initial hypoperfusion, trauma, or even indirect endotoxaemic damage. This endothelial damage perpetuates the inflammatory response. Therefore, it is likely that the use of tonometry to detect splanchnic endothelial damage is effectively making the diagnosis too late for clinical intervention to then alter the progress of the septic process.

Therefore, it is very likely that the gut does have a significant role in the generation of sepsis; current monitoring of this organ using tonometry may be used to predict outcome but not necessarily alter outcome once there are indications of endothelial damage.

Liver

The liver has a pivotal role in sepsis. It is well known that the liver has a dual blood supply from both the hepatic artery and the portal vein. The portal blood supply is of particular interest, as it carries blood from the splanchnic circulation, a region particularly prone to altered flow in sepsis and bacterial translocation during sepsis. In addition, the liver comprises a number of different cell types: hepatocytes, Kupffer cells and endothelial sinusoidal cells. All these have activity in immunity and protection from infection. The gut–liver axis is therefore key in the defence against sepsis, but may also be injured and altered by the septic process, due to either hypoperfusion from shock or bleeding from DIC.

Kupffer cells account for about 70 per cent of the total macrophage population of the body and are thought to be the primary defence against portal bacteraemia and endotoxinaemia. In animal studies, it has been shown that metabolites from an injected dose of endotoxin have been found in the bile duct and gallbladder. A large proportion (70 per cent) of active organisms injected into animals has also been found in the liver within 10 minutes. If liver function is decreased, systemic bacterial or endotoxin spillover may occur.

The liver is involved in both the uptake and clearance of IL-6. However, IL-6 in the liver results in the modulation of acute-phase protein production. The production of a number of acute-phase proteins is increased, including C-reactive protein, fibrinogen and prothrombin. Other acute-phase protein production is decreased, including protein C, antithrombin and albumin. This redistribution of the acute-phase proteins clearly contributes to a procoagulant state. C-reactive protein has a number of inflammatory actions, activating complement and promoting tissue factor expression by mononuclear cells and neutrophils.

Kidney

Acute renal failure induced by sepsis remains common (9–40 per cent of ICU admissions with sepsis), is relatively easily and safely treated by modern renal replacement therapies, and is commonly attributed to 'acute tubular necrosis'. Unfortunately, very few studies have explored the changes that take place in the kidney during sepsis, but none have found evidence of necrosis or tubular damage. Hypotension is clearly a contributing factor in septic shock because of the resulting decrease in the pressure gradient across the glomerulus. However, hypotension is not the sole cause of acute renal failure in sepsis, as this may still occur in the absence of haemodynamic changes. Therefore, the pathophysiology of renal failure in sepsis remains undefined.

It is now agreed by many authors that there is no evidence that either frusemide or dopamine have been shown convincingly to improve renal function or survival. Recovery of renal function may take several months, but is usually reversible to such a degree that most patients become independent of dialysis treatment. A recent audit of Scottish ICUs showed that the percentage of patients requiring long-term renal replacement therapy was just 1.6 in the absence of premorbid renal impairment.[5]

DIAGNOSIS AND MARKERS OF SEPSIS

The initial diagnosis is made by the patient fulfilling the sepsis criteria as above, and by exclusion of the causes of SIRS, as documented in Table 6.1. Establishing and localizing the presence of ongoing infection may be very difficult but is extremely important. The three commonest sites of infection are the respiratory tract, the abdomen and the bloodstream, and these need to be considered extremely carefully. More than 90 per cent of cases of sepsis are caused by bacteria, as discussed above. However, in intensive care unit patients the identification of the microorganism responsible may be complicated by multiple pathological processes occurring at the same time, and by the use of broad-spectrum antibiotics that makes microbiological diagnosis extremely difficult. Yet there is good evidence to support the belief that patients given appropriate therapy are more likely to survive than those given inappropriate treatment. If positive microbiology is achieved, colonization then needs to be separated from infection before it is concluded that the organism isolated is indeed responsible for the clinical picture.

In addition, the diagnosis of sepsis may not be simple. Patients may mask the signs of sepsis either because of concurrent medications (e.g. β-blockade resulting in a heart rate consistently less than 90 bpm, or recent paracetamol use decreasing core temperature to normal) or because of their physiology (fit young patients may hyperventilate by increasing tidal volume with minimal increases in respiratory rate).

Clinical findings

If a patient develops any of the signs of sepsis as outlined above they should receive a full clinical examination. This involves a full examination of the chest and abdomen. All surgical and traumatic wounds need to be exposed and examined for signs of infection. All vascular access sites need to be examined for signs of inflammation, and the duration of, and requirement for, central venous access needs to be evaluated. Urine may be purulent, or there may be evidence of diarrhoea.

Investigations

BLOOD TESTS

- The white cell count forms part of the diagnostic criteria, but a change in this value during a critically ill patient's stay in hospital is frequently difficult to interpret
- Platelet count frequently changes during sepsis and may increase or decrease
- Changes in liver and renal function tests may occur as a result of specific, localized sepsis and may help define the cause
- The erythrocyte sedimentation rate (ESR), levels of procalcitonin (PCT) and C-reactive protein (CRP) are all non-specific markers of infection and inflammation. PCT rises quickly after the onset of inflammation and levels may correlate with the severity of sepsis, and it has been suggested that it may correlate with mortality. CRP also correlates well with the degree of inflammation, and has been used in specific circumstances to determine the presence of infection, e.g. whether a pleural effusion is likely to be infected or not.

BLOOD CULTURES

These should be taken whenever an infective cause of sepsis is expected. Ideally, all patients in whom sepsis is suspected should have blood cultures taken prior to starting antibiotics. If the patient is already receiving antibiotics the blood cultures should be taken immediately prior to the next dose, when the blood antibiotic concentration is at its lowest. Wherever possible blood cultures should be taken as soon as possible after the onset of fever. Strict attention to detail should be paid when taking blood cultures, which should include:

- Handwashing and sterile gloves and field
- Strict skin disinfection with an iodine-containing solution
- Venepuncture from a fresh peripheral site
- Aspiration of an adequate volume of blood (10–30 mL per culture bottle)
- Additional culture from any suspected lines that may be infected.

OTHER INVESTIGATIONS

Clinical examination and results from blood tests, particularly if positive microbiology is obtained, may be used to guide other investigations. These may include lumbar puncture, chest X-rays, bronchoscopy, chest CT, abdominal CT, echocardiography (including a transoesophageal echo to exclude subacute bacterial endocarditis), biliary tract ultrasound and renal ultrasound.

Other microbiological specimens should be taken depending on the clinical findings. Pus aspirated from any site, and particularly any specimens obtained during surgery, should be sent for culture.

Candidal infection remains extremely difficult to diagnose accurately and a high index of suspicion needs to be maintained. Patients particularly susceptible to invasive candidal infection are those who have had prolonged hospital stays with long courses of broad-spectrum antibiotics. Clinical findings such as fluffy white intraophthalmic deposits on ophthalmoscopy are pathognomonic but are seen rarely. More commonly the patient has been treated for a long time with broad-spectrum antibiotics. Despite this, they continue to have a high white cell count, a high temperature, and may have evidence of superficial candida in the groins, armpits, buccal or vaginal mucosae. In these patients empirical antifungal therapy should be discussed with the microbiologist.

MANAGEMENT OF PATIENTS WITH SEPSIS

Recently, increased attention has been drawn to the importance of early aggressive management of patients presenting with sepsis through the publication of the Surviving Sepsis Campaign guidelines for the management of severe sepsis and septic shock.[6] The emphasis of the Surviving Sepsis Campaign is that rapid and timely intervention is critical to successful treatment. Therefore, assessment and treatment should occur simultaneously and the latter would normally include the use of fluids, antibiotics and source control. In addition, this Campaign has gained consensus from a large number of experts who have reviewed all the relevant literature and a 'care bundle' has been produced that incorporates all the current evidence-based guidance. In this section the various components of the Surviving Sepsis Campaign will be discussed.

Stabilization and assessment

The initial management of a patient presenting with sepsis should follow a standard protocol. This includes the following principles, as described fully in material such as the CCRiSP Manual published on behalf of the Royal College of Surgeons.[7]

- Assessment of the airway, with action taken to open and protect the airway as indicated
- Assessment of breathing, with action to support respiration as required – a minimum requirement should be the administration of high-concentration oxygen (60 per cent or more) via a face mask
- Assessment of the cardiovascular system, with action to give a fluid bolus to maintain blood pressure if this is low while considering the need for further monitoring, transfer to a higher level of care, and the potential need for vasoactive drug support
- An assessment of the conscious level should be made, and the AVPU (alert, responsive to verbal stimulus, responsive to painful stimulus or unconscious) scale is adequate at this stage to guide the management of the patient
- The patient should be exposed and examined with a view to determining the likely source of the sepsis. In surgical patients sepsis most commonly occurs in one of three sites: the abdomen, the chest or the urine. Physical examination must include an examination of any drains and indwelling line sites.

Once this is complete appropriate investigations should be organized, along with a full review of the patient's notes and any charts that are available. Targeted investigations may include a chest X-ray, abdominal ultrasound or CT and echocardiogram.

Once complete, a full plan should be written in the patient's notes and appropriate help should be summoned.

Source control

Early surgical debridement of an infected area or removal of infected lines etc. may also form an essential part of sepsis management. Long-term patients or those returning to the ward from higher care areas may well have indwelling vascular or urinary catheters which can act as a site of infection and sepsis.

CATHETER-RELATED BLOODSTREAM INFECTION (CRBSI)

Catheter-related bloodstream infections now occur at the rate of around 5.8 per 1000 catheter days, and it is estimated that in the USA there are of the order of 80 000 such infections

per year. The mortality attributed to CRBSI varies between 0 and 35 per cent, depending on the report. However, all reports appear to confirm that these infections are associated with increased duration of intensive care unit and hospital stay and increased cost of management. Following a large number of studies in this area the following recommendations have been made:[8]

- Strict attention to asepsis during insertion and use of any indwelling line. This includes the use of gown, gloves and mask during insertion, and sterile drapes should be placed over the whole patient
- Chlorhexidine-containing solutions should be used for skin cleansing in preference to iodine-containing solutions. The solution should be allowed to dry before proceeding
- Hands should be washed thoroughly before and after each contact with the line connections to prevent infection transit via the hubs
- Occlusive dressings should be applied over the line insertion site and changed immediately if they become detached
- The femoral vein should be avoided, the relative risk of infection being four times greater than with the subclavian route
- The subclavian route is associated with the lowest rate of CRBSI but has an increased complication rate in inexperienced hands, and these factors need to be weighed in the final choice of site
- There is no evidence to support specific line change intervals. When there is evidence of infection around a line site the line should be changed to an alternative site and not changed over a wire in the same position
- A variety of antimicrobial/antiseptic-impregnated catheters are available. There is some evidence to support the fact that catheters impregnated with either chlorhexidine/silver sulfadiazine or minocycline/rifampicin decrease the incidence of catheter-related sepsis. Catheters impregnated with silver/platinum are also available, but currently there is less evidence to support their use.

Surgical intervention

The use of antibiotics, fluids and the critical care management of sepsis described in this chapter are all relatively recent innovations. The surgical treatment of infection in terms of abscess drainage and debridement of dead tissue is recorded as occurring as far back as 4 BC. However, this age-old tradition of surgical management has resulted in much surgical intervention being based on traditional teaching and relatively little evidence base for many practices. Surgical intervention should only occur once basic resuscitation has started and the patient's condition stabilized, and in the majority of situations this should be regarded as urgent rather than emergency surgery.

Necrotizing soft tissue infection

This requires debridement of infected or non-bleeding tissue as rapidly as possible after early stabilization. Some reports have suggested that improved outcome is associated with surgical intervention within 3 or 12 h of admission.

Intra-abdominal collections

Drainage may be performed by either surgical or radiological intervention. Some authorities suggest that laparotomy should be reserved for those circumstances in which there are no well-defined collections, dead tissue that requires debridement, or residual collections that cannot be drained percutaneously. Clearly, the decision to drain percutaneously or perform open surgery will be based on a number of factors, which include local expertise and the availability of personnel; certainty of diagnosis; percutaneous access to the collection; and the condition of the patient. If a patient has had a laparotomy for an intra-abdominal collection and has ongoing signs of sepsis a second-look laparotomy should be considered. A planned re-laparotomy is indicated for patients with ischaemic bowel when intestinal viability is a concern, for patients with necrotizing pancreatitis when demarcation of necrotic tissue is not distinct, or when bleeding precludes complete debridement.

Examination of an abdomen in an unconscious, sedated critically ill patient may not yield classic physical signs. Factors that would point toward a potential intra-abdominal collection include:

- Raised serum lactate concentration
- Increasing base deficit
- Cessation of previously successful enteral feeding
- Intra-abdominal collection defined on CT/ultrasound
- Stoma no longer functioning.

ORGAN SYSTEM SUPPORT IN SEVERE SEPSIS

Cardiovascular support in sepsis

Maintenance of the normal systemic perfusion pressure is central to the critical care management of severe sepsis and septic shock. As discussed in Chapter 5, hypotension may occur because of either a decrease in cardiac output or systemic vascular resistance or both. Classically, sepsis is associated with peripheral vasodilation mediated by the cytokine and NO pathways discussed previously. In the majority of cases sepsis is associated with a significant increase in cardiac output, and therefore the first agent of choice is primarily an α receptor agonist. There remains considerable debate about which agent in this class should be the first-line choice: whereas some units around the world subscribe to dopamine in such cases, others would choose norepinephrine (noradrenaline).

In a proportion of patients there is coexisting cardiovascular disease limiting cardiac function in the face of decreased systemic resistance, and in another group the septic process itself may be adversely affecting cardiac function. The latter is classically seen in meningococcal sepsis, in which case the cardiac function may be severely depressed by the infective process per se. α-agonist drugs in the presence of a failing myocardium may further reduce the systemic perfusion pressure.

Thus, in some units in patients presenting with overt sepsis with no clear myocardial compromise α-agonist vasopressor agents such as norepinephrine will be commenced after appropriate fluid loading. If these actions do not result in an increase in blood pressure, cardiac output measurements will be obtained and the vasopressor may be changed to another agent, the dose further increased, or an inotropic agent such as dobutamine may be added to further stimulate cardiac contractility. If the patient has clear cardiac compromise in addition to systemic sepsis, cardiac output monitoring may be commenced earlier. If the patient is hypotensive and the diagnosis of sepsis remains unclear, an infusion of epinephrine with its combined α and β activities may often 'buy time' until cardiac output measurements can be made that may help clarify the principal cause of the hypotension.

The introduction of increasing numbers of monitors that allow cardiac output calculation without the need for intracardiac catheters, or for that matter any additional vascular access, has meant that cardiac output monitoring is again increasing in popularity.

Respiratory support in sepsis

If a patient presents with sepsis of non-respiratory origin, e.g. pancreatitis, oxygen exchange may be well within normal limits. If the patient has otherwise normal respiratory function CO_2 clearance may also be entirely normal, and young fit patients may be able to correct the metabolic acidosis attributed to their sepsis by hyperventilating to a remarkably low $PaCO_2$. However, even in young, fit patients the vast amount of work required to maintain this respiratory compensation is not sustainable for prolonged periods, and patients may need to be sedated and have their lungs ventilated for non-respiratory reasons. However, the application of mechanical ventilation in this situation is potentially hazardous. If the $PaCO_2$ is allowed to increase dramatically following institution of mechanical ventilation the pH will decrease significantly, with potentially life-threatening side effects. The appropriate $PaCO_2$ needs to be calculated for the bicarbonate that is present, and the CO_2 partial pressure can then be allowed to correct gradually as bicarbonate concentration increases. The expected $PaCO_2$ (in kPa) in metabolic acidosis may be given by:

$$\text{Expected } PaCO_2 = 0.2 \times HCO_3 + 1$$

Renal support in sepsis

Methods of renal replacement therapy in critically ill patients are discussed in Chapter 7. The concept of using haemofiltration to decrease the concentration of cytokines in the blood of septic patients has been assessed in a number of clinical and laboratory studies. Cytokines, soluble cytokine receptors, chemokines and other potentially harmful molecules, such as eicosanoids, platelet-activating factor, and complement factors C5a and C3a, are removed during continuous haemofiltration in humans. A significant decrease in plasminogen activator inhibitor type 1 (PAI-1) activity, an inhibitor of normal fibrinolysis, was identified in 40 patients with SIRS-associated acute renal failure treated with either continuous venovenous haemofiltration (CVVH) or haemodiafiltration. This may be of particular relevance because activated protein C stimulates fibrinolysis by decreasing the concentration of PAI-1, and this action is thought to be one of the underlying mechanisms for its efficacy in reducing mortality in severe sepsis.

The efficacy of a blood purification system in critically ill septic patients may be improved by unselective adsorption on a synthetic resin cartridge. Because there are currently no commercially available resins that can achieve effective adsorption of inflammatory mediators without significant problems with biocompatibility and immune cell activation, these filters have to be incorporated into a circuit in which plasma has been first separated from whole blood. Thus, plasma filtration can be coupled with plasma adsorption and conventional diffusion/convection, resulting in a device called coupled plasma filtration–adsorption.[9] In a recently reported small study this technique was used with some beneficial effect to improve haemodynamic stability, vasopressor requirement, pulmonary function and 28- and 90-day survival in patients with septic shock. However, much larger prospective randomized studies would be required before this technology could be incorporated in routine clinical practice.

Gut support in sepsis

IMMUNONUTRITION

The use of enteral rather than parenteral feeding in critically ill patients has gained widespread acceptance in recent years. One of the reasons behind this is that the concept of delivering substrate to the gut results in improved splanchnic blood flow and improved villous function, with decreased mucosal loss and subsequent translocation. More recently there has been an interest in developing immunonutrition. This is feed that contains extra L-arginine and sometimes glutamine, along with ω-3 fatty acids, vitamins and trace elements. Many studies have been performed seeking to show a mortality benefit from using immunonutrition in the critically ill, based on the immunity-enhancing properties that these feeds purport to offer. Recently a few publications have actually shown that when these are administered to patients with severe sepsis mortality is at best no better than that in patients receiving parenteral nutrition, but may actually be increased.[10] It is therefore reasonable at present to avoid immunonutrition in patients with severe sepsis.

SPECIFIC THERAPIES IN SEPSIS

Cytokine therapies

Many studies have been performed to examine the effects of either monoclonal antibodies to various cytokines, such as anti-TNF MAb (monoclonal antibodies) or cytokine receptor antagonists, e.g. IL-1ra, on the process of sepsis and septic shock. Typically, the first reports of these agents are in relatively small groups of patients (i.e. fewer than 250), and a significant effect is often demonstrated. At present all the large studies (over 250 patients) have shown no significant benefit from any of these therapies. The only MAb to reach the clinical arena was marketed as Centoxin (HA-1A). This was a monoclonal antibody directed at the lipid A part of endotoxin, but despite the initial benefits suggested from the early small reports this substance was subsequently withdrawn owing to increased mortality in some patients.

Antibiotic therapies

Antibiotics form an essential part of the management of sepsis, and their use can be divided into prophylactic and therapy. Prophylaxis should be applied in surgical patients wherever there is a risk of infected material being spilt, or where foreign material is being implanted. The exact prophylaxis used in these situations will depend on the nature of the surgery/implant, the local antibiotic formulary in use, and the local bacterial resistance and susceptibility patterns.

When antibiotics are used for treatment this should occur in one of the following situations:

- Wherever possible antibiotics should be targeted to specific organisms, as identified by microbiological investigations
- This standard is often not possible owing to the time taken for microbiological results to arrive; however, a Gram stain of infected material may guide appropriate antibiotic regimens
- At times it is not possible to obtain infected material until surgery, but this should not delay antibiotic administration. However, antibiotics should only be started after appropriate blood, sputum and urine cultures have been taken, and if broad-spectrum antibiotics are commenced these should be changed to specific therapy when microbiological results are available.

Prophylactic antibiotics and selective decontamination of the digestive tract (SDD)

Selective decontamination of the digestive tract was first introduced into critical care practice in the early 1980s. The objective is to eradicate colonization of aerobic, potentially pathogenic microorganisms from the oropharynx, stomach and gut in a selective way and to leave the indigenous (mostly anaerobic) flora largely undisturbed. The concept is based on two observations: colonization in the lower airways, bladder, skin and blood is almost always preceded by oropharyngeal and gastrointestinal colonization of disease-causing microorganisms; and the pathogenic potential of organisms varies to the point that some indigenous flora may support colonic enterocyte nutrition and limit aerobic microorganism overgrowth.

The technique involves the application of topical non-absorbable antimicrobials to the oropharynx and the administration of a parenteral agent that is excreted into the oropharynx during the first few days of the critical care stay.

A vast number of studies and meta-analyses have now been published examining this technique, with varying results.[11,12] The majority of studies conclude that SDD does result in a reduction in nosocomial infections, and in some studies there is at least a trend to a decrease in mortality. However, many concerns have been raised, including the emergence of resistant organisms, the difficulty of performing the techniques, the expense of the agents used, and the relatively small mortality effect. In addition, the studies compared in various meta-analyses have, unfortunately, used different inclusion criteria, different definitions, different antimicrobial regimens and different outcome measures.

The suggestion has been made that the outcome of a study is also particularly dependent on its methodological quality, with high-quality studies showing relatively less benefit. However, enthusiasts for SDD remain, but in general the technique is not in widespread use.

Glucose control

Hyperglycaemia is frequently seen in critically ill patients and has been attributed to increased insulin resistance. Although insulin administration will normally be commenced to maintain acceptable blood sugar levels, there is no consensus on the optimal plasma glucose. A recent prospective randomized study has examined the effects of maintaining blood sugar within a strictly normal range (4.5–6.1 mmol/L) or a restrictive insulin schedule where blood glucose was allowed to run between 10 and 12 mmol/L.[13] The patients managed with an intensive insulin schedule had an ICU mortality reduced by 43 per cent compared to those with a restrictive insulin schedule, and a hospital mortality reduced by 34 per cent. The mortality reduction was found to occur in the long-stay patients and was due to a reduced incidence of sepsis and multiple organ failure. Thus, it is possible that glucose control has a significant impact on the development of sepsis in critically ill patients. However, further studies examining the role of glucose control in a broader range of critically ill patients are awaited.

Anticoagulants

ACTIVATED PROTEIN C

In 2001 Bernard and co-workers published the results of a large randomized, double-blind placebo-controlled multi-centre trial in the *New England Journal of Medicine*.[14] In this study 1690 patients were randomized to receive an intravenous infusion of either recombinant human activated protein C or placebo for 96 hours after the diagnosis of systemic inflammation and organ failure due to acute infection. The mortality from all causes in the treated group was 24.7 per cent, compared to 30.8 per cent in the placebo group. This was statistically significant. However, activated protein C is a naturally occurring anticoagulant and the incidence of serious bleeding was higher in the activated protein C group than in the placebo group. The authors concluded that in the population studied, one additional life would be saved for every 16 patients treated; however, one additional serious bleeding event would occur for every 66 patients treated. This agent has subsequently been marketed in the UK, but the high cost of treatment has meant that it is not universally available at the time of writing.

This is the first time a single-agent treatment has been shown to result in a significant reduction in mortality in a study of this type, and therefore this represents a real advance in the management of sepsis.

ANTITHROMBIN III AND TISSUE FACTOR PATHWAY INHIBITOR

These naturally occurring anticoagulants have also been subject to repeated testing in the management of sepsis. However, the benefits of administration are much less marked than for activated protein C.

ANTITHROMBIN III

Antithrombin III is a naturally occurring glycoprotein which acts as a serine protease inhibitor and affects multiple components of the coagulation pathways. Animal work has shown that in supraphysiological doses antithrombin III possesses substantial anti-inflammatory as well as anticoagulant functions. The administration of heparin abolishes the actions of antithrombin III. In severe sepsis antithrombin III levels are decreased, and the KyberSept trial, published in 2001, was undertaken to determine the clinical efficacy of antithrombin III in this situation.[15] A total of 2314 adult patients with severe sepsis were randomized into two equal groups to receive either intravenous antithrombin III or placebo. There was no difference in the mortality between the groups, but there was a significant increase in the incidence of bleeding in the treatment group compared to controls.

TISSUE FACTOR PATHWAY INHIBITOR

Tissue factor pathway inhibitor 1 (TFPI-1) inhibits tissue factor in a two-stage process. First, TFPI-1 binds and inactivates Xa. In the second stage, TFPI-1 bound to Xa binds with the TF–factor VIIa complex, inhibiting thrombin generation and fibrin formation.

Under normal conditions, the majority of available TFPI-1 is found in the endothelial cells of the microvasculature but not larger vessels. A small fraction of TFPI-1 is stored in platelets or circulates in a free state in plasma. Fractionated and unfractionated heparin release TFPI-1 from the endothelial surface.

In sepsis, activation of the TF/VIIa pathway is a key process in the pathologic upregulation of the coagulation cascade. In bacterial sepsis, cytokines and endotoxins stimulate the expression of TF on circulating monocytes and endothelial cells. Human recombinant TFPI-1 (rTFPI-1) administered to animal models of severe sepsis resulted in a

significant reduction in mortality, an improvement in markers of coagulopathy, and a reduction in inflammatory markers such as IL-6. Several small phase 1 and 2 studies of rTFPI-1 in humans with sepsis have indicated that rTFPI can be given safely, with no increase in bleeding and a trend toward a reduction in all-cause mortality. In one multinational phase 2 study in 210 patients with severe sepsis, treatment with rTFPI reduced thrombin–antithrombin complexes and IL-6 levels, with no significant difference in adverse events. The study was not powered for a mortality outcome but showed a trend toward a reduction in 28-day mortality.

However, in July 2003 Abraham et al.[16] published a phase 3 clinical study which examined the use of recombinant TFPI in 1754 patients with severe sepsis. This study found no difference in mortality between the group of patients that received rTFPI and those that did not. However, the rate of serious adverse events due to bleeding was significantly increased in the treatment group compared to the placebo group.

Many papers have sought to address the question why activated protein C is a successful treatment for sepsis but antithrombin III and TFPI appear to have no effect. At present this remains unclear, but factors such as trial design, dosing and differences in anti-inflammatory properties have all been implicated.

Goal-directed therapies

Since the publication of a paper by Shoemaker in 1988[17] this has been an area of significant interest. In the original publication Shoemaker et al. showed that in high-risk surgical patients targeted use of the pulmonary artery catheter (PAC) to achieve an increased cardiac index and oxygen delivery resulted in a decrease in mortality. Since that time there have been in excess of 20 randomized clinical trials to determine whether this finding can be replicated in a variety of clinical situations. Many of these studies have found no improvement in mortality, and a number of reasons have been put forward for this. First, it appears that PAC-directed therapy needs to be instituted *before* the development of organ failure or sepsis. Second, if PAC-directed therapy is instituted in groups where the control mortality is less than 20 per cent, the differences are likely to be non-significant. Third, for PAC-directed therapy to be effective there needed to be measurable differences in the oxygen delivery between control and protocol groups. Thus, a more rational consensus to the use of goal-directed therapy seems to be developing, particularly in the management of surgical patients who have a very high predicted mortality and in whom targeted treatment can commence before surgery and be maintained throughout the perioperative period. In this situation the 'goals' that should be sought are a CI of $>4.5 \, \mathrm{L/min/m^{-2}}$ and a normal SvO_2 (>70 per cent). This should be done by placing a PAC to allow measurement of these parameters (in most institutions this will necessitate intensive care admission), and then titration of fluid and inotropes until these targets are met. The first-choice inotrope would usually be dobutamine, but there is some evidence supporting the use of dopexamine in preference to dobutamine in this setting.

Recently, Rivers *et al.* examined the use of goal-directed therapy in the early management of patients with severe sepsis.[18] In this study they randomized 263 patients admitted to the emergency department with severe sepsis or septic shock to either conventional treatment or early goal-directed therapy for the first 6 hours of management. In the treatment group, in addition to standard 'goals' for CVP, MAP and urine output, the central venous oxygenation saturation ($ScvO_2$) was maintained above 70 per cent, measured using a spectophotometric central venous catheter. They found that the in-hospital mortality rates were significantly higher (46.5 per cent) in the standard therapy group than in the early goal-directed therapy group (30.5 per cent). Although this was an unblinded study, the results may have a significant impact on the way severe sepsis is managed in the future.

Steroids

For over 50 years it has been proposed that corticosteroids may be useful in the management of sepsis. However, two systematic reviews of the literature have concluded that high-dose corticosteroids should not be used to treat patients with severe infection.[19,20] Also, there remains concern over the concepts of acute adrenal insufficiency and peripheral glucocorticoid resistance in catecholamine-dependent septic shock.

Acute adrenal insufficiency is probably best defined as a cortisol increment after a short corticotrophin test of $<9 \, \mu\mathrm{g/dL}$. Using this definition, the prevalence of occult adrenal insufficiency in severe sepsis has been estimated to be around 50 per cent. A peripheral glucocorticoid resistance syndrome may occur in patients with septic shock and be responsible for excessive immune-mediated inflammation.

Although two large randomized trials of large doses of corticosteroids have shown that reversal of shock may be achieved in over 50 per cent of patients, discontinuation of treatment was followed by increasing doses of vasopressor agents. Four placebo-controlled trials have now shown that in patients with catecholamine-dependent septic shock a prolonged treatment with low doses (approx. 300 mg daily) of hydrocortisone resulted in a significantly shorter duration of vasoactive drug administration than in patients not receiving steroid therapy.[21,22] The effect of steroids on mortality from septic shock remains more difficult to establish, but a beneficial effect may be seen in patients who do not respond to a short corticotrophin test.[21] Thus, in recent years the use of low-dose hydrocortisone in the management of patients with catecholamine-dependent shock has regained popularity.

NSAIDs

With arachidonic acid metabolism contributing significantly to mediators of sepsis it does appear to be logical that the administration of NSAIDs may decrease the systemic effects of sepsis. This was examined in a randomized, double-blind placebo-controlled trial of intravenous ibuprofen in 455 patients who met the criteria for sepsis conducted by Bernard and colleagues and published in 1997.[23] Despite the treatment group showing a decrease in urinary levels of prostacyclin and thromboxane, there was no reduction in the incidence or duration of shock or the acute respiratory distress syndrome, and the survival rate at 30 days was not significantly improved.

SUMMARY

Sepsis is the leading cause of death in critically ill patients. The diagnosis remains one that is made based on a large number of clinical signs and investigations. There is now clear evidence of a very close linkage between sepsis and DIC, and many of the biochemical pathways involved in these conditions are well elucidated. The majority of the management of patients with severe sepsis is supportive, but relatively recently the use of agents such as activated protein C has been associated with a significant decrease in mortality. The optimal management of these patients includes close liaison between microbiology, surgical teams and intensivists.

REFERENCES

1. Angus DC, Linde-Zwirble WT, Lidicker J, *et al.* Epidemiology of severe sepsis in the United States: analysis of incidence, outcome and associated costs of care. *Crit Care Med* 2001; **29**: 1303–10.
2. Levy MM, Fink MP, Marshall JC, *et al.* SCCM/ESICM/ACCP/ATS/SIS International Sepsis Definitions Conference. *Intensive Care Med* 2003; **29**: 530–8.

3. Marshall JC, Cook DJ, Christou NV, *et al.* Multiple organ dysfunction score: a reliable descriptor of a complex clinical outcome. *Crit Care Med* 1995; **23**: 1638–52.

4. Ferreira FL, Bota DP, Bross A, *et al.* Serial evaluation of the SOFA score to predict outcome in critically ill patients. *JAMA* 2001; **286**: 1754–8.

5. Noble JS, MacKirdy FN, Donaldson SI, Howie RI. Renal and respiratory failure in Scottish ICUs. *Anaesthesia* 2001; **56**:124–9.

6. Dellinger RP, Carlet JM, Masur H, *et al.* Surviving Sepsis Campaign Management Guidelines Committee. *Crit Care Med* 2004; **32**: 858–73.

7. Anderson ID, Sayers RD (eds) on behalf of the Royal College of Surgeons. *Care of the critically ill surgical patient*, 2nd edn. London: Arnold, 2003.

8. Centers for Disease Control and Prevention. Guidelines for the prevention of intravascular catheter-related infections. *Morbidity and Mortality Weekly Report* 2002; **51**: 1–30.

9. Bellomo R, Tetta C, Ronco C. Coupled plasma filtration adsorption. *Intensive Care Medicine* 2003; **29**: 1222–8.

10. Bertolini G, Iapichino G, Radrizzani D, *et al.* Early enteral immunonutrition in patients with severe sepsis: results of an interim analysis of a randomized multicentre clinical trial. *Intensive Care Med* 2003; **29**: 834–40.

11. de Jonge E, Schultz MJ, Spanjaard L, *et al.* Effects of selective decontamination of digestive tract on mortality and acquisition of resistant bacteria in intensive care: a randomized controlled trial. *Lancet* 2003; **362**: 1011–16.

12. Krueger WA, Lenhart FP, Neeser G, *et al.* Influence of combined intravenous and topical antibiotic prophylaxis on the incidence of infections, organ dysfunctions, and mortality in critically ill surgical patients. *Am J Respir Crit Care Med* 2002; **166**: 1029–37.

13. Van den Berghe G, Wouters P, Weekers F, *et al.* Intensive insulin therapy in critically ill patients. *N Engl J Med* 2001; **345**: 1359–67.

14. Bernard GR, Vincent JL, Laterre PF, *et al.* Efficacy and safety of recombinant human activated protein C for severe sepsis. *N Engl J Med* 2001; **344**: 699–709.

15. Warren BL, Eid A, Singer P, *et al.* High dose antithrombin III in severe sepsis. *JAMA* 2001; **286**: 1869–78.

16. Abraham E, Reinhart K, Opal S, *et al.* Efficacy and safety of tifacogin (recombinant tissue factor pathway inhibitor) in severe sepsis. *JAMA* 2003; **290**: 238–47.

17. Shoemaker WC, Appel PL, Kram HB, *et al.* Prospective trial of supranormal values of survivors as therapeutic goals in high-risk surgical patients. *Chest* 1988; **94**: 1176–86.

18. Rivers E, Nguyen B, Havstad S, *et al.* Early goal-directed therapy in the treatment of severe sepsis and septic shock. *N Engl J Med* 2001; **345**: 1368–77.

19. Lefering R, Neugebauer EA. Steroid controversy in sepsis and septic shock: A meta-analysis. *Crit Care Med* 1995; **23**: 1294–303.

20. Cronin L, Cook DJ, Carlet J, *et al.* Corticosteroid treatment for sepsis: A critical appraisal and meta-analysis of the literature. *Crit Care Med* 1995; **23**: 1430–9.

21. Annanne D, Sebille V, Charpentier C, *et al.* Effect of treatment with low doses of hydrocortisone and fludrocortisone on mortality in patients with septic shock. *JAMA* 2002; **288**: 862–71.

22. Bollaert PE, Charpentier C, Levy B, *et al.* Reversal of late septic shock with supraphysiologic doses of hydrocortisone. *Crit Care Med* 1998; **26**: 645–50.

23. Bernard GR, Wheeler AP, Russell JA, *et al.* The effects of ibuprofen on the physiology and survival of patients with sepsis. The Ibuprofen in Sepsis Study Group. *N Engl J Med* 1997; **336**: 912–18.

7 Renal support therapy

DAVID SELWYN & JAMES LOW

Viva topics

- What is the best management of incipient acute renal failure?
- Is intra-abdominal hypertension relevant to ARF?
- What indicates failed medical treatment of ARF?
- What are the differences between haemodialysis and haemofiltration?
- Which is more efficient at clearing urea, CVVH or intermittent haemodialysis?

Table 7.1 *RIFLE criteria for acute renal dysfunction*

	GFR criteria	Urine output criteria
Risk	Increased creatinine × 1.5 or GFR decrease >25 per cent	UO < 0.5 mL/kg/h for 6 hours
Injury	Increased creatinine × 2 or GFR decrease >50 per cent	UO < 0.5 mL/kg/h for 12 hours
Failure	Increased creatinine × 3 or GFR decrease >75 per cent	UO < 0.3 mL/kg/h for 24 hours or anuria for 12 hours
Loss	Persistent ARF = complete loss of renal function >4 weeks	
ESRD	End-stage renal disease	

Table 7.2 *ARF in intensive care patients*

- Incidence 7–23 per cent
- Associated with multiple organ failure
- Mortality 60–90 per cent
- Long-term requirement for RRT 1.6 per cent

INTRODUCTION

Despite vast improvements in the understanding of renal failure in critically ill surgical patients, the incidence of acute renal impairment requiring dialysis remains at *50–200 cases per million population*.[1,2] Modest degrees of acute renal failure (ARF) not resulting in dialysis treatment have been reported as increasing the risk of death approximately five-fold.[3] Specific surgical conditions are related to a higher incidence of ARF: for example, after cardiac surgery it has been reported to be as high as 30 per cent,[4] whereas abdominal aortic surgery is associated with an incidence of oliguric renal failure of 2–7 per cent and an associated mortality of 50–90 per cent.[5,6]

Compounding the exact incidence are imprecise definitions of ARF, for example: 'An acute and usually reversible deterioration of renal function, which develops over a period of days or weeks, and results in uraemia'. Although a marked reduction in urine volume is usual it is not invariable, and clearly, in the surgical population, if established acute renal failure is left untreated the patient will die. The mortality associated with the condition in isolation is 8 per cent; unfortunately, the patients who develop ARF while on the critical care unit do so as a part of generalized multiple organ failure (MOF), when the mortality increases to between 60 and 90 per cent.

Because critically ill patients develop acute renal failure as part of MOF, the traditional nephrology definitions for acute renal failure are, unfortunately, not applicable to this patient population. A simple statement definition, such as: 'A sudden and potentially reversible reduction in renal function, from which, if renal replacement is not provided, the patient will die'[3] may be more helpful. More specific standards, such as the RIFLE criteria (Table 7.1), have now been accepted as consensus definitions.[7]

The high incidence of ARF developing as a consequence of MOF has led to the suggestion that the kidney has replaced the splanchnic circulation as the 'new' forgotten organ of the critically ill (Table 7.2). This is contributed to by the lack of sophisticated functional tests and primitive treatment, which centres on an obsession with blood pressure and volume manipulation, despite well-recognized limitations of central venous pressure measurement. In addition, there are no widely available real-time monitoring systems capable of predicting incipient renal failure, or for that matter any well-proven medical treatment to alter the clinical course of ARF once it has become established.

The kidney has become the forgotten organ for largely historical reasons: traditional teaching has classified ARF according to prerenal, intrinsic renal and postrenal causes. This remains unhelpful in describing the multifactorial condition that affects critically ill patients. The kidney of the critically ill patient is subjected to a series of insults or 'multiple hits'. These may occur simultaneously or in series, with each additional insult increasing the chance of ARF development.

ARF may be classified according to the volume of urine produced each day, non-oliguric or oliguric renal failure being <400 mL urine per day. Oliguric failure implies a more severe insult to the kidney than non-oliguric failure, and anuria is defined as <100 mL of urine per day.

PATHOPHYSIOLOGY

Renal blood flow represents 25 per cent of the resting cardiac output and the circulating blood volume is filtered and reabsorbed twice per hour. The oxygen requirements of the kidney relate to the energy-rich concentrating mechanisms of the tubular cells. Renal perfusion, blood flow and glomerular filtration are governed by a complex series of renal vasculature afferent and efferent control mechanisms, the autoregulation mechanisms of which are well described. These phenomena occur independently of neuronal input and will occur in denervated renal vascular beds. Numerous well-defined mediators have been shown to be involved in this process, including the renin–angiotensin system, the sympathetic nervous system, prostaglandins and nitric oxide pathways.

The pathological changes that occur in this complex arrangement during multiorgan failure are less well understood. Well-perfused cortical nephrons are rarely at risk of ischaemic damage, whereas the high-energy salt-regulating juxtaglomerular nephrons are threatened by minimal changes in blood flow and oxygen supply. It remains a paradox that the highest energy-dependent nephrons are those with the most critical blood supply.

Inevitably, the cause of functional failure is a combination of ischaemic acute tubular necrosis with or without additional nephrotoxic injury and sepsis-derived mediator impairment. Usually there are minimal histological findings with acute tubular necrosis, the damage being predominantly focal and

Table 7.3 *Functions of the kidney*

- Regulation of blood pressure and plasma volume
- Regulation of sodium and potassium
- Acid-base balance
- Excretion of drugs
- Metabolism of drugs
- Regulation of calcium and phosphate
- Erythropoietin

Table 7.4 *Patients at risk of ARF*

- ALL surgical patients
- Cardiac surgery
- Vascular surgery
- Diabetic
- Contrast studies
- Trauma

localized to specific areas of the nephron. These marginal histological findings are at odds with the observed profound functional derangement. However, although there is a lag time to recovery of renal function, which outlives the disease process of MOF, complete resolution of renal impairment function would be usually expected. The long-term requirement for renal replacement therapy (RRT) is reported to be only 1.6 per cent.[8]

Rhabdomyolysis is a specific renal insult that occurs as a result of massive muscle damage, usually from trauma, although it may also be as a result of prolonged fits, hyperpyrexia, severe sepsis, compartment syndrome or drug toxicity. The release of cellular breakdown contents precipitates metabolic mayhem, with nephrotoxic damage occurring as a result of myoglobin exposure. The myoglobin molecule is readily filtered and deposited in the renal tubules. Measured intratubular pressures are normal,[9] demonstrating that the predominant cause of damage is not obstruction, nor the release of iron, but free radical activation and subsequent activity on cell membrane arachidonic acids.[10] In addition, myoglobin causes vasoconstriction both directly and via mediators such as thromboxane. Table 7.3 lists the various functions of the kidney.

PREVENTION OF ACUTE RENAL FAILURE

Instituting a therapeutic intervention to either prevent or reverse deteriorating renal function could have a significant impact on outcome; however, the mainstay of prevention continues to rely on preoperative identification of at-risk patients (Table 7.4). Because the only parameter amenable

Table 7.5 *Urinalysis and biochemistry of ARF*

	Hypovolaemia	ATN	Acute interstitial nephritis	Glomerulonephritis	Obstruction
Sediment	Bland	Broad, brownish granular casts	White blood cells, eosinophils, cellular casts	Red blood cells, red blood cell casts	Bland or bloody
Protein	None or low	None or low	Minimal. May be increased with NSAIDs	Increased, >100 mg/dL	Low
Urine sodium mEq/L	<20	>30	>30	<20	<20 (Acute) >40 (Few days)
Urine osmolality mmol/kg	>400	<350	<350	>400	<350
Fractional excretion of sodium (%)	<1	>1	Varies	<1	<1 (Acute) >1 (Few days)

Fractional excretion of sodium: is the urine to plasma (U/P) of sodium divided by U/P of creatinine $\times$ 100

to intervention remains renal perfusion pressure, established methods of preventing ARF remain fluid loading and maintenance of adequate perfusion pressure or cardiac output. This is achieved by maintenance of adequate intravascular volume pre-, peri- and postoperatively. Postoperative trauma patients have been shown to have a reduced need for renal support and a lower mortality following aggressive fluid management.[11] In addition, attention should be given to the general avoidance of physiological and pharmacological renal insults.

Postoperatively, the differential diagnosis will lie between prerenal failure and multiple-insult acute tubular necrosis (ATN). Initial therapy should be serial fluid challenges and appropriate monitoring in a suitable environment. Table 7.5 describes the urinalysis and biochemistry of ARF.

DRUG THERAPY AIMED AT PREVENTING ARF (TABLE 7.6)

Mannitol

This osmotic diuretic is thought to increase renal blood flow as a result of actions on intrarenal prostaglandins, atrial naturietic peptide (ANP) and a reduction in renin production. It has been suggested that mannitol can reduce tubular obstruction and act as a free radical scavenger. There is some experimental evidence that it can protect against ischaemic injury when administered pre insult. Mannitol has been advocated as a prophylactic agent in major surgery, including biliary surgery, vascular surgery and radiocontrast studies.

Unfortunately, there is no Grade 1 evidence that mannitol has any benefit. Three randomized studies using mannitol and fluid expansion in renal transplant patients suggested that it reduced the incidence of postoperative renal failure,[12–14]

Table 7.6 *Pharmacological therapy*

- Mannitol
- Furosemide
- Dopamine
- Dobutamine
- Norepinephrine (noradrenaline)
- Dopexamine
- ANP
- Aminophylline
- NAC
- Fenaldopam
- Renal rescue techniques

but this may have been related to fluid hydration alone. Small controlled studies have suggested a prophylactic role in general vascular surgery.

Mannitol has also been traditionally used to help prevent rhabdomyolysis-induced renal failure; however, fluid loading with or without alkalinization has been described as equally efficous.[15]

Although the debate for its use either prophylactically or therapeutically continues, there remains evidence that mannitol itself is a potent renal toxin. This may be due in part to severe renal vasoconstriction.[16]

Furosemide

Compared to anuric renal failure, polyuric renal failure is associated with an improved outcome. Consequently there is great attraction in using large doses of loop diuretics in a theoretical role influencing the natural clinical course of the disease. Unfortunately, there is little evidence to suggest that developing renal failure can be influenced in this way.

Probably patients that respond with polyuria represent those who continue to have a measure of renal reserve allowing a response, rather than those who can be influenced to follow a particular clinical disease course. Quite clearly there is grave concern that diuretic use in the absence of adequate fluid resuscitation and renal perfusion would only exacerbate impending renal failure.

The majority of studies have been in patients with established ARF. There remain a limited number of prophylactic studies. High-dose furosemide has been reported to reduce the duration of oliguria and the need for dialysis, yet it has no effect on mortality.[17] In another study increased urine output had no effect on duration of oliguria, dialysis or mortality.[18,19] Furosemide has shown no benefit in cardiac surgery, in radiocontrast-induced nephrotoxicity[20,21] or in combination with dopamine.

The administration of loop diuretics may have a protective effect in reducing the energy requirements of the ascending loop of Henle,[22] thereby increasing its resistance to ischaemia, and some centres use it in this capacity. Continuous infusions are better than single large doses, and the recommended treatment regimen would commence with an initial bolus dose of 10 mg followed by an infusion of 1–10 mg/h.

Dopamine

There has been enormous debate over the past 20 years as to the exact place for this non-specific dopamine receptor-1 (DA_1) and DA_2 agonist. Despite previous strong support, after recent publications such as the ANZICS trial and the latest meta-analysis, it now seems clear that dopamine has at best no effect, and seems to have significant deleterious side effects.[23–25] The ANZICS trial recruited 328 patients in 23 intensive care units given either placebo or dopamine at 2 μg/kg/min. The primary endpoint was serum creatinine, with surrogate endpoints of requirement for renal replacement therapy, ICU and hospital length of stay and mortality. There was no significant difference in any of these outcome variables.

A meta-analysis of 58 studies in over 2140 patients using dopamine in ARF also failed to show any benefit.[24] Any perceived effect on urine output is secondary to changes in cardiac output, and in view of the good evidence related to the harmful effects of dopamine on gut perfusion and critical pituitary-released stress hormones, there is no current therapeutic place for this agent.

Norepinephrine and dobutamine

In order to provide adequate renal perfusion pressure the aim should be to provide a mean arterial pressure (MAP)

which is normal for that patient. The patient's normal blood pressure should be determined (usually by examining existing medical records), and after any necessary fluid resuscitation, vasopressor therapy used to achieve this pressure. Patients with chronic hypertension will require a higher MAP to provide an adequate renal perfusion pressure than normotensive patients. In these patients renal autoregulation has been shifted to the right, resulting in the need for a higher MAP to maintain a normal renal blood flow. Some authors have recommended a trial of glyceryl trinitrate infusion prior to starting vasopressor therapy in an attempt to ensure maximal vasodilatation and optimized right-sided filling.

Early studies suggesting that renal function could be improved following norepinephrine infusion in septic shock were directly related to a pure vasopressor action on mean arterial pressure,[26,27] rather than any specific action on the kidney. Similarly, work suggesting that dobutamine improves quality but not quantity of urine (little effect on urine output, but some improvement in creatinine clearance)[28] is also related to an enhancement in mean arterial pressure and cardiac output.

Dopexamine

Dopexamine is a potent dopaminergic agonist as well as exhibiting β_2 activity. It increases cardiac output as a result of increased stroke volume and a reduction in systemic vascular resistance. Renal blood flow is increased only slightly. Small-scale studies to date have been conducted in infrarenal aortic surgery, orthotopic liver transplantation and coronary artery bypass grafting. This agent remains under investigation, but there is insufficient evidence yet to recommend its use as a renal salvage agent. There remains interest in its use as a free radical scavenging agent.

Aminophylline

Adenosine produced from ATP under ischaemic conditions has been recognized as a potent mediator of vasoconstriction. Adenosine acts as a non-specific antagonist of adenosine, and experimental and small-scale clinical work has suggested that aminophylline may prevent ischaemic injury.[29] There are no randomized controlled trials, although this is currently under investigation.

Atrial naturetic peptide

Another agent that has been used in an attempt to attenuate the course of ARF is atrial natriuretic peptide. In the early

1980s the natriuretic effect of an extract of mammalian atrial myocytes was reported. This active substance was characterized as a 28-amino acid polypeptide. It has a short half-life of approximately 5 minutes and is cleared via the lung, liver and kidney by neutral endopeptidase. ANP's action on the kidney is that of inhibition of sodium and water reabsorbtion in the distal nephron, vasodilating the afferent arteriole and vasoconstricting the efferent arteriole, thus improving glomerular filtration rate (GFR) without affecting renal blood flow. Although initial small-scale studies showed an improved clearance and a reduction in dialysis requirements, follow-up large-scale trials did not confirm this. In addition, there was no demonstrated effect on mortality.

Fenaldopam

Fenaldopam mesylate is a selective dopamine (DA_1 receptor) analogue that stimulates renal blood flow, natriuresis and urine output. It is six times more potent than dopamine in producing renal vasodilatation. It is currently approved for use in malignant hypertensive crisis. A number of non-randomized and one randomized study have suggested a reduced incidence of contrast nephropathy with fenoldopam and fluid compared to controls. Initial work has also suggested effective prevention of renal failure after abdominal aortic aneurysm and coronary artery bypass grafting;[30–32] larger multicentre trials are currently taking place.

N-acetylcysteine

There remains a 10 per cent incidence of hospital-acquired ARF caused by radiographic contrast. Two trials using a combination of oral acetylcysteine with 0.45 per cent saline have shown a reduction in contrast nephropathy in patients with chronic renal insufficiency. In patients undergoing CT scans a 90 per cent risk reduction was shown, and in coronary angiograms a risk reduction of 82 per cent occurred. There continues to be debate about the choice of fluids, yet it seems reasonable to administer oral acetylcysteine the day before and on the contrast study day, probably with 0.45 per cent saline at 1 mL/kg for 6–12 hours prior to study.

INCREASED INTRA-ABDOMINAL PRESSURE (TABLE 7.7)

The abdominal compartment syndrome may result from intra-abdominal haemorrhage or haematoma, intestinal ileus and ascites. Intra-abdominal hypertension reduces abdominal perfusion pressure and consequently results in

Table 7.7 *Increased intra-abdominal pressure*

- Causes abdominal compartment syndrome
- Easily measured using urinary bladder pressure technique
- Normal mean value 6.5 mmHg
- Elevated by intra-abdominal haemorrhage or haematoma, ascites or ileus
- Consider abdominal decompression if >25 mmHg

end-organ hypoperfusion.[33] Normal intra-abdominal pressure (IAP) varies between 0 and 17 mmHg, with a mean value of 6.5 mmHg; an elevation of IAP to 25 mmHg has been shown to reduce GFR and is refractory to fluid loading and increased cardiac output. Unless urgent abdominal decompression occurs when IAP reaches 25 mmHg, acute renal failure will result.[34–37]

TREATMENT OF ESTABLISHED ARF

The management of the metabolic and biochemical consequences of established ARF is still debated. Evidence suggests that instituting renal replacement therapy early, with more aggressive control of biochemical parameters, may improve outcome. The following indications for initiating renal replacement therapy (RRT) have been suggested.

Absolute indications

- Uncontrollable non-lactic metabolic acidosis
- A rapidly rising urea, or any urea level resulting in uraemic symptoms (e.g. pericarditis)
- Fluid overload not amenable to other forms of medical therapy (e.g. deterioration in PaO_2/FiO_2 ratio in excess of 20 per cent)
- Uncontrollable hyperkalaemia
- Urea > 35 mmol/L.

'Relative' indications

- Progressively rising urea
- Persistent oliguria despite adequate fluid resuscitation with a rising serum urea
- Metabolic acidosis (lactic or non-lactic)
- Vasopressor-refractory septic shock.

There is little evidence to support the 'relative indications', although a beneficial effect is biologically plausible.

However, before instituting RRT the significant risks and costs must be considered. The major considerations are listed below:

- Mortality and morbidity related to venous cannulation
- Mortality and morbidity related to the use of anticoagulation and mechanical effects of the extracorporeal system
- Mortality and morbidity related to technical/human failure (e.g. air embolism, disconnection)
- Mortality and morbidity related to fluid and electrolyte shifts (e.g. cerebral oedema)
- Cost
- High nursing skill requirements.

The problems of major fluid shifts and severe cardiovascular instability have to a large extent been removed with modern continuous venous filtration techniques, but fluid shifts at a cellular level can still cause considerable problems. The decision about how and when to institute RRT is usually customized to each individual clinical situation.

Treating renal failure in critically ill patients has a high mortality rate. Early, aggressive RRT may improve mortality and reduce the duration of ARF.

Absolute indications for RRT are:

- Urea > 35 and creatinine > 350 μmol
- Uraemic symptoms
- Fluid overload not responsive to diuretics
- Uncontrollable acidosis and hyperkalaemia.

BOX 7.1 KEY POINTS
- Identify at-risk patients early
- Institute appropriate monitoring in these patients in an appropriately clinical area
- Low threshold for invasive CVP and arterial pressure monitoring if oliguria fails to respond to simple measures
- Think obstructed cause if sudden cessation of urine flow
- Do the simple things well
- Furosemide and dopamine may cause harm

Failed medical therapy: criteria for initiation of RRT in critically ill patients

- Serum creatinine > 350 μmol/L
- Plasma urea > 35 mmol/L
- Persistent metabolic acidosis (pH < 7.2)
- Hyperkalaemia K > 6.5 mmol/L
- Pulmonary oedema unresponsive to conventional therapy

- Uraemic encephalopathy
- Uraemic pericarditis
- Uraemic neuropathy.

MODES OF RENAL REPLACEMENT

Peritoneal dialysis

This mode of RRT is seldom used in adult intensive care but is still frequently used in paediatric ICUs. A dialysis catheter, similar to that used for peritoneal lavage, is inserted, usually below the umbilicus, in the midline and directed towards either iliac fossa. Dialysis fluid is then infused into the peritoneum, left in situ for a period and then drained out, and with the development of automated machines the reliability of fluid balance has improved. This method uses the patient's peritoneal membrane as the dialysis membrane and removes solute by allowing diffusion into the dialysis fluid. It is not efficient at removing solute or fluid in adults, but still has limited use because of its simplicity and lack of requirement for anticoagulation. It can also be a useful adjuvant to active rewarming in severely hypothermic patients.

Although a recent laparotomy is not necessarily a contraindication to peritoneal dialysis, many surgical patients are not suitable for this form of RRT because of intra-abdominal sepsis. Recent evidence suggests that patients with ARF secondary to sepsis who are treated with peritoneal dialysis have a higher mortality rate than those treated with venous filtration.

Continuous renal replacement therapy

Now universally accepted as the mainstay of renal support in the critically ill patient, continuous renal replacement therapy is the most common form of RRT in the UK. Continuous therapy can either be arteriovenous (Figure 7.1) or venovenous (Figure 7.2). Arteriovenous filtration does not require a pump to drive blood through the filter, instead depending on the patient's arterial blood pressure to do this. Venovenous filtration pumps blood through the filter and works independently of the patient's blood pressure. It is, however, dependent on the quality of venous access to allow the pump to generate high blood flow rates.

Solute and fluid can be removed from blood in three ways:

- Filtration
- Dialysis
- Diafiltration.

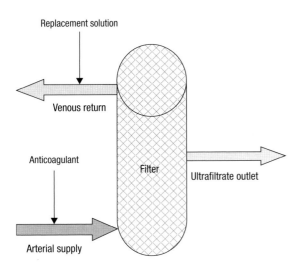

Figure 7.1 Schematic diagram of continuous arteriovenous haemofiltration. Arterial blood, driven by the patient's own blood pressure, passes through the filter. The filter removes ultrafiltrate and replacement fluid is added to the remaining blood before it returns to the patient

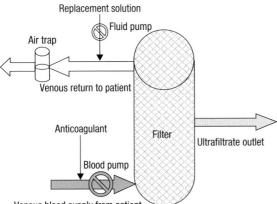

Figure 7.2 Schematic diagram of continuous venovenous haemofiltration. Venous blood is pumped from the patient through the filter. Once again, ultrafiltrate is removed and replacement fluid is added to the blood before it returns to the patient (post dilution)

FILTRATION

Blood is passed through a filter with a pressure being applied across the filter membrane (transmembrane pressure). Fluid moves across the membrane by convection (filtrate), taking with it electrolytes and small solute molecules such as urea, forming a yellow ultrafiltrate which is then collected and discarded. The filtration pressure is dependent entirely on the driving pressure or blood flow, the membrane surface area and pore size, and any back-pressure on the ultrafiltrate.

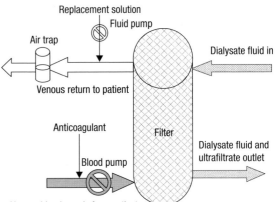

Figure 7.3 Schematic diagram of continuous venovenous haemodiafiltration. As for Figure 7.2, except that the dialysate fluid is passed through the filter on the opposite side of the membrane to the blood, resulting in diafiltration

This ultrafiltrate fluid is then replaced with a replacement solution that has an electrolyte concentration similar to that of normal plasma (without containing any urea). Adjusting the relative amounts of fluid removed and replaced controls the overall fluid balance. Patients are said to have a zero balance if the amounts of fluid removed and replaced are equal. The more filtrate removed, the greater the clearance of solute. Performing filtration over a long period of time allows large volumes of fluid to be removed slowly, and therefore without rapid changes in fluid balance and consequently cardiovascular parameters.

DIALYSIS

Blood is passed through a filter in one direction and fluid with a similar concentration of electrolytes to plasma (dialysis solution) is passed in the other direction. A semipermeable membrane separates the fluid and blood. The membrane allows electrolytes, metabolites and water to move along a concentration gradient by diffusion. Dialysis is very efficient at removing solute, that is, it provides the most efficient reduction in urea, but is usually completed in a 2–4-hour timescale and is generally associated with dramatic fluid shifts, which are poorly tolerated in the critically ill.

DIAFILTRATION

This is a combination of the above methods whereby not only is the blood 'squeezed' through the filter membrane, but dialysis solution is pumped in the opposite direction, creating a countercurrent mechanism and 'pulling' fluid and electrolytes out of the blood (Figure 7.3). Theoretically it offers improved clearance of solute, but in reality a very rapid clearance of solute is not required in critically ill patients. It does, however, have the advantage of reducing electrolyte loss by virtue of the countercurrent mechanism. The greater complexity does also increase the cost of RRT.

> **BOX 7.2**
> - CVVHF is the most common form of continuous renal replacement therapy in the UK
> - Filtration relies solely on convection to clear solute and is very efficient at maintaining fluid balance
> - CVVH is associated with minimal cardiovascular instability and functions independently of patients' MAP
> - Filtration combined with dialysis (CVVHDF) will increase the efficiency of solute clearance at the expense of increased complexity
> - The role of techniques such as slow continuous ultrafiltration (SCUF) and continuous venovenous haemodialysis (CVVHD) is mainly within the renal unit

The advantages of continuous as opposed to intermittent RRT are:

- Better control of fluid balance
- Improved control of renal biochemistry
- Steady-state anticoagulation
- Less risk of cardiovascular instability.

The advantages of intermittent as opposed to continuous RRT are:

- RRT-free periods allow procedures and investigation to be performed
- Reduced levels of nursing skill for part of the shift when the patient is not on the filter
- Less time spent fully anticoagulated.

VENOUS ACCESS

Large-diameter reliable central venous access is required for efficient RRT. This is usually placed in either the internal jugular, subclavian or femoral veins using a 'Seldinger' or 'cutdown' technique. Ideally an ultrasound imaging device should be available to aid the identification of venous structures, as line complications are a major contributory factor to the mortality and morbidity associated with RRT. If in doubt, a blood gas measurement should be used to confirm that the needle and guidewire are placed in a central vein or a pressure wave transduced, prior to dilating a tract and inserting the catheter. The catheters usually have two or three lumina and are constructed as coaxial or lumen-by-lumen,

each being associated with differing flow characteristics. The preferred site has been widely debated: internal jugular lines may allow better flow rates than subclavian lines, but there is a lower infection rate and superior patient comfort associated with subclavian lines. Femoral line catheters possibly need to be longer to allow good blood flow, and once the patient is awake, bending of the legs will cause repeated machine alarms. They are also associated with a higher infection rate than subclavian lines. It is important to flush the catheter thoroughly once it is inserted, as thrombus formation will reduce the efficacy of the line.

PRESCRIBING CONTINUOUS VENOVENOUS HAEMOFILTRATION

The following parameters need to be considered:

- **Fluid balance** This is usually prescribed for a predetermined cycle, such as 4 or 12 hours, and all fluids given to the patient must be considered, e.g. drugs, TPN etc. If fluid is to be removed then usually a target balance for each hour is set, e.g. 100 mL removed per hour. Usually on the initial cycle a neutral or zero balance is prescribed, and this is also used if the patient is cardiovascularly unstable and unable to tolerate fluid loss on the filter.
- **Type of replacement solution** Two major types of replacement solution are available:
  - Replacement fluid with lactate as a buffer
  - Replacement fluid without lactate as a buffer.

One of the major functions of the kidney is to reabsorb and regenerate bicarbonate. It is therefore essential to either provide bicarbonate or a substitute when performing RRT. Bicarbonate is very unstable in solution and until recently was not commercially available as the buffer in replacement solutions. Lactate is more stable and is consequently usually used as buffer. Lactate is metabolized in a hydrogen ion-accepting process and allows HCO^{3-} to be formed by pushing the equation below to the right.

$$CO_2 + H_2O \leftrightarrow HCO^{3-} + H^+$$
$$CA$$

In some patients with severe lactataemia or lactic acidosis, lactate may not be metabolized and the serum lactate will rise, with a deteriorating metabolic acidosis. This is seen in patients with acute liver failure or post cardiac surgery, and in these patients a lactate-free replacement solution may be used. As lactate is provided as sodium lactate the replacement solution that is lactate free has a low (122 mmol/L) sodium concentration. When using lactate-free solutions a buffer such as sodium bicarbonate must be infused at the same time to replace both the bicarbonate and the sodium.

- **Potassium replacement** Replacement solutions do not usually have potassium in them. This allows high serum potassium levels to be corrected very rapidly. All patients having CVVHF will require potassium replacement after the initial cycle. It is usual to add 20 mmol of KCL to each 5-litre bag, thereby giving a 4 mmol/L concentration. Patients often have other potassium losses or shifts and may require more replacement than this, which is usually supplemented as a parenteral infusion.
- **Phosphate replacement** There is no phosphate in replacement solutions and hypophosphataemia often develops. Phosphate cannot be added to the bag as it would interact with the calcium content and precipitate out. Phosphate levels should be monitored, and supplements should be prescribed by intravenous or oral routes.
- **Dosage of RRT** This is the amount of replacement solution that is to be given to the patient per hour. Variable doses between 15 and 70 mL/kg/h (ideal body weight) have been suggested. One study has suggested that the optimal dose is about 35 mL/kg/h, or just over 2000 mL/h for a 70 kg patient, demonstrating a significant improvement in survival.[38] Increasing the dosage of RRT (i.e. the volume of replacement fluid given to the patient) will either require a change in the fluid balance (allowing the patient to receive more fluid than is removed) or increased removal of filtrate, to allow this. The more fluid that is being removed, the higher the flow rates through the filter that will be required. This may indeed be the rate-limiting step in determining the dose of RRT that can be given, as flow rates through the filter are determined by the venous access. If the access is poor then the high blood flow rates – in excess of 250 mL/min through the filter – will not be achieved.
- **Membranes** Membranes have traditionally been manufactured from cuprophane, a polysaccharide-based membrane obtained from pressed cotton. Increasingly a systemic inflammatory response syndrome has been recognized, caused by blood activation as its passes through this bioincompatible membrane. Modern synthetic biocompatible membranes have been developed from polysulfone, polymethyl methylacrylate, polyamide and polyacrylonitrile.[39,40] Artificial kidney membranes have also been constructed as flat plate membranes, in addition to the more universal hollow-fibre cylindrical membranes.
- **Anticoagulation** The primary aims of anticoagulation are to prolong the life of the filter and thereby improve its function, as well as avoiding thrombus formation in the whole of the extracorporeal circuit. The requirement for

anticoagulation must be balanced against the potentially fatal complications that can occur. Several methods are available to reduce the coagulation of blood passing through a filter. These are listed below:
- Decreased activation of the intrinsic and common clotting cascade
- Decreased blood viscosity passing through the filter by predilution
- Decreased platelet adhesion
- A combination of the above
- No anticoagulation.

DECREASED ACTIVATION OF THE INTRINSIC AND COMMON CLOTTING CASCADE

Unfractionated heparin has traditionally been used to prolong the partial thromboplastin time (PTT) to 60–90 seconds or an activated clotting time (ACT) of 180–200 seconds. Heparin is usually given as a bolus followed by a continuous infusion. The infusion can either be added to the venous limb of the filter (filter anticoagulation) or be given systemically (systemic heparinization). Both methods will cause prolongation of the PTT, and although it makes more sense to primarily anticoagulate the filter and not the patient, the majority of units perform systemic anticoagulation. It is possible to conduct regional heparinization by anticoagulating blood entering the filter with heparin, and then reversing it with protamine as it leaves the filter before returning to the patient. Excess doses of protamine can, however, cause further anticoagulation and vasodilatation, making this a more difficult technique to manage.

Critically ill patients often have abnormalities of coagulation prior to starting RRT. A consumptive coagulopathy may be present, with a degree of heparin resistance. This combination can result in poor filter anticoagulation and fluctuating coagulation blood results. Heparin-induced thrombocytopenia (HIT) can also occur, with a reported incidence of 5–30 per cent.[41] A decreasing platelet count is common with RRT and can make HIT difficult to exclude except by specific antibody testing. Danaparoid, a heparinoid product (a mixture of glycosaminoglycans), may be used if HIT is suspected, but has a cross-reactivity of 10 per cent. Hirudin, a specific thrombin inhibitor, is a useful alternative that does not cause HIT.

Low molecular weight heparins (LMWH) are also used, but although the pharmacodynamics of these drugs during RRT has not yet been established, recently published data have shown good filter life and safety profile.[42]

Some patients will be autoanticoagulated and will not require any further anticoagulation, and excellent filter life and urea clearance may be achieved using no additional anticoagulant.

Regional citrate is becoming increasingly popular as a form of anticoagulation, particularly in post-cardiac bypass renal failure patients and those at a high risk of life-threatening haemorrhagic complications. There are a number of substantial technical challenges involved in citrate anticoagulation, and industry development of standardized stable citrate and calcium reversal solutions is required. Debate continues about the advantages of post-filter citrate anticoagulation compared to pre-filter administration, although it seems likely that this will become a more popular form of extracorporeal anticoagulation.

DECREASED BLOOD VISCOSITY PASSING THROUGH THE FILTER

The viscosity of the blood increases as it passes through the filter because fluid is moving out of the blood, causing the haematocrit to rise. The blood is most viscous when it exits the filter before any replacement solution is added. If the replacement solution is added before the blood enters the filter then the viscosity of the blood will be decreased and the blood less likely to clot. This is the principle behind pre-filter fluid dilution or 'predilution'. The major disadvantage is that removal of patient solute is decreased and so less efficient filtration is achieved. However, it has very little effect on the patient's coagulation, and can be useful if patients are at high risk of a serious complication if anticoagulation is used. Optimal levels for pre- and postfilter dilution remain undecided.

DECREASED PLATELET ADHESION

Prostacycline, a potent inhibitor of platelet function, is usually used. The advantages are that it has a very short half-life and a reversible effect on platelet function. Unfortunately, it may cause profound vasodilatation and can aggravate hypotension in patients who are cardiovascularly unstable. It also increases shunt by pulmonary vasodilatation of underventilated areas of lung, and remains relatively expensive. It is administered as an infusion, usually into the blood before it enters the filter.

A COMBINATION OF THE ABOVE

Heparin is usually used first and predilution or prostacycline added if this is not sufficient. The choice of second-line agent will depend on the patient's condition and the risk: benefit ratio for the chosen agent.

CURRENT PRACTICE

At present continuous venovenous filtration is the standard method of providing renal support. Recently, following suggestions of improved survival, there has been a trend towards earlier, higher volume filtration with more emphasis on tighter control of serum urea.[43,44] Therapy is given continuously at high blood flow rates, with aggressive ultrafiltration replacement at 35 mL/kg/h, until the patient's clinical condition improves or intrinsic renal function has returned.

BOX 7.3

- High-flow (large diameter) venous access is required for efficient filtration
- Large-diameter venous access for RRT is a significant cause of mortality and morbidity
- All patients receiving CVVH for more than a few hours will require potassium replacement
- Dosage of RRT is determined by the patient's lean mass and is about 35 mL/kg/h
- The type of fluid used will depend on the clinical condition of the patient
- Fluid balance must be considered when prescribing the dosage of RRT, as an equivalent volume of fluid will need to be removed from the patient to prevent fluid accumulating
- Anticoagulation protocols will minimize filter loss and bleeding.

FUTURE TRENDS

Unfortunately, there are no drugs currently available that are able to prevent ARF, and so improved early detection remains imperative, ideally using more sensitive and specific real-time renal monitors. Once renal failure has become established then technological advances in venous catheter design are essential to allow increased blood flow, and membrane composition and surface area are also likely to alter. It seems that bicarbonate buffer solutions have gone full circle and now are no longer in favour, but there is increasing interest in regional citrate anticoagulation and this may become more common.

The vision of removal of specific inflammatory cytokines using filtration membranes, and in so doing attenuating or stopping the inflammatory process, remains. Medium-sized trials are starting to appear suggesting improved survival in SIRS/sepsis using plasmapheresis, and development continues on dual filtration–adsorption systems.

REFERENCES

1. Feest TG, Round A, Hamad S. Incidence of severe acute renal failure in adults: results of a community based study. *BMJ* 1993; **306**: 481–3.

2. Liano F, Pascual J. The Madrid Acute Renal Failure Study Group. Epidemiology of acute renal failure: a prospective, multicentre, community-based study. *Kidney Int* 1996; **50**: 811–18.

3. Levy EM, Viscoli CM, Horwitz RI. The effect of acute renal failure on mortality: a cohort analysis. *JAMA* 1996; **275**: 1489–94.

4. Block CA, Manning HL. Prevention of acute renal failure in the critically ill. *Am J Respir Crit Care Med* 2002; **165**: 320–4.

5. The Standards and Audit Subcommittee of the Renal Association on behalf of the Renal Association and the Royal College of Physicians. Treatment of adult patients with renal failure: recommended standards and audit measures, 2nd edn. *J R Coll Physicians Lond* 1995; **29**: 190–1.

6. Bertolissi M. Prevention of acute renal failure in major vascular surgery. *Minerva Anestesiol* 1999; **65**: 867–77.

7. Palevsky PM, Metnitz PGH, Piccinni P, Vinsonneau C. Selection of endpoints for clinical trials of acute renal failure in critically ill patients. *Curr Opin Crit Care* 2002; **8**: 515–18.

8. Noble JS, MacKirdy FN, Donaldson SI, Howie RI. Renal and respiratory failure in Scottish ICUs. *Anaesthesia* 2001; **56**: 124–9.

9. Oken DE, DiBona GF, McDonald FD. Micropuncture studies of the recovery phase of myohemoglobinuric acute renal failure in the rat. *J Clin Invest* 1970; **49**: 730–7.

10. Holt SG. Rhabdomyolysis. In: Galley H. (ed.) *Critical care focus volume 1: renal failure.* London: BMJ Books/Intensive Care Society, 1999.

11. Shin B, Mackenzie CF. Postoperative renal failure in trauma patients. *Anesthesiology* 1979; **51**: 218–21.

12. Tiggeler RGW, Berden JHM, Hotsma AJ, Koene RAP. Prevention of acute tubular necrosis in cadaveric kidney transplantation by combined use of mannitol and moderate hydration. *Ann Surg* 1985; **201**: 246–51.

13. Weimar W, Geerlings W, Bijnen AB, *et al.* A controlled study on the effect of mannitol on immediate renal function after cadaveric donor kidney transplantation. *Transplantation* 1983; **35**: 99–101.

14. Van Valenberg PL, Hoitsma AJ, Tiggeler RG, *et al.* Mannitol as an indispensable constituent of an intraoperative hydration protocol for the prevention of acute renal failure after renal cadaveric transplantation. *Transplantation* 1987; **44**: 784–8.

15. Horrsi E, Barreiro MF, Orlando JM, Higa EM. Prophylaxis of acute renal failure in patients with rhabdomyolysis. *Renal Failure* 1997; **19**: 283–8.

16. Perez-Perez AJ, Pazos B, Sobrado J, *et al.* Acute renal failure following massive mannitol infusion. *Am J Nephrol* 2002; **22**: 573–5.

17. Cantarovich F, Galli C, Benedetti L, *et al.* High dose frusemide in established acute renal failure. *BMJ* 1973; **4**: 449–50.

18. Brown CB, Ogg CS, Cameron JS. High dose frusemide in acute renal failure: a controlled trial. *Clin Nephrol* 1981; **15**: 90–6.

19. Kleinknecht D, Ganeval D, Gonzalez-Duque LA, Fermanian J. Furosemide in acute oliguric renal failure. A controlled trial. *Nephron* 1976; **17**: 51–8.

20. Nuutinen LS, Kairaluoma M, Tumonen S, Larmi TKI. The effect of frusemide on renal function in open heart surgery. *J Cardiovasc Surg* 1978; **19**: 471–9.

21. Solomon R, Werner C, Mann D, *et al.* Effects of saline, mannitol and furosemide on acute decreases in renal function by radiocontrast agents. *N Engl J Med* 1994; **331**: 1414–16.

22. Brezis M, Rozen S, Silva P, Epstein FH. Transport activity modifies thick ascending limb damage in the isolated perfused kidney. *Kidney Int* 1984; **25**: 65–72.

23. Bellomo R, Chapman M, Finfer S, *et al.* Low-dose dopamine in patients with early renal dysfunction: a placebo-controlled randomized trial. Australian and New Zealand Intensive Care Society (ANZICS) Clinical Trials Group. *Lancet* 2000; **356**: 2139–43.

24. Kellum JA, Decker J. Use of dopamine in acute renal failure: a meta-analysis. *Crit Care Med* 2001; **29**: 1526–31.

25. Galley HF. Renal-dose dopamine: will the message now get through? *Lancet* 2000; **356**: 2112–13.

26. Redl-Wenzl EM, Armbruster C, Edelmann G, *et al.* The effects of norepinephrine on hemodynamics and renal function in severe septic shock states. *Intensive Care Med* 1993; **19**: 151–4.

27. Marin C, Eon B, Saux P, *et al.* Renal effects of norepinephrine used to treat septic shock patients. *Crit Care Med* 1990; **18**: 282–5.

28. Duke GJ, Briedis JH, Weaver RA. Renal support in critically ill patients: Low-dose dopamine or low dose dobutamine? *Crit Care Med* 1994; **22**: 1919–25.

29. Abizaid AS, Clark CE, Mintz GS, *et al.* Effects of dopamine and aminophylline on contrast induced renal failure after coronary angiography in patients with pre-existing renal insufficiency. *Am J Cardiol* 1999; **83**: 260–3.

30. Gilbert TB, Hasnain JU, Flinn WR, *et al.* Fenoldopam infusion associated with preserving renal function after aortic cross clamping for aneurysm repair. *J Cardiovasc Pharmacol Ther* 2001; **6**: 31–6.

31. Halpenny M, Lakshmi S, O'Donnell A, *et al.* Fenoldopam: renal and splanchnic effects in patients undergoing coronary artery bypass grafting. *Anaesthesia* 2001; **56**: 953–60.

32. Tumulin J, Wang A, Murray P, Mathur V. Fenoldopam mesylate blocks reduction in renal plasma flow after radiocontrast dye infusion: a pilot trial in the prevention of contrast nephropathy. *Am Heart J* 2002; **143**: 894–903.

33. Richards WO, Scovill W, Shin B, Reed W. Acute renal failure associated with increased intra-abdominal pressure. *Ann Surg* 1983; **197**: 183–7.

34. Sugrue M. Intra-abdominal pressure: time for clinical practice guidelines? *Intensive Care Med* 2002; **28**: 389–91.

35. Harman PK, Kron IL, McLachlan HD. Elevated intra-abdominal pressure and renal function. *Ann Surg* 1982; **196**: 594–7.

36. Burch JM, Moore EE, Moore FA, Franciose R. The abdominal compartment syndrome. *Surg Clin North Am* 1996; **76**: 833–42.

37. Sugre M, Jones F, Deane SA, *et al.* Intra-abdominal hypertension is an independent cause of postoperative renal impairment. *Arch Surg* 1999; **134**: 1082–5.

38. Ronco C, Bellomo R, Homel P, *et al.* Effects of different doses on continuous veno-venous haemofiltration on outcomes of acute renal failure: a prospective randomised trial. *Lancet* 2000; **356**: 26–30.

39. Gastaldello K, Melot C, Kahn RJ. Comparison of cellulose diacetate and polysulfone membranes in the outcome of acute renal failure. A prospective randomised study. *Nephrol Dial Transplant* 2000; **15**: 224–30.

40. Subramanian S, Venkataraman, Kellum JA. Influence of dialysis membranes on outcomes in acute renal failure: a meta-analysis. *Kidney Int* 2002; **62**: 1819–23.

41. Pravinkumar E, Webster NR. HIT/HITT and alternative anticoagulation: current concepts. *Br J Anaesth* 2003; **90**: 676–85.

42. Knight D, Selwyn D, Harvey R, Girling K. Dalteparin anticoagulation for continuous veno-venous haemofiltration in a teaching hospital intensive care unit – one year's experience. *Br J Anaesth* 2003; **90**: 558.

43. Bouman CSC, Oudemans-van Straaten HM, Tijssen JGP, *et al.* Effects of early high-volume continuous venovenous hemofiltration on survival and recovery of renal function in intensive care patients with acute renal failure: A prospective, randomised trial. *Crit Care Med* 2002; **30**: 2205–11.

44. Misset B, Timsit JF, Chevret S, *et al.* A randomised cross-over comparison of the hemodynamic response to intermittent hemodialysis and continuous hemofiltration in ICU patients with acute renal failure. *Intensive Care Med* 1996; **22**: 742–6.

8 Nutritional and metabolic care

SIMON ALLISON & DILEEP LOBO

Viva topics

- Describe the typical metabolic response to injury.
- How would you assess the nutritional status of a patient prior to surgery?
- How would you support the case for early, as opposed to late, feeding in the postoperative period?
- What are the normal daily nutritional requirements for a critically ill patient?
- What do you understand by the term 'immune enhancing diet'? What is the role of this material in nutrition in the critically ill?

INTRODUCTION

The heterogeneity of the patient population passing through intensive care units makes it impossible to give a universal prescription for nutritional and metabolic care that covers all situations, from the transient problem of status asthmaticus to the more prolonged and varied problems encountered by patients with major trauma and sepsis. Nutritional and metabolic care must also be considered in relation to other aspects of management, as there are close interactions between these, e.g. between metabolism and respiration, between fluid and electrolyte balance and gastrointestinal function, and between protein metabolism and immobility. We should therefore speak of *integrated care*, in which each aspect is balanced in relation to the whole.

PATIENT GROUPS

It is useful to classify patient groups according to their needs.

- **Group 1. Well-nourished patients** who spend less than 5 days in the intensive care unit and whose clinical course is uncomplicated. There is no clear evidence that such patients benefit, in terms of survival or outcome, from artificial nutritional support. In cases where outcome is uncertain, nutritional support should be started within 24–48 hours after admission and discontinued as soon as oral intake is established.

- **Group 2. Patients with malnutrition prior to admission, without severe catabolism** Up to 40 per cent of patients admitted to hospital have significant undernutrition, as defined by anthropometric measurements (see Screening and Assessment) and continue to lose weight during their stay unless attention is paid to their nutritional care.[1,2] This group should receive nutritional support as early as possible.

- **Group 3. Patients who have undergone elective or emergency surgery and who are unable to eat normally for more than 7 days postoperatively due to complications** These patients should receive enteral and/or parenteral nutrition without further delay.[3]

- **Group 4. Elective surgical patients** These should undergo nutritional screening prior to admission,[2] and, if significantly undernourished (see below), should receive nutritional supplementation for 7–10 days preoperatively.[3,4] The traditional preoperative 12-hour fast is deleterious both metabolically and clinically. Bringing patients to surgery in a metabolically fed state, with a glucose drink or infusion within 4 hours preoperatively, reduces postoperative insulin resistance and the catabolic response to injury, and accelerates recovery.[5–7] Oral intake should be resumed as soon as possible after surgery. After colorectal surgery, for example, oral intake can be resumed in most patients within 24 hours. In patients with prior malnutrition and impaired gastrointestinal (GI) function, artificial feeding, preferably by the enteral route, should be resumed as soon as possible postoperatively.[8] This is an integral part of the ERAS (enhanced recovery after surgery) programme being developed by Scandinavian surgeons.[7]

- **Group 5. Patients with or without prior malnutrition suffering from acute catabolic illness, e.g. trauma, burns, sepsis, pancreatitis** Such patients often spend prolonged periods in the ICU and run a complicated subsequent course.[9] They suffer from the combined effects of starvation,[2] immobility[10] and increased metabolic rate, with consequent catabolic loss of lean mass (see below).

These patients may pass through a complex series of stages in their illness:

– Shock phase of cardiorespiratory resuscitation
– SIRS (systemic inflammatory response syndrome), during which the initial inflammatory and immune surge takes place; in its extreme form this may overwhelm the patient, causing death; alternatively, it may respond to treatment and lead to rapid recovery. An intermediate phase may occur where there is a compensatory anti-inflammatory response syndrome (CARS), during which the patient's immune responses are suppressed although catabolism continues. At this stage patients are vulnerable to nosocomial and secondary infections as well as multiple organ failure, which may result in death. Although these phases are useful conceptually, they represent an overlapping and continuous disease process with considerable variation. On theoretical grounds, therefore, substrates such as ω3 fatty acids, which reduce inflammation, glutamine, which is an enhancer of immunity and is an antioxidant precursor, and arginine, which is a precursor of nitric oxide as well as enhancing immunity, may each have beneficial, harmful or neutral effects according to their dosage and the phase of illness in which they are administered. Different outcomes might also be expected according to genotype, which determines the degree of the inflammatory response.[11]

DISEASE-RELATED MALNUTRITION

Prevalence

Not only is there a 15–40 per cent prevalence of malnutrition among patients admitted to hospital, but they continue to lose an average of 7 per cent of residual weight during their stay[1,2] unless nutritional care is adequate.

Causes[2]

These are threefold:

- Anorexia and decreased food intake, due either to the disease or its treatment.
- The response to injury,[12] which increases metabolic rate and causes preferential wasting of lean mass. Even obese individuals may lose considerable lean mass before much loss of fat is apparent. In most ICU patients metabolic rate rises by 10–30 per cent, being offset by a reduction of similar order due to immobility. A rise in body temperature of 1°C increases metabolic rate by 13 per cent. Severe

sepsis, pancreatitis or burns may increase metabolic rate by more than 30 per cent.
- Immobility. Muscles not subject to mechanical forces waste away, so that being paralysed on a ventilator leads to loss of lean mass, although passive stretching may ameliorate this.[10] Studies of healthy individuals immobilized in bed have shown large negative nitrogen balances despite feeding.[13] Conversely, early mobilization prevents muscle wasting and enhances anabolism.

Consequences[2,14–20]

Some loss of fat is of little significance, but loss of body cell mass upon which function is dependent is a striking feature of illness, during which the normal protein-conserving mechanisms of starvation fail to operate. With 5 per cent involuntary weight loss over a short time measurable impairments of function occur, and become clinically marked at 15 per cent weight loss, corresponding to 20 per cent loss of body protein. Mental changes include depression, apathy and loss of vigour. Muscle weakness (particularly of the respiratory muscles) develops, thermoregulation is impaired, and immune responses are blunted. With further weight loss, digestive and cardiovascular functions begin to deteriorate. Severe malnutrition and weight loss also cause a reduction in resting metabolic rate and body temperature, with failure to develop fever in response to infection. The catabolic response to injury is also blunted by a reduction in substrate reserves. With adequate nutritional support, these functions begin to improve even before there is a significant gain in cell mass. With malnutrition, mortality from illness is increased, complications, particularly infections, are more numerous, recovery and rehabilitation are prolonged, and length of stay and costs are increased. Appropriate nutritional support may improve all these outcomes.

RESPONSE TO INJURY[14,20–22]

This can be divided into three phases:

- A brief shock or ebb phase, when metabolic activity is reduced.
- The flow or catabolic phase, during which metabolic rate rises and substrates are diverted from normal activity to meet the needs of the inflammatory and immune response. Glycogen is mobilized to release glucose and muscle protein is broken down to meet the needs for healing, and for hepatic gluconeogenesis. At the same time, intracellular potassium linked to protein and glycogen is released and excreted. During this phase salt and water are retained,

causing expansion of the extracellular fluid volume –
Moore's 'sodium retention phase' of injury, during which
patients are easily overloaded with crystalloids.[22]

- The convalescent or anabolic phase, during which lost
tissue is restored as protein and glycogen are resynthesized,
with cellular uptake of potassium and phosphate. At this
time the capacity to excrete a salt and water load returns –
the 'sodium diuresis phase' of injury.

MEDIATION OF THE RESPONSE

Neuroendocrine[14,21–24]

Afferent neural signals reach the hypothalamus via peripheral nerves and the spinal cord, stimulating catecholamine
and ACTH secretion and a rise in levels of cortisol and
glucagon. In the shock phase there is α-adrenergic suppression of insulin secretion, followed in the flow phase by a prolonged period of insulin resistance. These changes return to
normal during convalescence. The response to lower-body
injury may be modified by blocking neural afferent signals
with epidural analgesia.[24]

Cytokines[11]

The cytokines interleukin (IL)-6, IL-1 and tumour necrosis
factor (TNF) are released by cells at the site of injury in an
inflammatory cascade. They act locally to produce inflammation, at the hypothalamus to induce fever and enhance the
neuroendocrine response, and directly on tissues to enhance
catabolism. This sequence is then followed by the production
of counterregulatory cytokines to limit the extent of inflammation. These cytokine balances are genetically determined,
so that the severity of the inflammatory response – and hence
survival – depends partly on inherited factors.

EFFECTS OF THE RESPONSE[14,20–23,25,26]

Carbohydrate, protein and fat

To have evolved at all, the metabolic response must have
had beneficial effects on survival, focusing metabolism on the
processes needed for healing. Not only are amino acids
needed for the immune response and for repairing damaged
tissues, but wounds have an obligatory requirement for glucose, which is respired anaerobically. In patients who had acci-
dentally burned one limb, Wilmore[25] found that the injured
limb had four times the glucose uptake and lactate output

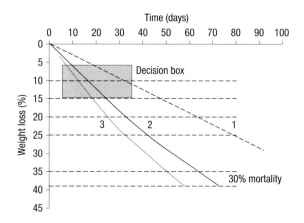

Figure 8.1 Percentage weight loss against time with 1) semistarvation
at 20 per cent energy; 2) total starvation hunger strikers; and
3) during starvation after injury or during illness (from Ref. 17, with
permission)

of other limbs, the latter being recycled through hepatic
gluconeogenesis, an energy-consuming process. Accelerated
gluconeogenesis also provides substrates for other glucose-
dependent tissues, such as the brain, once glycogen reserves
have been exhausted in the first 24 hours. Apart from its gly-
cerol component, fat cannot be converted to glucose; the only
other sources of gluconeogenic precursors are amino acids
from muscle protein and lactate from glycolysis. The consequence is that the injury response accelerates loss of body cell
mass, prolonging recovery time and threatening survival. The
relative rates of weight loss between normal subjects on
hunger strike, semistarved volunteers and starved patients
with acute illness or injury are shown in Figure 8.1,[17] and
indicate that the time taken to reach fatal weight loss is short-
est in injured patients. The 'decision box' indicates the degree
of weight loss at which significant impairment of function
begins and when the decision to give nutritional support
needs to be taken.

The response also causes intolerance to infused glucose, and
hyperglycaemia which predisposes to infection.[27] Shortage of
conditionally essential amino acids such as glutamine and
arginine may also occur, and oedema from salt and water
retention is easily induced. Lipolysis is increased, releasing
fatty acids, to meet 80–90 per cent of energy needs. In the anabolic or convalescent phase these changes are reversed, and
both hypokalaemia and hypophosphataemia may be induced
by refeeding as the cells resynthesize protein and glycogen.

Minerals, micronutrients and antioxidants[28]

Critical illness is associated with increased production of free
radicals, which are atoms or molecules with one or more

unpaired electrons, classified as reactive oxygen species (ROS), e.g. O_2^-, H_2O_2 or OH, and nitric oxide species (NOS), e.g. NO. ROS are produced by white blood cells, and are responsible for bacterial defence. NOS are produced in epithelial cells and govern vascular tone and permeability. These compounds are therefore essential to survival, but in excess can cause tissue damage and threaten survival. Antioxidants such as glutathione (formed from glutamine), vitamins C and E, and minerals selenium and zinc, normally balance ROS production but, if lacking during illness, allow a low antioxidant status to develop unopposed. A number of studies[27] have shown beneficial effects on outcome in critical illness from supplementation with selenium, vitamins C and E, copper and zinc. There may also be increased requirements for folate and vitamin B. The differences between the requirements of this class of nutrients in health and disease continue to be studied. All patients should receive at least the recommended daily intakes, supplemented in severe illness according to published evidence.

The gut[29,30]

Critical illness and its treatment are associated with changes in bowel microorganisms, in mucosal permeability to toxins and bacteria, and in the function of gut-associated lymphatic tissue (GALT). These changes may contribute to the development of septic complications, and much attention is being paid to the possible role of pre- and probiotics, enteral versus parenteral feeding, and special substrates to restore normal gut function and improve outcome.

MEASUREMENT OF NUTRITIONAL STATUS[2,31]

The probability of clinically significant malnutrition being present or the risk of its development can be detected by rapid screening on admission, or preferably in the preadmission assessment clinic. Those screened at risk may then be referred for more detailed assessment as necessary. Emergency admissions should be assessed as soon as possible after admission. Continuing monitoring of nutritional status is also important. Assessment should in all cases lead to appropriate action and protocols of care.

Screening

An example of a rapid screening tool used by the authors is shown in Figure 8.2. This depends on measuring current body mass index (BMI, wt kg/ht^2 m), percentage weight loss over 3 months, change in appetite and food intake, and severity of illness. If it is not possible to measure height and weight (e.g. in emergencies), the mid-arm circumference (measured halfway between the olecranon and the acromium) is a useful surrogate measure of body composition which can be related to percentile reference values for age and sex.

Assessment

This involves a more detailed clinical history and examination with some assessment of functional changes and laboratory values in patients screened at risk.

Laboratory values

SERUM PROTEINS[32]

The serum albumin is often mistakenly quoted as a nutritional marker. In health, albumin leaks out of the circulation into the interstitial space at a rate of 5 per cent per hour, and is restored to the circulation via the lymphatic system. Following major surgery the albumin escape rate increases three- to fivefold, returning to normal in 10 days. Similar changes may occur in major illness. As the albumin escape rate is ten times its synthesis rate, the serum albumin concentration will be more affected by redistribution than by nutritional status, and can be regarded as the reciprocal of the acute-phase reactants. It is therefore a measure of disease severity and hence of risk rather than nutrition. The infusion of 2 L of 0.9 per cent saline over 1 hour in normal subjects reduces the serum albumin by 20 per cent.[33] Clearing of oedema in the post-ICU phase is also associated with a rise in serum albumin of 1 g/L for every kilogram loss of excess fluid.[34] Dilution is also therefore a major factor in hypoalbuminaemia. Correction of plasma volume deficits in the post-acute phase is the main indication for using concentrated salt-poor albumin infusions, but these should not be used just to correct hypoalbuminaemia per se. Continuing losses of plasma from inflamed bowel or wounds also contributes and may lead to plasma volume deficit as well as hypoalbuminaemia.

During convalescence, the recovery of serum albumin to normal may be enhanced by feeding in malnourished patients. Measured serially over several weeks it may be a useful measure of recovery as well as response to feeding. The shorter half-life proteins, such as thyroid-binding prealbumin, behave in a similar way and the same considerations apply.[35]

SERUM CREATININE

This not only measures renal function but also reflects lean mass, and in wasted individuals is low.

Is YOUR patient at nutritional risk?		

Q1 a Height

☐ . ☐☐ metres

Q1 b ☐ Estimated or
☐ Measured

Q2 a Weight

☐☐ . ☐ kg

Q2 b ☐ Estimated or
☐ Measured

Q3 Body Mass Index (BMI) = kg/m^2 (refer to ready-reckoner)

☐☐

		Score
Greater than 20	☐	0
18 to 20	☐	2
Less than 18	☐	3

Q4 Food intake – has this decreased over the last month prior to admission or since the last review (or is the patient NBM)?

		Score
No	☐	0
Yes	☐	1
Not known	☐	2

Q5 Has the patient **unintentionally lost weight** over the last 3 months or since the last review?

			Score
	No	☐	0
Up to ½ stone (3 kg)	**A little**	☐	1
More than ½ stone (3 kg)	**A lot**	☐	2

Q6 Stress factor/severity of illness

				Score
None		**None**	☐	0
Moderate	Minor or uncomplicated surgery, minor infection, chronic disease, pressure sores, CVA, inflammatory bowel disease, other gastrointestinal disease, cirrhosis, renal failure, COPD, diabetes	**Moderate**	☐	1
Severe	Multiple injuries, multiple fractures, burns, head injury, multiple deep pressure sores, severe sepsis, malignant disease, severe dysphagia, pancreatitis, post-op complications	**Severe**	☐	2

TOTAL SCORE ☐

Review patient in 3 days

Action

If score	0–2	Repeat screening within 7 days	☐
If score	3–4	Keep food record charts and start supplements if food intake poor	☐
If score	≥5	Refer for expert advice	☐

Figure 8.2 Example of a screening tool used at Queen's Medical Centre, Nottingham, UK

SERUM UREA

Serum urea reflects renal function, and also protein turnover and net catabolism. Urea production rate is increased in catabolic patients and decreased in cachexia.

MINERALS AND ELECTROLYTES

These are of particular value in patients who have or are likely to have excess losses or changes in physiology, e.g. K^+ and PO_4^{2-} concentrations.

MONITORING

All measurements should be recorded on serial data charts, so that serial changes as well as the interrelationship between the various parameters can easily be observed and interpreted.

TREATMENT

Goals

Wolfe and colleagues[36] have described the goal of nutritional management of the critically ill as follows: 'The goal of nutritional management of critically ill patients is to promote wound healing and resistance to infection while preventing loss of muscle protein, since survival of critically-ill patients is inversely correlated with loss of lean mass'.

Soon after his description of the metabolic response to injury, however, Cuthbertson[20] observed that injury catabolism could not be reversed by feeding alone, and that the best that could be achieved was to treat the starvation element and to reduce but not abolish the rate of tissue loss. Campbell[37] has summarized the problem: 'In the severely septic and injured patient, an improvement of nutritional status or increase of lean body mass by nutritional support alone is likely to be impossible. The most one can hope for is to slow the rate of decline. If lean body mass is to be maintained, it is likely that pharmacological methods will have to be found for doing so.'

Early efforts through hyperalimentation with high glucose loads to bludgeon the catabolic patient into positive nitrogen balance not only failed, but also caused toxicity through excess nutrients. On the other hand, despite some tissue loss, nutritional support can help to preserve function, including muscle strength, weaning from ventilators and immunity.[38] It can also correct and prevent imbalances of minerals and micronutrients.[28] The use of special substrates, antioxidants, drugs and hormones may help to lessen the severity of the illness.[9] Goals of treatment have therefore changed over the years, with steps to reduce the severity of the catabolic stimulus (Table 8.1) combined with a more conservative nutritional regimen (see below), increasing intake as the patient becomes mobile during convalescence and can utilize a higher food intake to restore lost tissue.

Some of our daily energy expenditure goes to maintain core temperature within a narrow range around 37°C. In an environmental temperature between 29° and 30°C normal subjects are in their thermoneutral zone, at which metabolic expenditure to maintain body temperature is minimal.[39] During illness the zone may rise to 32°C or above.[22] Nursing patients in a warm environment can therefore reduce metabolic demands. Similarly, pain, anorexia and fever all increase

Table 8.1 *Steps to reduce catabolic stimulus*

Better control of infection

Improved fluid management

Nursing in a thermoneutral environment

Better control of pain – epidural analgesia

Improved surgical and anaesthetic techniques, e.g. early debridement and grafting of burns

Adequate oxygenation

metabolic rate and protein catabolism. Optimal management of these also reduces metabolic requirements, emphasizing the importance of integrating nutrition and metabolic care within the overall framework of management.

THE CLINICAL DECISION TO TREAT

This is based on assessment of the initial nutritional state of the patient and on the likely natural history of their condition. The risks of enteral or parenteral nutrition, as described in the literature, need to be weighed against the published benefits of particular feeding regimens.

TIMING OF TREATMENT[9]

Evidence is accumulating that the earlier optimal treatment, including nutritional, is achieved, the better the outcome in relation to subsequent complications such as multiple organ failure (MOF) and to survival and rate of recovery. Early adequate and appropriate feeding may well show benefits which are only apparent after discharge from the ICU. It is therefore important to assess the outcome of interventions over a period of several months.

NUTRITIONAL REQUIREMENTS

Energy[40]

A full range of oral, enteral and parenteral feeds are now available which allow the use of a balanced proportion of protein 15 per cent, fat 30–40 per cent and carbohydrate 55–60 per cent of energy intake. Excessive administration of energy is prevented by oral or enteral tolerance, but is only too easy to achieve by the parenteral route. Confusion is sometimes caused by authors failing to make clear whether they are discussing total or non-protein energy. Energy intake should be calculated to include protein according to nutritional science. It may, however, be useful to consider non-protein

Table 8.2 *Calculation of energy expenditure using Schofield equations*[42]

Age (yrs)	RMR (male)	RMR (female)
15–18	$17.6 \times Wt + 656$	$13.3 \times Wt + 690$
18–30	$15.0 \times Wt + 690$	$14.8 \times Wt + 485$
30–60	$11.4 \times Wt + 870$	$8.1 \times Wt + 842$
>60	$11.7 \times Wt + 585$	$9.0 \times Wt + 656$

Weight (Wt) in kg; resting metabolic rate (RMR) in kcal/24 h

calorie-to-nitrogen (g) ratios, which should be in the range 125–150 in critically ill patients, although optimum utilization of nitrogen in health may be achieved with a ratio as high as 300:1. The general consensus is to start feeding with a total energy intake of $1.0 \times$ resting metabolic rate (RMR) according to Harris-Benedict[41] or Schofield[42] (Table 8.2), increasing to 1.2–$1.3 \times$ resting expenditure over the first week. This usually means 20–25 kcal/kg body weight to start with, increasing to 30–35 kcal/kg over a few days (see Table 8.2).

Although good clinical practice can be achieved by prescribing energy intakes based on estimated resting metabolic expenditure from Harris-Benedict or Schofield, it should be remembered that estimated and measured resting metabolic rate in critically ill patients may differ from each other by as much as 30–50 per cent and vary from day to day.[37,43] The ideal, therefore, is to measure metabolic rate daily by indirect calorimetry and adjust intake accordingly, but this is technically demanding, and available in only a few centres. It is unlikely to become a routine assessment in clinical practice.

Carbohydrate[23,44–47]

Infusion of glucose at a rate in excess of 6 mg/kg/min or 7.8 g/kg/day increases oxygen consumption and CO_2 production, with corresponding strains upon ventilation. Fatty liver, abnormal liver function and increased adipose tissue may also occur without any corresponding improvement in nitrogen balance. It is usual, therefore, to limit glucose infusion rates to 5 mg/kg/day or less.

Fat [47–49]

Lipid emulsions should not be infused intravenously at a rate which gives more than 1.5 g/kg/day, in order to avoid hyperlipidaemia and other side effects. Long-chain triglycerides (LCT) in excess have been implicated in immune impairment, and also in pulmonary and hepatic complications in children. Too-rapid administration also causes hyperlipidaemia by exceeding lipolytic capacity. There may be some advantage in giving a mixture of LCT and MCT (medium-chain triglycerides), as medium-chain fatty acids can bypass the mitochondrial carnitine shuttle and be more rapidly metabolized. Mixtures of LCT, MCT and $\omega 3$ fatty acids have also been developed.

Protein[40,50]

Intake is usually expressed as grams of nitrogen (N), 1.0 g of N being equivalent to 6.25 g protein. In oral or enteral feeds nitrogen is usually given as whole protein, although peptides may be useful in some cases of malabsorption. In parenteral feeds, however, nitrogen is always given as amino acids, in optimal combination as judged against egg protein. Certain amino acids are excluded, however, because of instability, e.g. glutamine, or insolubility, e.g. cysteine, and can only be satisfactorily stored in solution as dipeptides, although glutamine can be given as a last-minute addition to the feed.

Nitrogen balance is dependent not only on adequate N intake but also on meeting energy needs to allow the nitrogen to be used for protein synthesis. Studies in ICU patients have shown that if energy needs are met, nitrogen balance improves up to a dose of 0.25 g/kg/day. Above this it is simply converted to urea and excreted. Normally, 80 per cent of waste nitrogen is excreted as urea, although with starvation, and the response to injury or acidosis, this fraction falls, owing to the formation of ammonia and other waste products. Although some ICUs measure nitrogen balance by the Kjeldahl method once or twice weekly, the authors regard this as a research tool and not particularly useful clinically. It has already been pointed out that a positive nitrogen balance is not achievable in any meaningful sense during catabolic illness, although during convalescence the body with depleted lean mass responds like the growing child and will tolerate and utilize high rates of energy and protein intake. The consensus therefore is that N intake in the critically ill should be 0.2–0.25 g/kg/day or 1.25–1.5 g protein per kg per day. Starting doses for both enteral and parenteral feeding may be lower, increasing gradually as tolerated to achieve the target. These figures may be compared to the consensus requirement for N in health, which is 0.8 g/kg/day, although elderly persons have been shown to stay in better health with 1.0 g/day.

ROUTES OF FEEDING

Oral

Although most patients in ICU, being on ventilators, are unable to take food by mouth, those in high-dependency and other step-down facilities should be given appetizing energy- and protein-dense food by mouth as soon as possible. More rapid recovery from surgery can be achieved by early oral intake,[7] accompanied if necessary by proprietary oral supplements to achieve the desired target intake.[51] Oral intake has the advantage over enteral tube feeding that it includes the cephalic phase of digestion, with the secretion of saliva, which contains potent antibacterial substances.

Enteral[52]

Small bowel function usually recovers before gastric emptying. Nasogastric feeding should therefore be initiated using a Ryle's tube to allow 4-hourly aspiration. Start at 20 mL/h, which can be increased if the aspirated gastric residual does not exceed 300 mL, and the wider tube replaced by a fine-bore feeding tube. Alternatively, with persistent delay in gastric emptying a nasojejunal tube may be passed or the problem anticipated by insertion of a jejunostomy tube at the time of operation. The risk of aspiration and chest infection can be minimized by ensuring that large gastric residues do not accumulate and by nursing the patient in the semirecumbent position. Aspiration risks are not reduced by jejunal compared to nasogastric feeding. Although, rightly, the enteral route is regarded as optimal, in practice only 20–50 per cent of target intakes may be achieved, resulting in considerable underfeeding.[9]

Complications of enteral feeding

- Wide-bore tubes cause reflux oesophagitis.
- Reflux and aspiration pneumonia. Prevented by slowing rate of feed, avoiding large gastric residues and nursing patient at a 30–40° angle.
- Bloating and discomfort, with abdominal distension pressing on diaphragm and impairing ventilation. Prevented by slowing feed rate and/or metoclopramide.
- Diarrhoea. Largely due to associated antibiotics. Prevented by stopping antibiotics (check for *Clostridium difficile*), slowing feed rate, in some cases adding fibre-containing feed, use of codeine/loperamide syrup.
- Rarely bowel necrosis, especially in infants, when poorly perfused bowel is infused with excessive feed rates.

Parenteral[8,9,52,53]

This technique, using peripheral or central veins, is sometimes discussed erroneously as though it were competitive to enteral feeding. It is in fact the treatment of partial or complete gastrointestinal failure, as dialysis is of renal failure or ventilation of respiratory failure, and is an effective way of delivering adequate amounts of nutrients. The downside of this is that it is easy to give excess substrate or fluids, or to cause septicaemia and venous thrombosis. Enteral feeding should always be used where possible for its effects on gut function and immunity, but it may need to be supplemented or replaced by parenteral feeding in the many patients where insufficient feed can be delivered enterally. The two technologies are therefore complementary, not competitive. Indeed, studies in which parenteral and enteral feeding were combined have shown superior or similar results to enteral feeding alone. The careful protocols needed for the safe insertion and care of central lines have been fully described elsewhere. A polyurethane or Silastic catheter is inserted via the subclavian or internal jugular vein and its tip (checked by chest X-ray) placed at the junction of the superior vena cava and right atrium. Connecting and disconnecting feed lines – or indeed any contact with the catheter or its hub – should be a surgically sterile procedure. Catheter infection rates can be reduced from 30 per cent or more to less than 1 per cent when such protocols are employed by properly trained staff. Reductions in metabolic and mechanical complications can be similarly reduced in expert hands. Standards of care should be closely monitored and audited.

SPECIAL SUBSTRATES[9]

These have been given as isolated preparations or as cocktails in the form of so-called immune-enhancing diets (IED).

Immune-enhancing diets

These enteral feeds consist of various mixtures of arginine, ω3 fatty acids, glutamine and nucleotides, given with the aim of reducing excessive inflammation, enhancing antioxidant status and reducing infection by preventing immunosuppression. The most impressive results have been seen when IEDs are given preoperatively as well as postoperatively to patients undergoing major upper gastrointestinal surgery. Benefits have included reduced infections, reduced mortality and shorter hospital stay. The results of their use in other ICU patients are conflicting, with some studies showing increased mortality in the treated groups. One study of major abdominal injuries showed a striking benefit in terms of nutritional complications.[54] The balance of evidence does not currently favour the routine use of IED in the ICU population, although there is good evidence to support their use in major elective surgery and in some cases of trauma.

Glutamine and ornithine α-ketoglutarate [9,55–57]

Used as single substrates, each of these has been shown to be beneficial in critically ill patients to improve healing and to reduce secondary infections, multiple organ failure and overall mortality. The two compounds are closely related metabolically, α-ketoglutarate being converted to glutamine via transamination. Both therefore address the problem of decreased glutamine availability and its conditionally essential nature in severe illness, as a substrate for immune cells and the gut mucosa, and as glutathione precursors to improve antioxidant status. Their use has improved outcome in patients suffering burns, major injuries and marrow transplants. Glutamine is more effectively administered intravenously, as much enterally administered glutamine is taken up and metabolized in the upper gastrointestinal tract and does not reach the circulation. A study in which glutamine was given in high doses (30 g) enterally did, however, show striking benefits in terms of outcome.[57]

Fibre[30]

The addition of soluble fibre to enteral feeds in septic patients has been shown to reduce the incidence of diarrhoea. It also acts as a prebiotic substrate for the large bowel flora, helping to maintain a more normal and less pathogenic bacterial population and protecting mucosal and immune function.

Future developments

Individual substrates rather than cocktail mixtures need more detailed evaluation in terms of timing, dosage, and their benefits in different diagnostic groups.

HORMONES AND DRUGS[9,23,58–60]

Insulin

In the 1960s and 1970s we advocated the use of insulin not just for its effects in controlling hyperglycaemia in catabolic patients, but for its protein-sparing effects (Figure 8.3) and effects on cell membrane function. These benefits were confirmed by others, but not until recently has insulin been shown to have striking beneficial effects on clinical outcome. Van den Berghe and colleagues[58] showed that giving intensive insulin therapy to maintain normoglycaemia reduced infections, polyneuropathy, mortality, time on ventilators and length of hospital stay. These effects are mainly due to

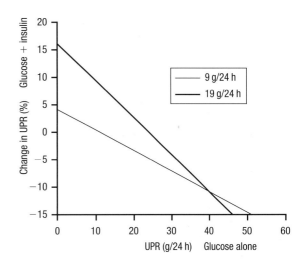

Figure 8.3 Comparison between infusion of glucose alone and glucose + insulin on urea production rate at two levels of nitrogen administration. UPR: urea production rate (mmol/24 h), N: nitrogen. Adapted from Woolfson[61]

the maintenance of normoglycaemia and normal triglyceride concentrations, but the other effects of insulin may also contribute. Other studies of insulin treatment have shown improved healing and better outcome in burned patients. A useful algorithm to guide insulin dosage according to blood glucose monitoring was devised by Woolfson.[61]

Growth hormone

This has been shown to have anabolic and protein-sparing effects, although when applied to a general ICU population, two trials showed that it increased mortality. It may still have a place, however, in burned patients, particularly in children, in whom it maintains growth, reduces negative nitrogen balance, and accelerates healing.

Anabolic steroids

Sex steroid levels are reduced in severe injury and malnutrition. The use of both testosterone and oxandralone has been shown to have protein anabolic effects in burned patients.

α and β blockers

These have been shown to reduce cardiovascular and metabolic load in burned patients and to significantly reduce loss of lean mass.

SUMMARY

- The ICU population is heterogeneous and there is no universal formula for nutrition and metabolic care.
- Nutritional and metabolic care must be integrated with other aspects of the patient's pathology and treatment, from which they are independent.
- Nutritional screening and assessment are essential to clinical decision-making concerning feeding, its appropriate timing, route and amount.
- Optimizing treatment of infections, wounds, fluid balance and pain, as well as nursing in a thermoneutral environment, reduces metabolic demands.
- Nutrition during the catabolic phase of illness should be adequate but not excessive. Too much carbohydrate, protein or fat has toxic and undesirable effects. Sufficient energy is supplied to most patients by giving 1.2–1.3 times estimated resting expenditure and 0.15–0.25 g N/kg body weight per day, although individual patients may need more or less.
- Nutrition and early muscle stimulation or mobilization aims to reduce the loss of lean mass during critical illness. During mobilization and convalescence, much larger amounts of feed may be consumed with benefit.
- Special substrates such as glutamine may confer specific benefits in the critically ill. The value of pre- and probiotics is beginning to be evaluated. Immune-enhancing diets are of established benefit pre- and postoperatively in major elective surgery, and in some cases of trauma. Their general use in the ICU population remains controversial.
- The use of hormones and drugs, particularly insulin, has benefits in terms of metabolism and clinical outcome.
- Early nutritional and metabolic interventions may have benefits which are not seen until later in the evolution of illness.

REFERENCES

1. McWhirter JP, Pennington CR. Incidence and recognition of malnutrition in hospital. *BMJ* 1994; **308**: 945–8.
2. Stratton RJ, Green CJ, Elia M. *Disease related malnutrition – an evidence-based approach to treatment.* Oxford: CAB International, 2003.
3. ASPEN. Standards for nutrition support: hospitalised patients. *Nutr Clin Pract* 1995; **10**: 208–18.
4. Satyanarayana R, Klein S. Clinical efficacy of perioperative nutrition support. *Curr Opin Clin Nutr Metab Care* 1998; **1**: 51–8.
5. Thorell A, Nygren J, Ljungqvist O. Insulin resistance, a marker of stress. *Curr Opin Clin Nutr Metab Care* 1999; **2**: 69–78.
6. Hessov I, Ljungqvist O. Perioperative oral nutrition. *Curr Opin Clin Nutr Metab Care* 1998; **1**: 29–33.
7. Nygren J. Accelerated recovery from surgery. *Clin Nutr* 2002; **21**: 171–3.
8. Allison SP. Perioperative nutrition in elective surgery. In: Pichard C, Kudsk KA. (eds) *From nutrition support to pharmacologic nutrition in the ICU. Update in intensive care and emergency medicine.* Berlin: Springer Verlag, 2000.
9. Griffiths RD. Nutrition support in critically ill septic patients. *Curr Opin Clin Nutr Metab Care* 2003; **6**: 1–8.
10. Griffiths RD. Effect of passive stretching on the wasting of muscle in the critically ill: background. *Nutrition* 1997; **13**: 70–4.
11. Grimble RF. Stress proteins in disease: metabolism on a knife edge. *Clin Nutr* 2001; **20**: 469–76.
12. Elia M. Organ and tissue contribution to metabolic rate. In: Kinney JM, Tucker HN. (eds) *Energy metabolism, tissue determinants and cellular corollaries.* New York: Raven Press, 1992.
13. Schønheyder F, Heilskov NSC, Olesen K. Isotopic studies on mechanism of negative nitrogen balance produced by immobilization. *Scand J Clin Lab Invest* 1954; **6**: 178–88.
14. Hill GL. *Disorders of nutrition and metabolism in clinical surgery.* Edinburgh: Churchill Livingstone, 1992.
15. Hill GL. Body composition research: Implications for the practice of clinical nutrition. *J Parenter Enteral Nutr* 1992; **16**: 197–218.
16. Jeejeebhoy KN. Bulk or bounce – the object of nutritional support. *J Parenter Enteral Nutr* 1988; **12**: 539–49.
17. Allison SP. The uses and limitations of nutritional support. *Clin Nutr* 1992; **11**: 319–30.
18. Keys A, Brozek J, Henschel A. *The biology of human starvation.* Minneapolis: University of Minnesota Press, 1988.
19. Tucker H. Cost containment through nutrition intervention. *Nutr Rev* 1996; **54**: 111–21.
20. Cuthbertson DP. Post-shock metabolic response. *Lancet* 1942; **1**: 433.
21. Moore FD. *Metabolic care of the surgical patient.* Philadelphia: Saunders, 1959.
22. Wilmore DW. *The metabolic management of the critically ill.* New York: Plenum, 1977.
23. Martinez-Riquelme AE, Allison SP. Insulin revisited. *Clin Nutr* 2003; **22**: 7–15.
24. Holte K, Kehlet H. Epidural anaesthesia and analgesia – effects on surgical stress responses and implications for postoperative nutrition. *Clin Nutr* 2002; **21**: 199–206.
25. Wilmore DW. The wound as an organ. In: Little RA, Frayn KN. (eds) *The scientific basis for the care of the critically ill.* Manchester: Manchester University Press, 1986.
26. Long JM, Wilmore DW, Mason AD, Pruitt BA Jr. Effect of carbohydrate and fat intake on nitrogen excretion during total intravenous feeding. *Ann Surg* 1977; **185**: 417.
27. Khaodhiar L, McCowen K, Bistrian B. Perioperative hyperglycaemia, infection or risk. *Curr Opin Clin Nutr Metab Care* 1999; **2**: 79–82.
28. Berger M, Chiolero RL. *Key vitamins and trace elements in the critically ill.* Nestlé Nutrition Workshop Series Clinical and Performance Programme 2003; **8**: 99–111; discussion 111–17.

29. Bengmark S. Gut microenvironment and immune function. *Curr Opin Clin Nutr Metab Care* 1999; **2**: 83–5.

30. Bengmark S. Progress in perioperative enteral tube feeding. *Clin Nutr* 1998; **17**: 1–8.

31. Gibson RS. *Principles of nutritional assessment*. New York: Oxford University Press, 1990.

32. Allison SP, Lobo DN, Stanga Z. The treatment of hypoalbuminaemia. *Clin Nutr* 2001; **3**: 275–9.

33. Lobo DN, Stanga Z, Simpson AD, *et al*. Dilution and redistribution effects of rapid 2-litre infusions of 0.9 per cent (w/v) saline and 5 per cent (w/v) dextrose on haematological parameters and serum biochemistry in normal subjects: a double-blind crossover study. *Clin Sci* 2001; **101**: 173–9.

34. Lobo DN, Bjarnason K, Field J, *et al*. Changes in weight, fluid balance and serum albumin in patients referred for nutritional support. *Clin Nutr* 1999; **18**: 197–201.

35. Bastow MD, Rawlings J, Allison SP. Benefits of supplementary tube feeding after fractured neck of femur: a randomised controlled trial. *BMJ* 1983; **287**: 1589–92.

36. Sakurai Y, Aarsland A, Herndon DN, *et al*. Stimulation of muscle protein synthesis by long-term insulin infusion in severely burned patients. *Ann Surg* 1995; **222**: 283–97.

37. Campbell IT. Limitations of nutrient intake. The effect of stressors: trauma, sepsis and multiple organ failure *Eur J Clin Nutr* 1999; **53**: 143.

38. Allison SP. Nutritional support. In: Healy TEJ, Knight PR. (eds) *A practice of anesthesia*, 7th edn. London: Hodder Arnold, 2003.

39. Brengelmann GL, Savage MV. Thermoregulation in the neutral zone. In: Kinney MJ, Tucker HN. (eds) *Physiology, stress and malnutrition: functional correlates, nutritional intervention*. Philadelphia: Lippincott-Raven, 1997.

40. Bursztein S, Elwyn DH, Askanazi J, Kinney JM. *Energy metabolism, indirect calorimetry and nutrition*. Baltimore: Williams Wilkins, 1993.

41. Harris JA, Benedict FG. *A biometric study of basal metabolism in man*. Washington: Carnegie Institute, 1919. Publication No. 279.

42. Schofield WN. Predicting basal metabolic rate, new standards and review of previous work. *Hum Nutr Clin Nutr* 1985; **39C**: 41.

43. Shaw-Delanty SN, Elwyn DH, Askanazi J, *et al*. Resting metabolic expenditure in injured septic and malnourished adult patients on intravenous diets. *Clin Nutr* 1990; **9**: 305–12.

44. Askanazi J, Rosenbaum SH, Hyman AI, *et al*. Respiratory changes induced by large glucose loads of total parenteral nutrition. *JAMA* 1980; **243**: 1444.

45. Covelli HD, Waylon-Black J, Olsen MS, Beekman JF. Respiratory failure precipitated by high carbohydrate loads. *Ann Int Med* 1981; **95**: 579.

46. Burke JF, Wolfe RR, Mullaney CJ, *et al*. Glucose requirements following burn injury. *Ann Surg* 1979; **190**: 274–85.

47. Tappy L, Chiolero R. Carbohydrate and fat as energetic fuels in intensive care unit patients. In: Pichard C, Kudsk KA. (eds) *From nutritional support to pharmacologic nutrition in the ICU. Update in intensive care and emergency medicine*. Berlin: Springer-Verlag, 2000.

48. Carpentier YA, Dupont IE. Fatty acids, lipoproteins and lipid emulsions. In: Pichard C, Kudsk KA. (eds) *From nutritional support to pharmacologic nutrition in the ICU. Update in Intensive care and emergency medicine*. Berlin: Springer-Verlag, 2000.

49. Calder PC, *Lipids and the critically ill patients*. Nestlé Nutrition Workshop Series Clinical and Performance Programme 2003; **8**: 75–91; discussion 91–8.

50. Furst P, Kuhn KS, Stehle P. New nitrogen containing substrates in artificial nutrition. In: Pichard C, Kudsk KA. (eds) *From nutritional support to pharmacologic nutrition in the ICU. Update in intensive care and emergency medicine*. Berlin: Springer-Verlag, 2000.

51. Rana SK, Bray J, Menzies Gow N, *et al*. Short term benefits of postoperative oral dietary supplements in surgical patients. *Clin Nutr* 1992; **11**: 337–44.

52. Silk DBA, Green CJ. Perioperative nutrition: parenteral versus enteral. *Curr Opin Clin Nutr Metab Care* 1998; **1**: 21–7.

53. Elia M. Artificial nutritional support in clinical practice. *J R Coll Physicians Lond* 1993; **27**: 8–15.

54. Kudsk KA, Minard G, Groce MA, *et al*. A randomized trial of isonitrogenous enteral diets after severe trauma. An immune-enhancing diet reduces septic complications. *Ann Surg* 1996; **224**: 531–43.

55. Donati L, Ziegler F, Pongelli G, Signorini MS. Nutritional and clinical efficacy of ornithine α-ketoglutarate in severe burns. *Clin Nutr* 1999; **18**: 307–11.

56. Moukarzel A, Goulet O, Cynober L, Ricour C. Positive effects of ornithine α-ketoglutarate in paediatric patients on parenteral nutrition and failure to thrive. *Clin Nutr* 1993; **12**: 59–60.

57. Ziegler TR. L-glutamine enriched parenteral nutrition in catabolic patients. *Clin Nutr* 1993; **12**: 65–6.

58. Van den Berghe G, Wouters P, Weekers F, *et al*. Intensive insulin therapy in critically ill patients. *N Engl J Med* 2001; **345**: 1359–67.

59. Proceedings ASPEN's 23rd Clinical Congress Research Workshop. Anabolic hormones in nutrition support. *J Parenter Enteral Nutr* 1999; **23**: No. 6, supplement.

60. Lee JO, Herndon DN. *Modulation of the post burn hypermetabolic state*. Nestlé Nutrition Workshop Series Clinical and Performance Programme 2003; **8**: 39–49; discussion 49–56.

61. Woolfson AMJ. An improved method for blood glucose control during nutritional support. *J Parenter Enteral Nutr* 1981; **5**: 436–40.

9 Infection in critical care

HILARY HUMPHREYS

Viva topics

- Common infections in the ICU and how they are acquired.
- Important ICU pathogens.
- Diagnostic approaches.
- Empirical antibiotic treatment.
- Principles of infection prevention.

INTRODUCTION

The prevalence of infection in the intensive care unit (ICU) is greater than in most other parts of the hospital. Bloodstream infection, sometimes resulting in septic shock, and ventilator-associated pneumonia are the most important, and the presence of antibiotic resistance limits the options for therapy. The diagnosis of infection is made more difficult by the severity of underlying disease and the presence of organ dysfunction in many ICU patients. Consequently, a multidisciplinary approach to diagnosis is essential. Methicillin-resistant *Staphylococcus aureus* (MRSA), vancomycin-resistant enterococci (VRE), *Clostridium difficile* diarrhoea and systemic fungal infections are increasing challenges in terms of prevention and treatment. Many patients require antibiotics, but restricting their use to those who are infected and curtailing the duration of therapy will greatly assist in preventing antibiotic resistance. In particular, it is often preferred to investigate and observe a patient with possible infection, if stable, until the results of investigations are available, as this may avoid the use of unnecessary antibiotics if infection is subsequently excluded. Controversy remains about the role of antibiotic prophylaxis in the form of routine selective decontamination of the digestive tract (SDD) because of concerns about promoting the emergence of antibiotic resistance. The cornerstone of infection prevention in the ICU is compliance with handwashing practice, early detection of infection, especially when caused by antibiotic-resistant bacteria, adequate space to care for patients, patient isolation where feasible, and adequate staff numbers to care for patients. Developments in the future may include the use of molecular techniques such

as the polymerase chain reaction (PCR) to provide a more rapid diagnosis, and developments in enhancing compliance with routine infection prevention strategies through human behaviour modification, but it seems likely that there will be no major breakthrough in the development of new antimicrobial agents.

BACKGROUND

Infection remains an important indication for admission to the ICU and a complication of intensive care for the severely ill patient. Although a proportion of patients who are ill with infection, such as severe community-acquired pneumonia or meningococcal septicaemia, may require admission to the ICU, many infections are diagnosed there following multiple trauma, major surgery, or severe debilitating disease such as neoplasia.

The pathophysiology of sepsis is now well described.[1] Diagnosing and controlling the source of infection is a major challenge and warrants a combined clinical, laboratory and radiological approach.[2] The critically ill patient requires repeated assessments and investigations, both to exclude infection and to identify the cause of infection as a prelude to effective management. In the UK, there is an increasing requirement of hospitals to undertake prospective surveillance and to collect data on important infections such as MRSA bacteraemia.[3] Many of these infections occur in the ICU and contribute significantly to overall hospital data.

Because the ICU has a higher proportion of patients with infection than other parts of the hospital, hospital-wide infection prevention strategies focus on the ICU, where measures such as handwashing, patient isolation, the use of protective clothing and the rational and sensible use of antibiotics are a priority.

EPIDEMIOLOGY AND RISK FACTORS

During the last decade it has been easier to study the epidemiology of infection in the ICU following the standardization of case definitions such as 'sepsis,' 'sepsis syndrome' and 'septic shock'. It is estimated that in the USA the incidence of sepsis has increased from 73.6 per 1 000 000 patients in 1979 to 175.9 per 100 000 in 1989,[4] and since then it is likely to have increased further. It is, none the less, difficult to generalize, as hospitals differ considerably and ICUs admit a mix of patients that may vary considerably, from patients admitted to a local hospital to those admitted to the ICU in a major tertiary referral centre. Even within the same ICU the patient population is quite heterogeneous. Therefore, the prevalence of specific infections, e.g. bloodstream infection, urinary infection, ventilator-associated pneumonia (VAP) etc., will vary depending on the type of ICU. For example, the prevalence of VAP is considerably higher in neurosurgical ICUs than in medical or coronary ICUs, but the incidence of bloodstream infection secondary to line-associated infection is higher in paediatric ICUs.[5]

There is considerable variation in patient mortality, depending on risk factors and the patient group. Patients with sepsis, however, have a high mortality, and this varies from 40 to 80 per cent.[4] Mortality can be correlated with various clinical assessments of the patient's state, e.g. APACHE score, and the presence of two or more dysfunctional organs. There has been considerable research in recent years in trying to identify risk factors for those patients particularly at risk of sepsis and of dying from sepsis, in order to target interventions that might improve outcome.[1,4] Polymorphism in the gene for tumour necrosis factor (TNF), cytokine levels at the time of presentation and the specific pathogen causing infection, are believed to be important.[4]

Respiratory tract infection, urinary tract infection, bloodstream infection and surgical site infection were found to be the commonest categories of infection documented in the most recent Europe-wide survey.[6] The most frequently reported pathogens were enterobacteriaceae (34 per cent), *Staphylococcus aureus* (30 per cent), *Pseudomonas aeruginosa* (29 per cent), coagulase-negative staphylococci (19 per cent) and fungi (17 per cent). Although criticisms can be made of this study because of the definitions used to diagnose infection, the relatively high proportion of infections caused by fungi is an increasing finding in patients in the ICU (see below). Bloodstream infection and VAP are the infections most likely to be associated with a poor outcome. In a study of over 1900 patients, the incidence of bloodstream infection was 2.67 per 100 admissions.[7] The most common causes were coagulase-negative staphylococci, and the attributable mortality was 35 per cent with an additional duration of ICU stay of 8 days.[7]

In most countries ICUs are faced with the increasingly rapid emergence and spread of antibiotic-resistant bacteria that have arisen as a result of the prolonged length of ICU stay,

the presence of invasive devices such as endotracheal tubes, and the need to use broad-spectrum antibiotics.[8] There is a financial and clinical cost associated with such antibiotic resistance, as the available agents are often more expensive than first-line drugs and may be less potent than those available to treat antibiotic-susceptible pathogens. International comparisons of resistance in ICUs show considerable variation in prevalence. In a study that examined consecutive clinical specimens, increased antibiotic resistance, across all species and agents, was highest in Portuguese ICUs, followed by French, Spanish, Belgian and Swedish.[9] The majority of strains of *Staphylococcus aureus* isolated in most European ICUs are methicillin resistant, but in general methicillin resistance is less likely to be found in ICUs in Germany, Switzerland and the Netherlands.[10] The use or overuse of antibiotics is a common theme in studies looking at risk factors for the presence of specific antibiotic-resistant bacteria. For example, in a model controlling for type of ICU when assessing rates of vancomycin-resistant enterococci (VRE), vancomycin use itself and the use of third-generation cephalosporins were independently associated with VRE prevalence.[11]

DIAGNOSIS OF INFECTION

Continuous patient assessment, together with the judicious use of laboratory, radiological and other investigations, is the key to diagnosing infection early and reducing mortality. A team approach involving intensivists, ICU nurses, microbiologists or infectious disease physicians, and radiologists should combine on a daily basis to maximize diagnostic acumen.[12] This is required not only to diagnose infection but to exclude non-infectious causes of fever, such as drug-induced fever, deep vein thrombosis, myocardial infarction etc.,[1] and therefore also help reduce the use of unnecessary antibiotics. In a retrospective study of over 500 patients, the introduction of an infectious disease consultation service was associated with a 49 per cent increased odds that a diagnosis of infection was microbiologically based, and there was also a 57 per cent reduction of antibiotic costs per hospitalized patient.[13]

Although the critically ill patient is often pyrexial, bloodstream infection may not be associated with an obvious spike or rise in temperature and a leukocytosis. Consequently, regular blood cultures, often twice a day taken from a peripheral site and from a central line (to exclude line-associated infection), are important to confirm a diagnosis and guide appropriate antibiotic therapy.

The diagnosis of VAP is particularly difficult as clinical and radiological criteria alone can be misleading. There is some controversy on the usefulness of invasive specimens such as bronchoalveolar lavage (BAL) and protected brush specimens (PBS) to identify a pathogen. In addition, quantitative cultures of endotracheal aspirates may be as effective. None the less, the use of such investigations can help to ensure that appropriate antibiotics are started earlier, and this may have an effect on mortality.[14]

Recent years have seen the publication of a number of studies assessing the usefulness of biochemical and/or other markers of infection, e.g. erythrocyte sedimentation rate (ESR), C-reactive protein (CRP) or a combination of cytokines. Although studies have demonstrated that cytokinaemia and elevated levels of procalcitonin and CRP are associated with infection and correlate with an adverse outcome,[4] such findings are not exclusive to infection and the routine measurement of cytokines does not necessarily further enhance clinical judgement.[15]

RESISTANT BACTERIA AND EMERGING PATHOGENS

Although the challenges posed by antibiotic-resistant bacteria will vary from unit to unit, Gram-positive bacteria have probably achieved a greater profile in recent years than multiantibiotic-resistant Gram-negative bacilli.

Methicillin-resistant *Staph. aureus* (MRSA)

MRSA is endemic in many UK hospitals and elsewhere. In the majority of cases patients are merely colonized and do not require specific antibiotic therapy. However, approximately a quarter to a third of patients may become infected and treatment may be difficult, as the drugs of choice for MRSA, i.e. the glycopeptides, are less effective than antistaphylococcal penicillins such as flucloxacillin. In a recent study from London in which 97 of 305 patients admitted to an ICU for longer than 48 hours were colonized on admission or became colonized shortly after admission, 53 patients developed 56 episodes of infection.[16] Although the mortality rates were similar in the MRA-colonized, MRSA-infected and non-MRSA patients, the length of stay was increased in both colonized and infected patients.[16] The most recent UK guidelines, which are due to be updated shortly, emphasize the importance of focusing on those most at risk of becoming infected, such as patients in intensive care, patients undergoing organ transplantation, orthopaedic patients etc. These are the areas of the hospital where the consequences of MRSA infection are likely to be greatest.[17] The essential elements of control are early identification of colonized patients, patient isolation and decontamination (where possible), and handwashing.

Table 9.1 *Multivariate analyses of risk factors for MRSA in an adult ICU (Adapted from reference 18)*

	Clustered cases		Sporadic cases	
	Relative risk	*p* value	Relative risk	*p* value
Urgent admissions	2.16	0.08	3.5	0.01
APACHE II score at 24 h	1.04	0.2	1.07	0.04
Bronchoscopy	1.62	0.45	3.68	0.01
Staff shortages	1.05	0.001	0.98	0.56

Compliance with handwashing or hand hygiene regimens is *the* single most important infection prevention measure. A recent elegant study from Nottingham which combined genetic analysis of MRSA isolates with cluster analysis of cases during a 12-month period revealed the presence of three clusters of cases and 59 per cent compliance with hand-disinfection procedures (an increase of 12 per cent in hand hygiene would have limited transmission), but on multivariate analysis (Table 9.1) only shortages of staff were associated with clusters.[18] Improved compliance with hand hygiene procedures and ensuring that staff deficiencies are reduced to a minimum would be key elements in improving the control of MRSA, and indeed many other nosocomial pathogens, in the ICU. Therefore, even though a more relaxed approach to the control of MRSA may be taken in other areas of the hospital, such as long-stay care of the elderly wards, this does not apply in this clinical setting. Such an aggressive approach becomes especially important with the recent description of isolates of *Staph. aureus* resistant to vancomycin in the USA.

VANCOMYCIN-RESISTANT ENTEROCOCCI (VRE)

Enterococci are normal inhabitants of the gastrointestinal tract, and apart from causing urinary tract infection in the community are not considered primary pathogens. However, in the acutely ill patient whose normal intestinal flora is disturbed, translocation to the bloodstream or the peritoneum following perforation of a viscus may result in systemic infection requiring treatment. Where isolates are susceptible, ampicillin with or without an aminoglycoside is the drug of choice, but glycopeptides such as vancomycin and teicoplanin have remained the mainstay of treatment for those isolates not susceptible to ampicillin. However, many ICUs have by now experienced patients with VRE or outbreaks. Increased use or abuse of antibiotics is among the main risk factors for the acquisition of VRE.[11] In a study of ICU patients, additional risk factors were length of stay prior to ICU admission and a history of solid organ transplantation.[19] Although the proportion of patients colonized with VRE who develop infection is less than that of patients with MRSA, infection control measures are important to prevent spread, although there are no topical agents available for gastrointestinal or skin decolonization. The degree to which patients should routinely be screened for VRE remains controversial.

ANTIBIOTIC-ASSOCIATED DIARRHOEA

Diarrhoea arising from antibiotic use in hospitalized patients is increasingly prevalent and in the vast majority of cases is caused by toxins produced by *Clostridium difficile*. Almost all antibiotics, even where only a few doses have been administered, have been implicated, but those that especially disrupt the normal flora, e.g. cephalosporins, are associated with the highest incidence. A recent large prevalence study in five Swedish hospitals revealed that antibiotic-associated diarrhoea occurred in 4.9 per cent of 2462 patients on antibiotics, and that patients suffering from two or more concomitant illnesses had a greater risk of acquisition.[20] The recent or concurrent use of cephalosporins, clindamycin or broad-spectrum penicillins posed the highest risk, but treatment with antibiotics for less than 3 days was associated with a lower risk; therefore, of the patient subgroups analysed, orthopaedic patients had the lowest prevalence, as in this specialty short perioperative courses are often the norm.

Cl. difficile is common in the ICU, where antibiotic use is among the highest in the hospital and where many patients have concomitant illnesses. Furthermore, patients may be incontinent and this increases the risk of spread, especially as this bacterium can form spores and hence is resistant to commonly used disinfectants. Management includes, if possible, stopping the antibiotic causing the diarrhoea, rehydration, and oral metronidazole; intravenous metronidazole may be used in patients unable to take oral medication, but vancomycin is not the drug of first choice and its excess use may predispose to the emergence or spread of VRE. Effective prevention and control measures in the ICU and elsewhere include, where possible, choosing those antimicrobial agents least likely to induce diarrhoea, e.g. quinolones; restricting the duration to as short a period as compatible with other aspects of the patient's care; making a diagnosis early so that therapy can be instituted quickly, thereby reducing the possibility of spread; instituting enteric infection control precautions for symptomatic patients; and regular cleaning and disinfection of the ICU environment to prevent the persistence of clostridial spores.

FUNGAL INFECTION

Patients in the ICU have a number of well recognized risk factors for the development of fungal infection, e.g. candidaemia, such as recent or prolonged courses of antibiotics, invasive intravascular or other devices, total parenteral nutrition, and either immunosuppression or other major debilitating factors such as major surgery, burns, etc.[21] Although many patients may become colonized with *Candida*, definitive evidence of invasive infection can be difficult to confirm although the isolation of *Candida* from the bloodstream is significant and should almost always be treated. In particular, long lines, which are often the source of the problem, should be removed. Although there is no clear consensus on the use of prophylaxis to prevent candidal infection, antifungal therapy significantly improves outcome.[21] Other fungal infections that occur less frequently in the ICU include aspergillosis and cryptococcosis (particularly common where a high proportion of patients are HIV-positive). Although neutropenia is the major risk factor for invasive aspergillosis, ICU patients who are non-neutropenic may acquire aspergillosis either from the environment or perhaps even from person-to-person transmission. A recent report suggests that two patients who had undergone liver transplantation acquired a strain of *Aspergillus* from another patient, possibly arising from the debriding and dressing of wounds.[22] The future may see an increasing proportion of infections caused by fungi in the ICU and the emergence of rarer fungi not hitherto encountered very commonly, except in the bone marrow transplant or severely neutropenic patient, because of the major advances in organ support available in the ICU and the increasing use of immunosuppressive agents.

USE OF ANTIBIOTICS

Despite the threat of the emergence of multiply antibiotic-resistant bacteria in the ICU, critically ill patients with infection require immediate and effective antibiotic therapy. In particular, the ICU patient may need more than one agent and may require more than one course of antibiotics, especially if stay is prolonged or complicated. This, however, contributes to the high prevalence of antibiotic-resistant bacteria in the ICU compared to other parts of the hospital. The key element in the effective use of antibiotics in this setting is to have all the information available, such as clinical data, the results from microbiological investigations, radiological investigations and other sources, before starting or changing antibiotics. Preferably, such decisions should be made by all members of the multidisciplinary team working together. Because patients in the ICU are constantly monitored, it is feasible – and indeed advisable on many occasions – to simply observe patients who have a temperature if they are otherwise haemodynamically stable. The presence of a low-grade fever and leukocytosis is not an indication per se for antibiotic therapy.[1]

In the Netherlands, where the prevalence of antibiotic resistance is especially low, a study looking at the indications for antibiotic use in ICU patients revealed that antibiotics were prescribed in 61 per cent of admissions, the most common reason being respiratory tract infection.[23] The authors concluded that efforts to prevent respiratory tract infections would further reduce the indications for antibiotic use, but acknowledged that the relative lack of significant resistance among nosocomial pathogens in their ICU was as a result of a restrictive antibiotic policy. Such policies, especially when they are specifically directed to the ICU, greatly assist in the management of patients as well as helping reduce the emergence or spread of antibiotic resistance. The availability of more sophisticated information technology systems in the ICU should provide suitable prompts and guidance for those prescribing electronically, particularly out of hours. The main emphasis in such antibiotic policies should be to provide specific guidance for the treatment of specific infections, restrict the use of certain agents such as clindamycin, which may promote the emergence of antibiotic-associated diarrhoea, and also expensive agents such as meropenem, and reduce the overuse of third-generation cephalosporins.[24] Intensivists can also, by liaising closely with their colleagues in the operating theatre, ensure that patients receive appropriate antimicrobial prophylaxis and that this is not continued.[25] Most patients following multiple trauma will have a fever, and although prophylaxis is indicated for compound fractures or major injury, this does not need to be continued. Advice on specific antibiotics will be governed largely by local antibiotic resistance patterns, but certain key principles should guide their use in the ICU:

- If the patient is haemodynamically unstable and clearly septic, but without an obvious source, and the results of laboratory investigations are pending, potent antibiotics, including combination therapy, e.g. gentamicin and piperacillin-tazobactam, should be started.
- If investigations rule out infection, antibiotics should usually be stopped.
- Certain infections should be treated with specific narrow-spectrum agents that are also the most effective, e.g. methicillin-sensitive *Staphylococcus aureus* with flucloxacillin, β-haemolytic streptococci with benzylpenicillin.
- The presence of *Candida* in the blood is an indication for the changing of IV lines and the institution of antifungal

therapy such as fluconazole. Amphotericin B, especially new or more expensive formulations, should be reserved for those patients with fluconazole-resistant *Candida*, patients not responding to fluconazole, or those with *Aspergillus* infection.

- Except for patients with endocarditis, bone or joint infections, tuberculosis, and a few other specialized infections, most courses of antibiotic, i.e. antibacterial agents, can be kept to 7 days at most, especially if the patient has improved, the source of infection has been removed and the underlying disease or condition precipitating infection is resolving. Continuation of antibiotics beyond 7 days may result in the emergence of resistance or superinfection, such as candidiasis.
- In units where the proportion of isolates of *Staph. aureus* resistant to methicillin is significant, e.g. 30 per cent or more, empirical treatment of suspected *Staph. aureus* should probably be treated with a glycopeptide such as vancomycin or teicoplanin. If the isolate is then confirmed as methicillin susceptible, therapy should be changed to flucloxacillin.
- Usually, most isolates of coagulase-negative staphylococci in the ICU are methicillin resistant, and hence empirical therapy should be a glycopeptide pending the results of antibiotic susceptibility testing.

The routine use of prophylactic antibiotics, both topically and parenterally, in the form of selective digestive tract decontamination (SDD), during the course of ICU stay has been advocated in the Netherlands and some other countries. The results from a well conducted recent prospective, stratified, randomized double-blind trial carried out in Germany on surgical/trauma patients, revealed that only 10 per cent of ICU patents were eligible for SDD, confirmed a reduction in both infection rates and acquired organ dysfunction, demonstrated a fall in mortality in patients with APACHE scores of 20–29 while in the ICU, and a reduction in the number of therapeutic interventions in patients on SDD, resulting in overall cost reductions.[26] Surveillance cultures carried out during the conduct of this trial did not show an increased incidence of antibiotic resistance, and although meta-analyses have shown a benefit in reducing the incidence of respiratory infection and mortality in patients on SDD, there is considerable concern that such a strategy may promote the emergence of resistance.[27] Therefore, many ICUs, where MRSA, VRE and resistant Gram-negative bacilli are endemic, are cautious about instituting SDD routinely. Large-scale multicentre studies with long-term surveillance are required to determine whether SDD predisposes to the emergence of antibiotic-resistant bacteria in ICUs where these are not normally prevalent, and whether this approach can be used safely in units where antibiotic resistance is endemic.

INFECTION PREVENTION AND CONTROL

Although the prevalence of infection is the ICU is higher than in other parts of the hospital, the principles of infection control and prevention are similar and have been well reviewed recently.[28] Measures include surveillance of infection, isolation precautions, standard precautions, i.e. the use of gloves for anticipated contact with blood, control of antimicrobial use as already discussed, and specific measures for individual infections, e.g. subglottic aspiration to prevent ventilator-associated pneumonia.[28] However, the environment in which the patient is being cared for, especially the availability of sufficient space, wash-hand basins, positively and negatively ventilated rooms for high-risk patients, and sufficient storage and utility space, is very important[29] but may not be optimal, especially in ICUs located in older hospitals. Handwashing, between patients and before invasive procedures, is the single most effective intervention, but compliance is poor, particularly among medical staff, even where facilities are adequate. However, a coordinated approach including education, and the availability of alcohol hand rubs, together with the investment of resources to support such a programme, has been shown to be effective in improving compliance and reducing infection.[30] Compliance with handwashing regimens and other examples of good practice is compromised by under-staffing, especially among nursing staff. In a case-control study of patients in a surgical ICU, an outbreak of central venous catheter-associated bloodstream infection was related to an increased patient-to-nurse ratio as well as parenteral nutrition and assisted ventilation.[31] Adequate numbers of staff as well as ongoing education programmes to decrease catheter-related bloodstream infections emphasize the importance of a multidisciplinary team approach.[32] A retrospective study conducted in France demonstrated a significant reduction in the percentage of patients with MRSA and a fall in total antibiotic costs from £98.70 to £62.70 after a focused programme of infection prevention.[33] The use of new molecular techniques to characterize organisms, and in particular to detect resistance earlier, e.g. the *MecA* gene for MRSA, would be advantageous as this would ensure earlier isolation of colonized or infected patients. Furthermore, discriminatory bacterial typing or fingerprinting techniques could provide a greater understanding of the dynamics of antibiotic resistance transmission in the ICU and elsewhere. When routine specimens were studied, and multiresistant Gram-negative bacilli and *Staph. aureus* were appropriately characterized and typed, interesting and important findings emerged, such as the presence of more than one strain of multiresistant Gram-negative bacilli but a single strain of MRSA.[34]

THE FUTURE

As improvements in organ replacement modalities continue, it seems likely that in the future increasingly vulnerable patients will be admitted to ICUs who will be at increased risk of infection. Improved and more rapid diagnostic approaches are needed, but molecular technology has not really delivered to date, except in the area of mycobacterial diseases and viral encephalomeningitis. A clinical and investigative protocol that rapidly differentiates infective from non-infective organ dysfunction is needed, and this might include multiplex polymerase chain reaction or gene arrays, or a battery of cytokine measurements, assuming the resources are available to implement this. This would greatly facilitate the management of infection and also help reduce the use of unnecessary antibiotics.

The emergence of bacteria for which there are no treatment agents available has not so far arisen, but the fear is that this may be imminent, and the recent description of strains of *Staph. aureus* resistant to vancomycin in the USA may presage this. Unlike in the 1970s and 1980s, there are relatively few new antibacterial agents being developed or launched by pharmaceutical companies, and those emerging are niche drugs that may have a defined but limited role. For example, linezolid, a new anti-Gram-positive agent, is increasingly indicated for the therapy of MRSA and VRE, but additional agents to treat infections caused by multiantibiotic-resistant Gram-negative bacteria such as *Serratia* species are needed. Alternatives to amphotericin B, such as voriconazole and caspofungin, are now available and may be followed by others.

Improved compliance with infection prevention strategies is the key to reducing the incidence of ICU-acquired infection, but changing human behaviour even among highly trained and intelligent healthcare staff remains problematical. The use of SDD in more clearly defined groups of patients, and probiotics to help minimize the impact of antibiotics and other interventions on normal flora, may assist in controlling antibiotic resistance and the therapy of diarrhoea due to *Cl. difficile*.

CONCLUSION

Infection in the ICU patient represents a major challenge, but effective management significantly improves morbidity and mortality. Those with responsibility for the diagnosis and management of infection must liaise closely with intensivists and intensive care nurses to optimize patient care. The appropriate and often-repeated microbiological investigation of acutely ill patients, together with the use of imaging, will help guide antibiotic use, which should be sensible and logical. Patients who are stable may be observed, and therefore preemptive antibiotics are often not indicated. Finally, sensible measures of infection control are mandatory and should be incorporated into good clinical practice. In particular, handwashing is the single most effective measure in preventing infection.

REFERENCES

1. Deitch EA, Vincent J-L, Windsor A. (eds) *Sepsis and multiple organ dysfunction. A multidisciplinary approach.* Edinburgh: WB Saunders, 2002.

2. Rizoli SB, Marshall JC. Saturday night fever: Finding and controlling the source of sepsis in critical illness. *Lancet Infect Dis* 2002; **2**: 137–44.

3. Department of Health. MRSA bacteraemia surveillance in acute NHS Trusts in England: April 2001 to March 2002. *Commun Dis Rep* 2002; **12**: 1–17.

4. Angus DC, Wax RS. Epidemiology of sepsis: An update. *Crit Care Med* 2001; **29**: S109–16.

5. Weber SJ, Raasch R, Rutala WA. Nosocomial infections in the ICU. The growing importance of antibiotic-resistant pathogens. *Chest* 1999; **115**: 34S–41S.

6. Vincent J-L, Bihari DJ, Suter PM, *et al.* The prevalence of nosocomial infection in intensive care units in Europe. Results of the European Prevalence of Infection in Intensive Care (EPIC) Study. *JAMA* 1995; **274**: 639–44.

7. Pittet D, Tara D, Wenzel RP. Nosocomial bloodstream infection in critically ill patients. Excess length of stay, extra costs and attributable mortality. *JAMA* 1994; **271**: 1598–601.

8. Kollef MH, Fraser VJ. Antibiotic resistance in the intensive care unit. *Ann Int Med* 2001; **134**: 298–314.

9. Hanberger H, Garcia-Rodriguez J-A, Gobernado M, *et al.* Antibiotic susceptibility among aerobic Gram-negative bacilli in intensive care units in 5 European countries. *JAMA* 1999; **281**: 67–71.

10. Hanberger H, Diekema D, Fluit A, *et al.* Surveillance of antibiotic resistance in European ICUs. *J Hosp Infect* 2001; **48**: 161–76.

11. Fridkin SK, Edwards JR, Courval JM, *et al.* The effect of vancomycin and third generation cephalosporins on the prevalence of vancomycin-resistant enterococci in 126 US adult intensive care units. *Ann Int Med* 2001; **135**: 175–83.

12. Humphreys H, Willatts, Vincent J-L. *Intensive care infections. A practical guide to diagnosis and management in adult patients.* London: WB Saunders, 2000.

13. Fox BC, Imrey PB, Voights MB, Norwood S. Infectious disease consultation and microbiologic surveillance for intensive care unit trauma patients: a pilot study. *Clin Infect Dis* 2001; **33**: 1981–9.

14. Koeman M, van der Ven AJAM, Ramsay G, *et al.* Ventilator-associated pneumonia: recent issues on pathogenesis, prevention and diagnosis. *J Hosp Infect* 2001; **49**: 155–62.

15. van Dissel JT. Procalcitonin and other markers of infection. What should be their role in clinical practice? *Clin Microbiol Infect* 2002; **8**: 70–3.

16. Theaker C, Ormond-Walshe S, Azadian B, Soni N. MRSA in the critically ill. *J Hosp Infect* 2001; **48**: 98–102.

17. Report of a combined working party of the British Society for Antimicrobial Chemotherapy, the Hospital Infection Society and the Infection Control Nurses Association. Revised guidelines for the control of methicillin-resistant *Staphylococcus aureus* infection in hospitals. *J Hosp Infect* 1998; **39**: 253–90.

18. Grundmann H, Hori S, Winter B, *et al.* Risk factors for the transmission of methicillin-resistant *Staphylococcus aureus* in an adult intensive care unit: fitting a model to the data. *J Infect Dis* 2002; **185**: 481–8.

19. Ostrowsky BE, Venkataraman L, D'Agata MC, *et al.* Vancomycin-resistant enterococci in intensive care units. High frequency of stool carriage in intensive care units. *Arch Intern Med* 1999; **159**: 1467–72.

20. Wiström J, Norrby SR, Myhre EB, *et al.* Frequency of antibiotic-associated diarrhoea in 2462 antibiotic-treated hospitalised patients; a prospective study. *J Antimicrob Chemother* 2001; **47**: 43–50.

21. Flanagan PG, Barnes RA. Fungal infection in the intensive care unit. *J Hosp Infect* 1998; **38**: 163–77.

22. Pegues DA, Lasker BA, McNeill MM, *et al.* Cluster of cases of invasive aspergillosis in a transplant intensive care unit: Evidence of person-to-person airborne transmission. *Clin Infect Dis* 2002; **34**: 412–16.

23. Bergmans DCJJ, Bonten MJM, Gaillard CA, *et al.* Indications for antibiotic use in ICU patients: a one-year prospective surveillance. *J Antimicrob Chemother* 1997; **39**: 527–35.

24. Kollef MH. Optimising antibiotic therapy in the intensive care unit setting. *Crit Care* 2001; **5**: 189–95.

25. Timms J, Humphreys H. Antimicrobial prophylaxis in the intensive care unit. *Curr Anaesth Crit Care* 1997; **8**: 133–8.

26. Krueger WA, Lenhart F-P, Neeser G, *et al.* Influence of combined intravenous and topical antibiotic prophylaxis on the incidence of infections, organ dysfunctions and mortality in critically ill patients. *Am J Respir Crit Care Med* 2002; **166**: 1029–37.

27. Ebner W, Kropec-Hübner A, Daschner FD. Bacterial resistance and overgrowth due to selective decontamination of the digestive tract. *Eur J Clin Microbiol Infect Dis* 2000; **19**: 243–7.

28. Eggimann P, Pittet D. Infection control and the ICU. *Chest* 2001; **120**: 2059–93.

29. O'Connell NH, Humphreys H. Intensive care unit design and environmental factors in the acquisition of infection. *J Hosp Infect* 2000; **45**: 255–62.

30. Pittet D, Hugonnet S, Harbarth S, *et al.* Effectiveness of a hospital-wide programme to improve compliance with hand hygiene. *Lancet* 2000; **356**: 1307–12.

31. Fridkin S, Pear SM, Williamson TH, *et al.* The role of understaffing in central venous catheter-associated bloodstream infections. *Infect Control Hosp Epidemiol* 1996; **17**: 150–8.

32. Coopersmith CM, Rebmann TL, Zack JE, *et al.* Effect of an education program on decreasing catheter-related bloodstream infections in the surgical intensive care unit. *Crit Care Med* 2002; **30**: 59–64.

33. Souweine B, Traore O, Aublet-Cuvelier B, *et al.* Role of infection control measures in limiting morbidity associated with multiresistant organisms in critically ill patients. *J Hosp Infect* 2000; **45**: 107–16.

34. Grundmann H, Hahn A, Ehrenstein B, *et al.* Detection of cross-transmission of multiresistant Gram-negative bacilli and *Staphylococcus aureus* in adult intensive care units by routine typing of clinical isolates. *Clin Microbiol Infect* 1999; **5**: 355–63.

10 Critical care of the trauma patient

ADAM BROOKS, PETER MAHONEY & C WILLIAM SCHWAB

Viva topics

- Critical care priorities in damage control.
- Intra-abdominal pressure and the abdominal compartment syndrome.

INTRODUCTION

The critical care management priorities for the severely injured patient are resuscitation, restoration of physiology, maintenance of tissue oxygen, continual monitoring, prevention of infection and the provision of organ system support. In the UK more than 25 000 people are seriously injured each year; this translates to approximately 2500 trauma patients who will require intensive care facilities each year. Experience from a busy British teaching hospital suggests that at any one time approximately 20 per cent of patients on a general intensive care unit (ICU) will be victims of trauma.

ADMISSION TO ICU

Injured patients must be managed in a facility that offers an appropriate level of support for their requirements. Formal criteria exist for the acute admission of a severely injured patient to intensive care. These include the requirement for airway protection, or ventilation for head and chest injury, active resuscitation following damage control procedures, and the correction of gross physiological disturbances. Trauma scoring systems, such as the TRISS score and injury severity score, have been developed to grade the severity of the injury. Some of these use physiological parameters only, whereas others use a combination of physiological derangement and anatomical injuries; however, they are usually not applicable in the acute phase of care and are not sufficient alone to determine the requirement for admission to ICU. In the early phases clinical judgement must also be used to anticipate the potential for instability, blood loss, hypothermia, the likelihood of complications and future deterioration. Table 10.1

provides a guide to the anatomical injuries and physiological derangements that require ICU admission. When the criteria for ICU management are not met, then high-dependency or intermediate care should be considered (Table 10.2).

PHASES OF TRAUMA CRITICAL CARE

The critical care management of the injured patient has been divided into four phases.[1]

Resuscitation phase (initial admission to 24 h)

The priorities during the initial 24 h following admission to critical care are fluid resuscitation, maintenance of tissue perfusion and oxygenation, monitoring and re-examination. Patients who have undergone damage control or abbreviated surgical procedures because of physiological instability will need correction of acidosis and coagulopathy, and reversal of hypothermia (see later). Several problems can occur during this phase, including urgent unplanned return to theatre for surgical bleeding, failure to achieve adequate endpoints of resuscitation despite maximal efforts, and continued clinical deterioration or, rarely, the identification of a life- or limb-threatening injury.

Early life support phase (24–72 h)

During the 72 h that follow resuscitation, management concentrates on the support of the major organ systems. Damage-control patients will return to theatre after 24–36 h, and a further period of resuscitation may be required after this. The major problems encountered during this phase are respiratory failure, progressive raised intracranial pressure, multiple organ dysfunction syndrome (MODS) and the development of the abdominal compartment syndrome (ACS).

Prolonged life support (>72 h)

The duration of prolonged life support depends on the severity of the injury and the development of complications. In severely

Table 10.1 *Criteria for ICU admission (Adapted from The Trauma Manual, Lippincott, Williams and Wilkins, Philadelphia, USA, with permission)*

Anatomical trauma	Physiological trauma	Condition
Multisystem injury	Respiratory failure requiring mechanical ventilation	Elderly >65 years
Severe head injury (GCS <8)	Ongoing shock or haemodynamic instability	Comorbidity, esp. heart disease
Cervical spinal cord injury	Massive transfusion	
Severe pulmonary contusion or flail chest	High base deficit	
Facial or neck trauma with threatened airway	Hypothermia	
Postoperative repair major vascular injury	Decreased renal function, coagulopathy	Substance abuse with altered mental status
Severe pelvic fracture with retroperitoneal haematoma	Seizures	
Blunt cardiac trauma with dysrhythmia or hypotension	Elderly patients, comorbidity, haemodynamic instability	Multiple fractures, long bone fracture
Crush injury		
Severe burns or smoke inhalation		

Table 10.2 *Indications for high-dependency care*

Isolated liver/spleen injuries (conservative management)
Uncomplicated anterior chest injury
Isolated multiple rib fractures or pulmonary contusion, with adequate oxygenation
Isolated thoracic spinal cord injury
Head injury GCS 11–14
Isolated extremity vascular injuries
Non-invasive ventilation following chest trauma

injured patients this phase may be quite protracted. The aim is to provide ongoing support for organ failure. Complications can occur and their impact on the patient must be minimized; however, organ dysfunction, MODS, SIRS and sepsis can supervene and progress to multiple organ failure and death.

Recovery phase (preparation for transfer to a lower level of support)

During the recovery phase the patient is weaned from organ support and invasive monitoring before transfer to a high-dependency unit or the ward.

This chapter will concentrate on the priorities of care during the initial and early phases of intensive care admission.

INITIAL (RESUSCITATIVE) PHASE

Damage control

Over the last decade, damage control has been introduced as a surgical strategy for the massively injured, exsanguinating

patient.[2] The concept that the cold, coagulopathic, acidotic patient does not benefit from the long procedures that are associated with traditional surgical techniques has gradually become accepted. Rather than allowing progressive physiological derangement, this group of severely injured patients, who comprise approximately 10 per cent of trauma patients, need short focused surgery aimed at stopping bleeding and controlling contamination. Improved survival has been demonstrated in a maximally injured subset of patients using this approach, and a collective review of over 1000 damage-control patients has demonstrated an improved survival against traditional approaches, with 50 per cent overall survival.[3]

Damage control should start during the prehospital and emergency department phases,[4] with early recognition of the patient who will benefit from short prehospital times, abbreviated initial resuscitation, rapid access to theatre and damage-control surgery (Table 10.3). This phase has been termed 'damage control ground zero', and by adhering to this strategy 90 per cent survival has been reported by one centre in a damage-controlled population.[4]

PHYSIOLOGICAL BASIS OF DAMAGE CONTROL

The triad of hypothermia, coagulopathy and metabolic acidosis forms the core physiological derangement in the injured trauma patient in extremis. Hypothermia, defined as a core temperature less than 35°C, is precipitated by exposure and hypovolaemic shock and is further aggravated by the infusion of cold resuscitation fluids and blood. The relationship between trauma mortality and hypothermia is well documented, and Jurkovich et al.[5] demonstrated a 60 per cent increase in mortality in patients with a temperature of 32°C or less, compared to those with a temperature of 34°C.

Table 10.3 *Triggers for damage control*

Preoperative triggers and injury complexes	Operative triggers
High energy blunt trauma	Severe metabolic acidosis pH 7.3
Multiple torso penetration	Hypothermia <35°C
Abdominal vascular injury and multiple visceral injury	Coagulopathy – non-surgical bleeding (elevated prothrombin and partial thromboplastin times)
Exsanguination from multiple sources with visceral injury	Operative time >90 minutes
Abdominal injury with competing injuries (head trauma, pelvic fracture etc.)	

Hypothermia exacerbates coagulopathy through platelet dysfunction and inhibition of the coagulation pathway.[6] In addition, hypothermia predisposes to arrhythmias, reduced cardiac output and a left shift in the oxygen saturation curve.

Profound hypoperfusion of tissue with anaerobic respiration and the production of lactic acid results in metabolic acidosis. The interaction of hypothermia and acidosis in concert with the dilution of clotting factors following fluid resuscitation, exacerbates the developing coagulopathy and is likely to be recognized clinically by non-surgical bleeding and oozing before there are significant changes in the coagulation blood tests. Bedside coagulation tests such as the thromboelastogram may provide an early indication of coagulopathy. Progressive derangement leads to platelet dysfunction and inhibition of both the intrinsic and extrinsic pathways, with prolongation of both PT (prothrombin time) and PTT (partial thromboplastin time) ratios. Laboratory investigations routinely performed at 37°C will markedly underestimate the degree of coagulopathy in these patients.

The objective of the surgical damage control sequence is the rapid control of haemorrhage and limitation of contamination. This is achieved through the ligature of non-essential vascular injury, temporary shunt of essential vessels for later definitive repair, and packing of hepatic injury. Bowel injury is addressed through stapled closure and resection, leaving anastomosis and stoma formation to the definitive surgery phase. Injured solid organs and dissected areas are packed and a temporary abdominal closure fashioned prior to transfer to the ICU.

On admission to intensive care the damage-controlled patient requires restoration of physiology through aggressive resuscitation, rewarming, correction of acidosis and reversal of coagulopathy. Adequate tissue perfusion through appropriate fluid resuscitation provides correction of the metabolic acidosis and the clearance of accumulated lactic acid, which has been shown to be prognostic of outcome.[7,8] Resuscitation should be directed by invasive monitoring; however, accurate markers for the endpoints of resuscitation and supranormalization are contentious and are discussed later in this chapter.

Immediate core rewarming improves perfusion and assists in reversing coagulopathy. Prolonged postoperative hypothermia correlates with increased mortality, and rewarming should be aggressive through active and passive measures such as the use of warmed fluids, hot-air convection blowers, blankets, and warming of the environment. Severe hypothermia may be addressed through gastric and pleural lavage or extracorporeal circulation.

Correction of coagulation requires the reversal of external factors – hypothermia and acidosis – in addition to the correction of the coagulation abnormalities through the administration of warm clotting products, fresh frozen plasma as directed by the PT and PTT, cryoprecipitate if the fibrinogen is low, and platelets. The role of recombinant factor VIIa is discussed later.

Planned return to theatre is usually timed for 36–48 h after the initial surgery, depending on the stability and physiological status of the patient. Definitive organ and vessel repair and, where possible, abdominal closure, are the goals of this phase of damage control. Continued instability or rapid deterioration during the resuscitative phase will require an urgent unscheduled return to theatre.

MASSIVE TRANSFUSION PROTOCOLS

The massively bleeding patient poses acute problems both to the surgeon attempting haemorrhage control and the anaesthetist replacing blood and blood products. Massive transfusion, variously defined as replacement of the patient's circulating blood volume in 24 h, or more than a 10-unit transfusion, is associated with severe physiological and metabolic disturbances that include hyperkalaemia, hypocalcaemia, hypomagnesaemia and hypothermia. Substantial blood loss and replacement result in severe coagulation disturbances that are complicated by hypothermia and acidosis. Expedient blood and early component therapy is required, and although these should be commenced during operative surgery, active measures need to be continued in the ICU.

Techniques to optimize massive transfusion and counteract the physiological disturbances have been developed. Blood transfusion warmers are capable of flow rates of 1000 mL/min and temperatures of up to 38°C, and should be an integral component of resuscitation to address core hypothermia. Autotransfusion using cell recovery technology (Cell-Saver Plus, Haemonectics Corporation, Braintree,

Table 10.4 *Massive transfusion pack*

10 units group O non-cross-matched packed red blood cells

6 units of platelets

4 units of thawed fresh frozen plasma

MA) is effective for scavenging of non-contaminated blood, e.g. from thoracic trauma, and return transfusion to the patient. Technological advances now allow components to be removed from the recovered blood, and the production of fibrin glue, which may be used as an adjunct to the management of liver trauma.

Institutional massive transfusion policies[4] have been developed for exsanguinating patients (Table 10.4). This initial response provides rapid component therapy in proportion to the blood use and is automatically repeated until discontinued by a senior physician.

RECOMBINANT FACTOR VIIa

Recombinant factor VIIa (RFVIIa) is a procoagulant that is active only in the presence of tissue factor. When tissue factor is exposed in the subendothelium following vessel injury, the RFVIIa rapidly initiates activation of the extrinsic clotting system without activating the systemic coagulation system. Evidence from the management of uncontrollable bleeding in haemophiliacs and a laboratory grade V liver injury model[9,10] suggests that RFVIIa reduces blood loss and restores coagulation function without adverse clinical effects. Case reports using RFVIIa in trauma patients support these findings. RFVIIa has been the subject of a randomized double-blind clinical trial investigating the treatment of bleeding in severely injured patients, the results of which are currently awaited.

ENDPOINTS OF RESUSCITATION

The traditional endpoints of resuscitation that are readily measured include blood pressure, urine output and heart rate. However, the use of these parameters will result in 50–80 per cent of patients remaining with occult hypoperfusion and inadequate tissue oxygenation despite having achieved apparently satisfactory endpoints.[11] The sequelae of inadequate resuscitation are infection, multiple organ failure and death. Numerous studies have attempted to define the ideal endpoints of resuscitation in critically ill trauma patients.[11,12] Other investigators prefer resuscitation to 'supranormal' values, which include cardiac index >4.5 L/min/m^2, oxygen delivery index >600 mL/min/m^2, and an oxygen consumption index >170 mL/min/m^2.[13] Although some of these studies showed improved survival in optimized patients, others revealed no difference between patients resuscitated to either optimized or normal values.[14]

Alternative endpoints, including lactate clearance, have been studied[14] and shown to correlate with mortality. The search for the ideal marker of resuscitation endpoint continues.

EARLY LIFE SUPPORT PHASE

Management in the 48 h that follow resuscitation focuses on post-traumatic respiratory failure, management of raised intracranial pressure (see Chapter 11), recognition of abdominal or extremity compartment syndromes, and evaluation for all occult injuries. Several conditions unique to the trauma patient must also be detected and addressed appropriately during this phase.

Respiratory management

Pulmonary contusion is the most common intrathoracic injury from blunt trauma, has an associated mortality of 10–25 per cent,[15] and is an independent predictor for pneumonia[16] and ARDS.[17] The early identification of contusion allows the recognition of patients at risk of deteriorating respiratory function who may benefit from early non-invasive ventilation. Lung injury severity scoring systems have been developed that use the initial chest X-ray and the PaO_2/FiO_2 ratio to predict high-risk patients who may require ventilation. Tyburski *et al.* demonstrated that a PaO_2/FiO_2 ratio of <300 on admission or within the first 24 h correlated with a need for ventilatory support.[18] Alternative systems using the extent of contusion volume on 3D CT reconstruction have also been used to predict pulmonary dysfunction,[19] although the technology required may not be widely available.

ARDS is prevalent in trauma patients, especially those with chest injury. A study from Tennessee showed that severe injury (injury severity score >25), pulmonary contusion, hypotension on admission, large-volume blood transfusion and age over 65 years were independent risk factors for the development of ARDS following blunt trauma.[20] Numerous ventilation strategies for the management of thoracic injury and pulmonary contusion have been advocated. Lung-protective strategies with stabilization of alveoli using positive end-expiratory pressure (PEEP) are associated with reduced lung injury[21] and have become widely accepted in the management of lung injury in trauma patients. This technique and others used for the management of lung injury and ARDS, such as prone positioning and high-frequency jet ventilation, are discussed in detail in the respiratory and ARDS chapters.

Flail chest and multiple rib fractures are associated with underlying lung contusion, but in addition pain can lead to physiological splinting of the ribs, inadequate ventilation and the development of pneumonia. Adequate analgesia is important, and this may be best delivered as a thoracic epidural, although coagulation deficits would preclude this (see Chapter 12).

MISSED INJURIES AND THE TERTIARY SURVEY

Despite the structured approach to the delivery of care in the resuscitation room that is provided by the Advanced Trauma Life Support (ATLS) guidelines, significant injuries can be missed in both the primary and secondary surveys. Injuries undetected during resuscitation have been reported to occur in 8–65 per cent of trauma patients and can lead to significant morbidity and mortality.[22–24] Up to 25 per cent of these missed injuries may be clinically significant and require additional surgical procedures. It is important that these occult injuries, especially those that are life threatening, are detected early during the ICU admission.

The tertiary survey is a comprehensive clinical examination, repetition of the primary and secondary surveys, and review of all the investigations, including blood tests and radiology during the first 24 h. A formal tertiary survey should be performed in all trauma patients, by an experienced clinician, within 24 h of admission to the ICU.

CLEARANCE OF SPINAL INJURIES

Trauma patients are at risk of spinal injuries from blunt injury where deceleration or rotational forces are applied to the spinal column. Prolonged spinal immobilization is associated with increased morbidity from raised intracranial pressure, pressure sores from the hard collar, increased infection and difficulties with nursing care; however, the risk from inadequate immobilization is iatrogenic spinal cord injury.

The clearance of spinal injuries in the unconscious patient in the ITU has provoked much debate. Current ATLS guidelines allow for the clinical clearance of the cervical spine in conscious patients (without distracting injuries) during the resuscitation. Clearing the cervical spine in an unconscious trauma patient is much more difficult, and all of these patients should be assumed to have an unstable spine until proved otherwise.

Thoracic and lumbar bony injury is adequately detected on plain X-ray, but this is not the situation in the cervical spine, where lateral X-ray has a sensitivity for the detection of bony injury of up to 85 per cent, and with the addition of three-view plain radiology (lateral, anteroposterior and peg views) the sensitivity increases up to 94 per cent.[25] Computed tomography (CT) imaging of C1 and C2 for all head-injured patients is recommended by the Eastern Association for the Surgery of Trauma (EAST)[26] and further increases the sensitivity of fracture detection. In the Oxford study[27] 15 per cent of the cervical injuries were first detected by CT scanning. The potential for ligamentous injury and missed bony injury still exists despite normal radiology, therefore the Oxford protocol and EAST guidelines suggest CT imaging of C1/C2 and C7/T1 for all unconscious patients as part of the CT head protocol, and advocate dynamic screening of flexion and extension views to assess for ligamentous instability. A meta-analysis has suggested that cervical injuries undetected by three-view plain radiology and CT will be diagnosed by fluoroscopic flexion and extension views in 2.2 per cent of patients.[26] Using this approach the Oxford group reported a 3.5 year experience of 210 patients assessed without missed injury and early removal of the collar in the majority. In two patients unsuspected fractures were detected, and instability was assessed in three patients with known fractures, but in only one was instability demonstrated.[27]

INTRA-ABDOMINAL PRESSURE AND THE ABDOMINAL COMPARTMENT SYNDROME

The incidence of raised intra-abdominal pressure in surgical critical care patients has been reported to be between 14 and 33 per cent.[28,29] Patients with abdominal trauma, intra-abdominal sepsis, pancreatitis and emergency abdominal aortic aneurysm repair are at high risk for the development of raised IAP. Table 10.5 lists the clinical sequelae of raised IAP. The value at which the IAP becomes clinically significant and the appropriate management of the abdominal compartment syndrome (ACS) remain controversial.

Damage-controlled patients with packed abdomens are at especially high risk of developing abdominal compartment syndrome (ACS), and associated tissue hypoperfusion will further exacerbate metabolic acidosis. These patients should be monitored every 4–6 h by bladder pressure measurements to identify high IAP and should undergo abdominal decompression if ACS or a high IAP is identified.

- **Raised intra-abdominal pressure** Bladder pressure measurements in excess of 18 mmHg
- **Abdominal compartment syndrome (ACS)** Raised intra-abdominal pressure of 25 mmHg or greater, resulting in systemic effects.

Table 10.5 *Clinical sequelae of raised IAP*

Reduced cardiac output	Decreased pulmonary compliance
Raised intracerebral pressure	Decreased oxygenation
Inaccurate CVP and PAOP	Increased peak inspiratory pressure
Oliguria/anuria	

Bladder pressure correlates well with IAP, and the measurement technique was originally described by Kron in 1984.[30] It involves the instillation of 50 mL of saline into the bladder, with the pressure measured using a transducer zeroed at the symphysis pubis. Cheatham[31] has described a closed system technique that allows repeated measurements. High-risk patients should have at least daily IAP monitoring; however, Sugrue[32] has recommended that IAP measurement should be undertaken routinely every 8 h in all postoperative ICU patients.

The early physiological sequela of raised IAP is visceral and renal ischaemia; however, the clinically significant value of IAP is contentious: pressures of 20 mmHg or greater in the majority of patients will be significant, but must be interpreted against the patient's overall condition. IAP values of 18, 25 and 30 mmHg have all been quoted in the literature, the latter two as triggers for abdominal decompression. We consider decompression in patients with ACS and IAP of >25 mmHg.

Surgical abdominal decompression and laparostomy is the currently accepted management of established ACS. Numerous techniques for temporary abdominal closure, including the Vac Pack (Figure 10.1)[33] and the Bogotá Bag, have been used and clear benefit has been demonstrated from decompression, although the ideal timing of surgery remains unclear. The benefits can be immediate, and a marked survival benefit from decompression has been demonstrated.

Crush injury and myonecrosis

Both crush injury and myonecrosis are associated with muscle breakdown, vessel thrombosis and the development of limb compartment syndrome. Myonecrosis following high-voltage injury is characterized by destruction of the muscle adjacent to the bone and, like crush injury, reperfusion of the limb can result in the release of toxic metabolites and rhabdomyolysis. Early wound debridement is necessary, and fasciotomy may be required.

If myoglobin is present in the urine in these conditions, early active fluid management is required to prevent the development of renal failure. A urine output of >1 mL/kg/h should be the goal. This may be augmented by mannitol (25 g IV 4–6-hourly) and sodium bicarbonate if the urinary pH is less than 7.

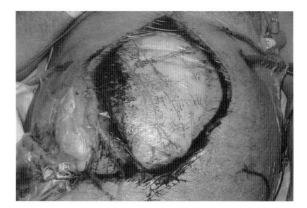

Figure 10.1 Temporary abdominal closure for abdominal compartment syndrome with modified Vac Pack closure

SUMMARY

This chapter has addressed key issues in the initial and early phases of critical care management of the severely injured patient. These patients will use the full resources of the ICU, and the management of their injuries and ensuing complications can require extensive critical care support and an integrated response from many hospital specialists.

FURTHER READING

American College of Surgeons. *Advanced trauma life support student course manual.* Chicago: American College of Surgeons, 1997

Botha A, Brooks A, Loosemore T. *Definitive surgical trauma skills.* London: Royal College of Surgeons of England, 2002

Peitzman AB, Rhodes M, Schwab CW, Yearly DM, Fabian TC. *Trauma manual.* Philadelphia: Lippincott, Williams and Wilkins, 2002

REFERENCES

1. Clancy KD, Darby JM. Priorities in the critical care of trauma patients. In: Peitzman AB, Rhodes M, Schwab CW, *et al.* (eds) *The trauma manual.* Philadelphia: Lippincott, Williams and Wilkins, 2002.

2. Rotondo MF, Schwab CW, McGonigal MD. Damage control: an approach for improved survival in exsanguinating penetrating abdominal injury. *J Trauma* 1993; **35**: 375–83.

3. Shapiro MB, Jenkins DH, Schwab CW, Rotondo MF. Damage control: collective review. *J Trauma* 2000; **49**: 969–78.

4. Johnson JW, Gracias VH, Schwab CW, *et al.* Evolution in damage control for exsanguinating penetrating abdominal injury. *J Trauma* 2001; **51**: 261–9; discussion 269–71.

5. Jurkovich GJ, Luterman GW, Curreri PW. Hypothermia in trauma victims: an ominous predictor of survival. *J Trauma* 1987; **27**: 1019–24.

6. Cosgriff N, Moore EE, Sauaia A, *et al.* Predicting life threatening coagulopathy in the massively transfused trauma patient: hypothermia and acidoses revisited. *J Trauma* 1997; **42**: 857–62.

7. Abramson D, Scalea TM, Hitchcock R. Lactate clearance and survival following injury. *J Trauma* 1993; **35**: 584–9.

8. McNelis J, Marini CP, Jurkiewicz A, *et al.* Prolonged lactate clearance is associated with increased mortality in the surgical intensive care unit. *Am J Surg* 2001; **182**: 481–5.

9. Schreiber MA, Holcomb JB, Hedner U, *et al.* The effect of recombinant factor VIIa on coagulopathic pigs with grade V liver injuries. *J Trauma* 2002; **53**: 252–7.

10. Martinowitz U, Holcomb JB, Pusateri AE, *et al.* Intravenous rFVIIa administered for hemorrhage control in hypothermic coagulopathic swine with grade V liver injuries. *J Trauma* 2001; **50**: 721–9.

11. Porter JM, Ivatury RR. In search of the optimal endpoints of resuscitation. *J Trauma* 1998; **44**: 908–14.

12. Shoemaker WC, Appel P, Kran H. Prospective trial of supernormal values of survivors as therapeutic goals in high-risk surgical patients. *Chest* 1983; **94**: 1176.

13. Velmahos GC, Demetriades DD, Shoemaker WC, *et al.* Endpoints of resuscitation of critically injured patients: normal or supranormal? *Ann Surg* 2000; **232**: 409–18.

14. Ahrns KS, Harkins DR. Initial resuscitation after burn injury: therapies, strategies, and controversies. *AACN Clin Issues* 1999; **10**: 46–60.

15. Hoff SJ, Shotts SD, Eddy VA, *et al.* Outcome of isolated pulmonary contusion in blunt trauma patients. *Am Surg* 1994; **60**: 138–42.

16. Antonelli M, Moro ML, Capelli O, *et al.* Risk factors for the early onset of pneumonia in trauma patients. *Chest* 1994; **105**: 224–8.

17. Croce MA, Fabian TC, Davis KA, *et al.* Early and late acute respiratory distress syndrome. *J Trauma* 1999; **46**: 361–8.

18. Tyburski JG, Collinge J, Wilson RF, Eachempati SR. Pulmonary contusions: quantifying the lesions on chest X-ray films and the factors affecting prognosis. *J Trauma* 1999; **46**: 833–8.

19. Miller PR, Croce MA, Bee TK, *et al.* ARDS after pulmonary contusion: accurate measurement of contusion volume identifies high-risk patients. *J Trauma* 2001; **51**: 223–8; discussion 229–30.

20. Miller PR, Croce MA, Kilgo PD, Scott J, Fabian TC. Acute respiratory distress syndrome in blunt trauma: identification of independent risk factors. *Am Surg* 2002; **68**: 845–50; discussion 850–1.

21. Offner PJ, Moore EE. Lung injury severity scoring in the era of lung protective ventilation. *J Trauma* 2001; **51**: 211.

22. Enderson BL, Reath DB, Meadors J, *et al.* The tertiary trauma survey: a prospective study of missed injury. *J Trauma* 1990; **30**: 666–9; discussion 669–70.

23. Janjua KJ, Sugrue M, Deane SA. Prospective evaluation of early missed injuries and the role of tertiary trauma survey. *J Trauma* 1998; **44**: 1000–6; discussion 1006–7.

24. Buduhan G, McRitchie DI. Missed injuries in patients with multiple trauma. *J Trauma* 2000; **49**: 600–5.

25. West OC, Anbari MM, Pilgrom TK, Wilson AJ. Acute cervical spine trauma: diagnostic performance of a single view versus three view radiographic screening. *Radiology* 1997; **204**: 819–23.

26. Marion D, Domeier R, Dunham CM, *et al. Determination of cervical spine stability in trauma patients.* Eastern Association for the Surgery of Trauma, 2000.

27. Brooks RA, Willett KM. Evaluation of the Oxford protocol for total spinal clearance in the unconscious trauma patient. *J Trauma* 2001; **50**: 862–7.

28. Meldrum DR, Moore FA, Moore EE, *et al.* Prospective characterization and selective management of the abdominal compartment syndrome. *Am J Surg* 1997; **174**: 667–72; discussion 672–3.

29. Sugrue M, Buist MD, Hourihan F, *et al.* Prospective study of intra-abdominal hypertension and renal function after laparotomy. *Br J Surg* 1995; **82**: 235–8.

30. Kron IL, Harman PK, Nolan SP. The measurement of intra-abdominal pressure as a criterion for abdominal re-exploration. *Ann Surg* 1984; **199**: 28–30.

31. Cheatham ML, Safcsak K. Intraabdominal pressure: a revised method for measurement. *J Am Coll Surg* 1998; **186**: 594–5.

32. Sugrue M. Intra-abdominal pressure: time for clinical practice guidelines? *Intensive Care Med* 2002; **28**: 389–91.

33. Barker DE, Kaufman HJ, Smith LA, *et al.* Vacuum pack technique of temporary abdominal closure: a 7-year experience with 112 patients. *J Trauma* 2000; **48**: 201–6; discussion 206–7.

11 Neurological critical care

KEITH GIRLING & BERNARD RILEY

Viva topics

- Describe the basic, early management principles for a patient following a severe traumatic brain injury.
- What is the purpose of ICP monitoring?
- Describe the tests required to fulfil the diagnosis of brainstem death.
- What are the principles of managing a patient following a subarachnoid haemorrhage?

INTRODUCTION

The last two decades have seen significant changes in the management of neurological conditions on the critical care unit. This has been due to the introduction of new therapies, new modalities of monitoring and imaging of the brain, and the appreciation that intensive monitoring and strict attention to detail in the management of this group of patients may have significant effects on the outcome of neurological conditions. This chapter will review the current management strategies for patients with traumatic brain injury, cerebrovascular disease and intracranial haemorrhage, and common neurological emergencies.

INTRACRANIAL PHYSIOLOGY

Some basic principles of intracranial physiology include:

- The adult skull is a rigid box which contains brain, blood and cerebrospinal fluid (CSF). If the volume of any one of these components increases, the volume of one of the others must decrease to maintain intracranial pressure in the normal range. If the volume of one component continues to increase the intracranial pressure will increase, as indicated in Figure 11.1.
- The cerebral blood flow in the normal state is autoregulated for pressure, as shown in Figure 11.2. Thus, fluctuations in arterial pressure between mean values of 60 and 130 mmHg will not result in changes in cerebral blood flow. The

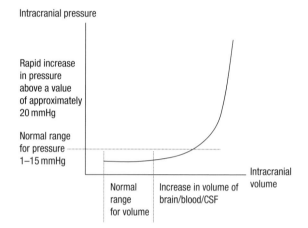

Figure 11.1 The relationship between intracranial pressure and volume

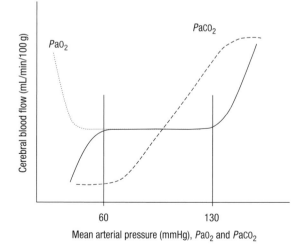

Figure 11.2 Changes in cerebral blood flow with mean arterial pressure, $PaCO_2$ and PaO_2

effects of changes in PaO_2 and $PaCO_2$ are also indicated in Figure 11.2.

- The cerebral blood flow is normally linearly related to the arterial carbon dioxide partial pressure, such that for a

1 kPa change in $PaCO_2$, cerebral blood flow changes by approximately 20 per cent (Figure 11.2).

- The brain tissue is an obligate glucose user. If a part of the brain is rendered ischaemic and blood concentrations of glucose are allowed to increase, metabolic activity will increase. This will result in an increase in local lactic acid concentrations and further cerebral ischaemia.

CRITICAL CARE MANAGEMENT OF TRAUMATIC BRAIN INJURY

The management of head-injured patients uses a vast amount of hospital resources. Approximately one million patients present, and more than 150 000 are admitted to hospitals each year following a head injury. Because of the difficulties in deciding which patients to admit and which require CT imaging, in June 2003 the National Institute for Clinical Excellence published guidelines on the early management of head injury in infants, children and adults.[1] These guidelines do not detail critical care management of these patients and are mainly concerned with prehospital care, imaging, observation and discharge of patients following a head injury. When considering only patients who have sustained a severe head injury (i.e. GCS <9), depending on the series, up to 85 per cent of survivors will remain disabled to some extent 1 year after the accident. Therefore, in addition to the personal and family costs, the social and economic effects of caring for these patients are massive.

Head injury classification

Head injuries and head-injured patients may be classified in a number of different ways using clinical or radiological criteria.

- The injury to the brain may be 'primary' or 'secondary'. A primary injury is that occurring at the scene at the time of the accident and it is generally not in the realm of the intensive care physician to influence this. Secondary injury is that injury occurring any time after the initial injury, and this may be influenced by doctors and ambulance staff at the scene, and doctors in the accident and emergency department and on the critical care unit
- Brain injury may be due to blunt or penetrating trauma. The type of trauma will vary with the location. In the UK at present penetrating brain trauma is still less common than blunt injury from road traffic accidents and falling downstairs
- Head injuries may be 'open' or 'closed', as for any other bony trauma. Recalling the physiology stated above, it should be remembered that open injuries may allow

Table 11.1 *Glasgow Coma Score*

Eye opening	Spontaneous	4
	To speech	3
	To pain	2
	Nil	1
Best motor response	Obeys commands	6
	Localizes pain	5
	Withdraws to pain	4
	Abnormal flexion	3
	Extensor response	2
	Nil	1
Verbal response	Oriented	5
	Confused conversation	4
	Inappropriate words	3
	Incomprehensible sounds	2
	Nil	1

decompression of the brain substance through the fracture site, which may permit survival but with severe disability.

The commonest scoring system used to assess head injury patients is the Glasgow Coma Score (GCS) (Table 11.1), as described by Teasdale and Jennet in 1974.[2] This 13-point scoring system (minimum value 3; see Table 11.1) has been well validated to allow prognosis to be estimated and has been incorporated into many other scoring systems, such as APACHE II (see Chapter 1). It is usual that a score of 13 or more indicates a minor head injury, 9–12 a moderate head injury, and less than 9 a severe head injury.

Other scoring systems include the Virginia Prediction Tree (see Chapter 1), which combines the type of injury with the age of the patient and surgical intervention to allow a prediction of likely outcome to be made.[3]

The Glasgow Outcome Score (GOS)[4] was developed to allow comparison of head-injured patients at intervals following the original incident. This scale divides patients into one of five groups:

- Death
- Vegetative state
- Severe disability (unable to support themselves for 24 hours in society)
- Moderate disability (significant restrictions in lifestyle or work capacity)
- Mild or no disability (resumed previous lifestyle).

Although this is a fairly crude clinical assessment it is important because it allows comparison of different treatment regimens on an objective outcome scoring system. The

GOS is normally applied at intervals between 3 and 12 months after the incident. Using this scale, Thornhill *et al.*[5] have shown that from a cohort of 73 severely head-injured patients, 1 year after the accident, 38 per cent were dead, 29 per cent had severe disability, 19 per cent had moderate disability, and 14 per cent had made a good recovery.

INTRACRANIAL PATHOLOGY FOLLOWING TRAUMATIC BRAIN INJURY

A traumatic brain injury may result in a wide range of pathological processes, some of which are amenable to neurosurgery and some of which are not. These include the following.

Cerebral contusions

These are essentially areas of 'bruising' within the brain tissue, with relatively localized cellular damage, haemorrhage and oedema. The size may vary from large haemorrhagic regions to small 'point' contusions. The effects of a contusion on outcome will depend on its location, size, and any pressure effect it may generate on local brain tissue. As with contusions elsewhere in the body the maximal swelling and bleeding associated with these is often not seen until up to 72 hours after the initial insult. Classically, a contusion is associated with a central area of damaged tissue surrounded by an area of oedema, termed a penumbra. The tissue in the penumbra is the region in which tissue viability is threatened but not actually lost. Secondary brain injury is often associated with extension of the central damaged tissue into the penumbra, with further loss of function. Thus, aggressive management techniques are aimed at preserving the function of the penumbra.

Diffuse axonal injury

This is depicted by loss of grey/white differentiation on the CT scan and is caused by widespread shearing forces that occur as the brain undergoes stresses such as rapid deceleration. It is a common finding in patients presenting with a severe head injury and constitutes around 50 per cent of all primary traumatic brain lesions. It is often associated with severe impairment of consciousness, starting from the moment of impact, and the clinical outcome is poor. The pathological lesions are small, multiple and bilateral, typically found in the white matter, corpus callosum and brainstem. The characteristic microscopic features are multiple intra-axonal retraction balls with numerous perivascular haemorrhages.

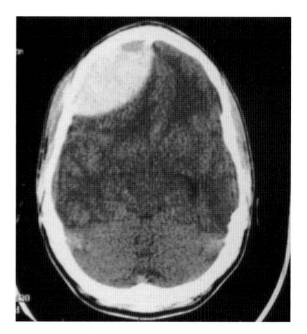

Figure 11.3 CT scan of extradural haematoma

Traumatic subarachnoid haemorrhage (SAH)

This is bleeding associated with tearing of an intracranial vessel caused by shaking of the brain tissue in a traumatic situation. This haemorrhage may be associated with vasospasm in the same way as non-traumatic SAH. Evidence for the beneficial effects of nimodipine in this situation has been limited by extremely poor-quality studies, and it cannot be recommended unless vasospasm has been demonstrated by angiography or alternative imaging techniques.

Extradural or subdural haematomata

These occur frequently following trauma, and if bilateral the associated localizing signs may be absent. Extradural haematomata (Figure 11.3) may have relatively little underlying associated 'brain damage', although if sufficiently large, brain compression and ischaemia may occur, and early evacuation is generally associated with a good outcome.

Subdural haematomata (Figure 11.4) develop within the potential space between the pia–arachnoid and the dura mater. Differential movement of the brain and adherent cortical veins with respect to the skull and attached dural sinuses, generates tensile and shear-strain forces which tear the cortical veins that bridge this potential space. The cortical bridging veins are especially vulnerable to rapid stretching, and for this reason subdural haematomata are particularly common in patients who have fallen, where head acceleration/deceleration

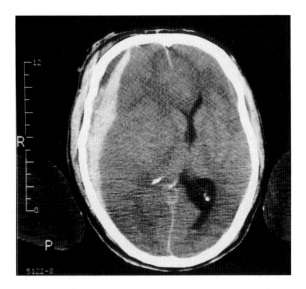

Figure 11.4 CT scan of subdural haematoma

is of brief duration and associated with a high-impact force. Because these haematomata are, by definition, under the dura there is frequent involvement of brain tissue and the prognosis is much worse than for extradural haematomata. Surgical evacuation will usually be performed if there is evidence of any mass effect or raised intracranial pressure (ICP) to which the haematoma may be contributing.

MANAGEMENT OF THE PATIENT WITH A SEVERE HEAD INJURY

Because the majority of patients with minor or moderate head injuries are not cared for on the intensive care unit only the management of the severely head-injured patient will be described in detail. However, many of the principles of management will also be applicable to the less injured patient. This chapter will concentrate on isolated head injuries; for details on multiple trauma management see Chapter 10. For the purposes of this chapter, management will be classified as either basic (applicable to any hospital in the UK) or advanced (generally only applicable to a neurointensive care unit).

Basic management of the severely head-injured patient

To a large extent, the basic management of a patient following a severe head injury should follow standard ATLS principles. Close attention needs to be paid to maintenance of the airway (with adequate cervical spine control), breathing and circulation. If a patient has a GCS less than 9 they are, by definition,

not able to protect their own airway and a definitive airway (endotracheal tube or tracheostomy) should be placed as soon as possible. Mechanical ventilation should be commenced at the earliest opportunity to maintain both adequate oxygenation and ventilation (carbon dioxide removal). It has been well documented that even transient periods of hypoxia may contribute to a significantly worse neurological outcome, and stringent attempts should be made to avoid this. Both hypercarbia and hypocarbia are also associated with detrimental cerebral effects, and the arterial carbon dioxide partial pressure should be maintained in the range of 4–5 kPa unless advanced monitoring indicates that this should be altered.

In cardiovascular system management, strict attention should be paid to avoiding hypotension and the maintenance of blood pressure within the normal range. Again, there is good evidence that even a single episode of hypotension (systolic BP <80 mmHg) is associated with a considerably worse outcome.

In addition to these basic 'ABC' principles, two additional factors require particular attention in the head-injured patient. These are maintenance of normoglycaemia and maintenance of normothermia. As noted above, the provision of glucose-containing solutions to an injured brain may result in increased metabolic activity without the ability to increase the local cerebral blood flow to supply adequate oxygenation, resulting in increased anaerobic respiration. This results in the increased production of lactic acid and a further local decrease in pH, worsening the tissue acidosis and increasing tissue damage. Clearly, hypoglycaemia should be avoided.

An increase in body temperature will result in an increase in cerebral metabolic activity and oxygen requirements. Thus, strict attention needs to be paid to maintaining normothermia.

Thus, the initial principles of head injury management can be summarized as the maintenance of normal PaO_2, $PaCO_2$, mean arterial pressure, blood sugar and temperature.

All patients admitted to hospital following a severe head injury should have a CT scan of the brain to identify the intracranial pathology. This allows the determination of surgically correctable lesions in addition to giving some information about prognosis. All severely head-injured patients transferred to the CT scanner should be accompanied by a suitably trained, airway-competent doctor who understands the essential principles of head injury management. During the transfer the patient should have adequate monitoring to ensure that the five basic principles of management can be maintained. However, if the patient does have other injuries, e.g. to the chest, abdomen or pelvis, it may be essential to manage these *before* imaging the brain to allow the basic principles to be maintained. In other words, no patient who is cardiovascularly unstable should be taken for brain imaging until the blood pressure has been stabilized. This may mean the patient having a laparotomy prior to the brain scan. Equally, following significant chest trauma a transport ventilator may not manage to ventilate the patient's lungs adequately, in which case they should be managed on an intensive care unit until such a time as safe transfer can be achieved.

Advanced management

Advanced management involves the use of alternative monitoring and management strategies, including neurosurgery. This therefore tends to be limited to centres that provide a neurosurgical service, and there is some evidence to support the fact that following a severe head injury the patient is likely to have a better outcome if managed in a unit that looks after a significant number of similar patients and has evidence-based protocols in use for each stage of management.[6]

ADDITIONAL MONITORING

Advanced management depends more on information gained from monitoring than on basic physiological parameters. Currently there are a number of devices available, as described below; however, the relative merits of these monitors, and whether combining information from multimodal monitoring results in a synergistic rather than an additive benefit, is difficult to define at present.

Intracranial pressure monitoring

Guidelines from the Brain Trauma Foundation[7] suggest that there are inadequate data to make intracranial pressure (ICP) monitoring a treatment standard in the early management of severe traumatic brain injury. However, the following guideline is suggested: 'Intracranial pressure monitoring is appropriate in patients with severe head injury with an abnormal admission CT scan. An abnormal CT scan of the head is one that reveals haematomas, contusions, oedema or compressed basal cisterns'.

Intracranial pressure may be monitored from various sites using different devices. A solid-state intraparenchymal monitor is associated with a reduced risk of intracranial infections, but whereas this is not true of an intraventricular catheter the latter will allow withdrawal of CSF and thereby provide an alternative method of ICP control. Subdural catheters have also been used but tend to carry the risk of infection without the potential benefits of CSF aspiration. Extradural monitoring is associated with a lower risk of infection, but the pressure reading may not be as accurate as with an intraparenchymal device. The preferred site for the ICP monitoring device is the right frontal lobe (non-dominant hemisphere, minimal essential brain tissue, away from the major cerebral venous sinuses). However, there may or may not be tissue involved in the head injury, and interpretation of the pressure readings may be difficult if the monitor is sited in the middle of an expanding contusion.

The principal uses of ICP monitoring are to guide therapies to control the ICP, to allow calculation and manipulation of a cerebral perfusion pressure (see CPP protocols below), and to identify patients in whom a significant increase in ICP over a short time may indicate a rapidly expanding haematoma that would be amenable to surgical intervention.

There is evidence to suggest that following a severe head injury, a high ICP is associated with a poorer outcome than a normal ICP. The critical ICP at which action should be taken to limit further rises is not clear and varies between 15 and 30 mmHg. However, 20 mmHg seems to be accepted as the treatment threshold by a large number of authorities. A management protocol for patients with an ICP >20 mmHg is discussed below.

However, it is possible that the combination of intracranial pressure and mean arterial pressure is more important than the ICP alone. Thus the cerebral perfusion pressure (CPP) may be a more appropriate measure (and target) than ICP, where CPP is taken as MAP − ICP.

ICP measurement has never been subjected to a randomized double-blind study, and to do so would be extremely difficult. However, there is a substantial body of evidence which suggests that monitoring helps in early detection of mass lesions (e.g. extradural or subdural haematomata), may limit the indiscriminate use of therapies to control ICP, which in themselves may be harmful, and may be helpful in determining prognosis. Because one of the main benefits of monitoring is to target early neurosurgical intervention, there is some debate about the place of monitoring the ICP in non-neurosurgical centres. This is not the place to discuss all the facets of this debate. Suffice to say, the protagonists suggest that ICP monitoring allows more appropriate management of severely head-injured patients; an increase in ICP that results in neurosurgical intervention occurs only relatively rarely; and local monitoring removes some of the requirements to transfer relatively unstable patients to over-burdened regional neurosurgical centres. Antagonists suggest that waiting for the ICP to increase and for a surgically amenable lesion to be identified prior to transfer puts these patients, even if a relatively small group, at an unnecessarily high risk of delaying potentially life-saving surgery.

Transcranial Doppler ultrasonography

The Doppler principle was described in 1842 by Christian Doppler to a meeting of the Royal Bohemian Society. One hundred years later, this principle was being used to develop ultrasound devices, and by the 1960s these were in regular medical use. However, it was only in the 1990s that Rune Aaslid made significant alterations to a Doppler device to allow assessment of intracranial blood flow velocity.

Transcranial Doppler ultrasonography (TCD) uses a 2 MHz pulsed wave signal applied to one of three 'acoustic windows'. These are the orbit, the foramen magnum or, most commonly, the temporal bone between the tragus of the ear and the lateral canthus of the eye above the zygoma. From these positions, all the basal cerebral arteries can be insonated; however, the middle cerebral artery (MCA) is the most common vessel studied. The normal MCA flow velocity is in the range of 30–70 cm/s. The signal returning to the ultrasound probe can be 'range gated', allowing its depth of origin to be determined by the operator. Normally the signal received from the MCA is approximately 4.5–5.5 cm from the probe. Each artery has specific Doppler characteristics that allow its identification. For example, when the MCA is studied from the ipsilateral temporal window, the flow is towards the probe, the vessel can be followed for at least 1 cm, and compression of the ipsilateral common carotid artery reduces the MCA flow velocity.

Interpretation of the MCA flow velocity may be confounded by a number of factors. These include movement of the probe with alteration of the insonation angle, significant changes in the patient's haemoglobin concentration, and changes in the diameter of the vessel being studied. If the vessel diameter remains constant, the increase in flow velocity is proportional to the increase in blood flow (true hyperaemia). If, however, the vessel diameter is decreased, the flow velocity will increase in proportion to the fourth power of the radius of the vessel (vasospasm). Thus, a small decrease in vessel diameter will result in a large increase in flow velocity.

TCD can be used to assess a number of features of the cerebral arterial circulation:

- **Vasospasm and hyperaemia** For reasons given above, TCD is a very sensitive method of detecting vasospasm. Traumatic subarachnoid haemorrhages following a severe brain injury are associated with vasospasm as occurs following non-traumatic SAH. However, following brain injury there is sometimes a state of increased cerebral perfusion (hyperaemia) in which blood flow is increased above its normal physiological requirement. In the case of true hyperaemia, the increase in cerebral blood flow may contribute to an increase in ICP and may be detrimental. A hyperaemic state may be controlled by elective hyperventilation to reduce the arterial carbon dioxide partial pressure to levels that are normally considered too low in brain injury management. However, allowing a

patient with vasospasm to be hyperventilated would be potentially very detrimental. Determining whether a high measured flow velocity (MCA flow velocity > 120 cm/s) is due to vasospasm or hyperaemia was the subject of some work by Lindegaard et al.[8] These authors proposed that if the flow velocity measured in the MCA is threefold or more greater than that measured in the internal carotid artery, the cause is most likely to be due to vasospasm. If the increased flow velocity in the MCA is less than three times greater than that measured in the internal carotid artery, the cause is most likely to be due to hyperaemia

- **Intracranial pressure** As the ICP increases, the flow velocity waveform changes in a characteristic way. First, diastolic flow velocity is decreased and then lost. Second, the systolic flow velocity is decreased, and is described as 'short systolic flow'. Third, reverberant flow is seen, with reverse flow being seen in diastole. Finally, the flow velocity waveform is lost completely. Unfortunately, although these changes follow a distinct pattern, they only start to occur at a relatively high ICP, probably >50 mmHg. Therefore, TCD cannot be used to determine ICP at levels that are within the normal clinical range. This may be useful, however, to corroborate the findings of an ICP monitor, if thought to be reading inappropriately high, or to determine the extent of intracranial hypertension following a CT scan which may avoid the placement of an ICP monitoring device

- **Estimated cerebral perfusion pressure** In view of the difficulty of using TCD to measure ICP, and the potential benefits of measuring CPP, Czosnyka and colleagues[9] have examined the use of TCD to estimate cerebral perfusion pressure. This calculation is given by the following equation:

$$eCPP = (BPm \cdot Vd/Vm) + 14$$

in which eCPP is the estimated CPP, BPm is the mean arterial blood pressure, Vd is the diastolic flow velocity and Vm the time-averaged mean flow velocity.

Using this formula, and comparing findings with the measured CPP, these workers found that the eCPP accurately reflected changes in measured CPP over time. They also found that the estimated CPP was less than 10 mmHg different from the measured CPP in 71 per cent of readings, and there was less than a 15 mmHg difference in 84 per cent of comparisons. Although this is not currently routine in clinical practice, the ability to predict CPP non-invasively is very attractive and is very likely to be developed in the future

- **Arterial cerebral pressure autoregulation** Normally, the blood flow to the brain remains constant over a wide range of perfusion pressures. Following a traumatic brain injury, the autoregulation curve is shifted to the right. Thus, the lower limit of pressure for maintaining a constant flow may be increased. In addition, the autoregulatory plateau may be shortened or lost altogether. It would seem intuitive that the brain would maintain more appropriate blood flow if autoregulation were to be preserved. TCD may be used to determine whether autoregulation is intact or not using one of two well-described techniques. Static autoregulation may be assessed by measuring the flow velocity at a baseline perfusion pressure. The perfusion pressure can then be increased by 20 per cent using drugs such as phenylephrine or norepinephrine, and a further estimation of MCA flow velocity can be made. If the flow velocity increases in proportion to the change in perfusion pressure, autoregulation is not intact. If flow velocity remains unchanged autoregulation is intact. Alternatively, dynamic autoregulation may be determined by compression of the ipsilateral common carotid artery for 10 s. During compression, in the normal state small vessel dilatation will occur, resulting in a transient hyperaemic response on release. The ratio of the flow velocity immediately following release compared to that immediately prior to compression may be used to assess the autoregulatory potential. A normal ratio would have a value of approximately 1.4, and autoregulation is impaired at values less than 1.2.

Although maintenance of autoregulation appears inherently sensible there are no reports in the literature confirming that this approach alters outcome following a severe brain injury.

In summary, TCD has the benefits of being a non-invasive bedside assessment of cerebral artery flow velocity. However, its use remains restricted by difficulty in interpreting the findings and lack of evidence to support management protocols based on the measured flow velocities.

JUGULAR VENOUS BULB OXIMETRY

This technique involves passing an oximetric catheter retrogradely into the internal jugular vein so that the tip sits in the jugular bulb. The mixed venous oxygen saturation ($SjvO_2$) of the blood passing through the bulb can then be measured. The accuracy of the technique depends on careful calibration of the device prior to insertion, and appropriate positioning of the catheter tip. The facial vein drains into the internal jugular vein in varying positions, but it may be as close as 5 cm to the jugular bulb. The oxygen saturation of blood from the facial vein clearly does not represent blood passing through the intracranial circulation. Thus, insertion of the catheter involves passing it as far as possible in a retrograde direction and then taking a lateral X-ray of the cervical spine to confirm that the tip of the catheter is lying opposite the body of the first cervical vertebra.

The estimation of $SjvO_2$ was introduced by Cruz and colleagues in the late 1980s and has been used as the basis of an algorithm to manipulate cerebral blood flow in patients with severe head injuries. In a review of use of jugular bulb oxygen saturation estimation over 10 years these authors compared the outcome of patients managed with manipulation of $SjvO_2$ with patients managed using a cerebral perfusion pressure maintenance protocol only (see below).[10] They found that the mortality in the group actively managed according to the $SjvO_2$ was 9 per cent, compared to 30 per cent in those managed with cerebral perfusion pressure maintenance only. Figures 11.5–11.8 summarize a model of cerebral microcirculatory and oxygen metabolic physiology. Using this model the management protocol using the $SjvO_2$ may be summarized as follows.

If the ICP was increased (>20 mmHg) and associated with normal or decreased cerebral extraction of oxygen (Figure 11.8), optimized hyperventilation was gradually increased to aim for simultaneous normalization of both oxygen extraction and ICP. If the ICP was increased with normal or increased cerebral oxygen extraction (Figure 11.7), mannitol boluses were administered until both parameters were normalized. If mannitol administration had resulted in hyperosmolality or hyperventilation had been optimized, additional management strategies included the administration of barbiturates or the institution of hypothermia. However, if all medical management methods failed the patients then underwent a decompressive craniectomy.

Although these results indicate the potential use of jugular bulb oxygen saturation monitoring in head-injured patients this technique is still not in universal use. This may be because of difficulty in ensuring that the catheter tip is in the correct position, concerns about the effect of facial vein oxygen confounding the findings, concerns about the reliability of the measurements over time, and the effects of the therapeutic interventions on the jugular bulb saturation. In addition, jugular bulb oximetry is only able to give a global guide to oxygenation and oxygen uptake, and local changes in the penumbra of a contusion may be completely obscured by the remainder of the brain tissue function.

BRAIN TISSUE OXYGEN PARTIAL PRESSURE MONITORING

Two sensors capable of monitoring brain tissue oxygen partial pressure are now available commercially: the Paratrend catheter (Diametrics Medical, High Wycombe, UK) and the Licox catheter (Gesellschaft fur medizinische Sondentechnik mbH, Kiel, Germany). These have been placed in brain tissue via a specialized ICP bolt and brain tissue oxygen partial pressures have been measured in a number of studies. The advantage of these measurement systems is that they allow continuous monitoring of cerebral oxygenation and early detection of ischaemia. The potential disadvantage is that

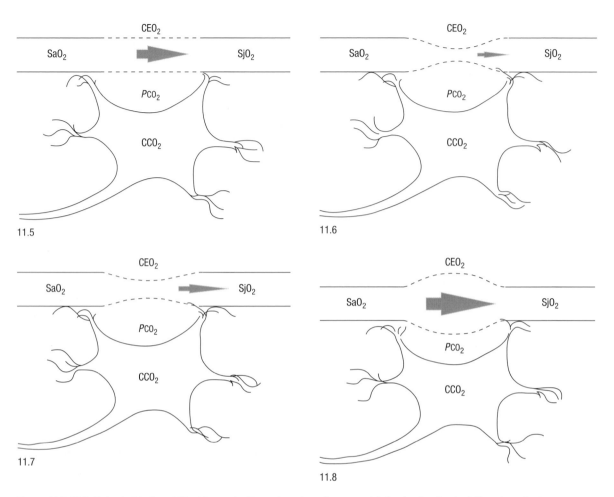

Figures 11.5–11.8 Clinicophysiologic model involving cerebral haemodynamics and oxygen metabolism in a functional unit. Normal coupling between cerebral blood flow and oxygen consumption in normal (awake) subjects. With normal neuronal aerobic metabolism, combined oxygen and glucose consumption lead to normal CO_2 production, which in turn mediates normal microcirculatory diameter. As cerebral blood flow and oxygen consumption are normally coupled, cerebral extraction of oxygen remains in the normal range. CCO_2, cerebral consumption of oxygen inside the neuron; PCO_2, partial tension of CO_2 in the interstitial and pericapillary space; SaO_2, arterial oxyhaemoglobin saturation; SjO_2, venous (also jugular) oxyhemoglobin saturation; CEO_2, cerebral extraction of oxygen, which represents the balance between cerebral consumption of oxygen and cerebral blood flow. Arrow represents cerebral blood flow. Republished with kind permission from: Cruz J. The first decade of continuous monitoring of jugular bulb oxyhemoglobinsaturation: management strategies and clinical outcome. *Crit Care Med* 1998; **26**(2): 344–51.

Figure 11.5 Normal coupling between cerebral blood flow and oxygen consumption in normal (awake) subjects. With normal neuronal aerobic metabolism, combined oxygen and glucose consumption lead to normal CO_2 production, which in turn mediates normal microcirculatory diameter. As cerebral blood flow and oxygen consumption are normally coupled, cerebral extraction of oxygen remains in the normal range.

Figures 11.6, 11.7 and 11.8 Illustrate the three conditions that may be found in patients presenting with acute traumatic coma, where cerebral consumption of oxygen is decreased. Accordingly, decreased neuronal aerobic metabolism and CO_2 production lead to a physiologic and proportional decrease in cerebral blood flow (intact metabolic autoregulation), and therefore the cerebral extraction of oxygen remains normal (Figure 11.6), indicating good balance between blood flow and oxygen consumption. If cerebral blood flow is low relative to decreased oxygen consumption, cerebral extraction of oxygen increases to compensate for the excessive decrease in cerebral blood flow (Figure 11.7). This latter condition has been termed 'oligaemic cerebral hypoxia'. Conversely, if cerebral blood flow is high relative to decreased oxygen consumption (defective metabolic autoregulation), cerebral extraction of oxygen decreases (Figure 11.8); this condition has been termed 'relative cerebral hyperperfusion,' or 'luxury perfusion'.

the tissue oxygen measurements made are extremely localized, within a few millimetres of the probe, which samples over approximately a 2 cm length. Both probes have a diameter of less than 1 mm. Both probes need time to stabilize in the brain tissue before accurate readings can be taken. This is normally achieved in under 2 hours. In patients with traumatic brain injury, low brain oxygen partial pressures ($PbrO_2$) have been recorded in more than 50 per cent of cases during the first 24 hours after injury.[11] The depth and duration of the tissue hypoxia recorded in this time are related to outcome and are independent predictors of both unfavourable outcome and death. These studies have defined that the critical lower limit for the $PbrO_2$ is 2 kPa, and the longer values remain lower than this the greater the likelihood of death. Many factors potentially affect the $PbrO_2$ measurement; they include: which probe is being used; whether the probe is positioned in normal or damaged tissue; arterial PO_2 and PCO_2 values; relative position of the probe in grey or white matter; and the presence of vasculature local to the probe, including local venules if functional shunting and microcirculatory disruption have occurred. Thus, the use of this technology remains in the very early stages of understanding the measurements that are being made and how to manipulate variables that will affect $PbrO_2$ and have a positive impact on outcome. However, it is very likely that many more studies will be published using this technology in the next few years.

MICRODIALYSIS

Cerebral microdialysis is a technique that has been developed in humans since the late 1980s. Until now it has been essentially a research tool, but recent advances in this technique mean that it may be used in routine clinical work before too long. The underlying principle of microdialysis is that a fine tube (<1 mm diameter) lined with a polyamide dialysis membrane is placed directly into the brain. A physiological salt solution is infused into the tube at extremely low flow rates (0.1–2.0 μL/min). At the distal end of the tube the salt solution passes back through the outer lumen lined with the dialysis membrane, and chemicals in the extracellular fluid of the brain are able to diffuse into the salt solution according to their molecular weight, charge and concentration. The resultant fluid is collected into vials that can be changed at 10–60-minute intervals. However, owing to the very low infusion rate extremely small volumes of fluid are obtained for analysis (<10 μL). Analysis can be performed by high-performance liquid chromatography but this is a slow laboratory-based technique. More recently, a commercial piece of equipment has been made available for microdialysis analysis (CMA600 Microdialysis Analyser, CMA Microdialysis,

Stockholm, Sweden) that allows online analysis of samples. Many chemicals can be measured using this technique, including lactate, glucose[12] and amino acids such as glutamate and aspartate (excitatory amino acids). These have been examined in patients following traumatic brain injury,[13] but currently the findings are all based on very small series. However, it is very likely that data obtained from this technology may affect head injury management in the near future.

Management protocols for severe traumatic brain injury

Two contrasting management protocols have been presented in the literature. The most commonly used is based on the maintenance of CPP. However, an alternative has been proposed by a team of doctors from Lund, Sweden, which has been suggested to have superior outcomes. When applying these algorithms to patient management it should be remembered that a traumatic brain injury is not a *static* event that occurs and resolves after a period of time; rather, it is an *evolving* event, i.e. the pathology and the pathophysiology change over time, from an initial period of hypoperfusion to relative hyperperfusion, prior to returning to a normal state. Thus, the proposed algorithms may both have appropriate uses at different stages of the evolution of the injury.

CEREBRAL PERFUSION PRESSURE MANAGEMENT (ROSNER)

In 1995 Rosner *et al.* published a study in which 158 patients with severe traumatic brain injury were managed with vasopressors (norepinephrine or phenylephrine) to maintain the CPP >70 mmHg.[14] The outcome of these patients was compared to that of ICP-based management protocol patients collected in the Traumatic Coma Data Bank (TCDB). The study found that in all GCS categories morbidity and mortality improved with CPP management compared to the TCDB data. The overall mortality in this group was 29 per cent, with 2 per cent remaining vegetative.

A number of studies have been performed to further validate this management protocol. However, there have been no randomized controlled studies allowing this to be confirmed as the optimal standard of care.

LUND

In 1998 neurocritical care physicians in Lund, Sweden, questioned the use of CPP-targeted treatment protocols.[15] They suggested that high CPP management may have the adverse effects of triggering the development of vasogenic brain oedema through forces striving toward the classic Starling equilibrium and causing an increase in ICP. The increase in

ICP will counteract the desired increase in CPP and the patient will come closer to a state of herniation. They also hypothesized that the use of vasopressor agents may enhance the vasoconstrictor response that is likely to be present following trauma. They proposed a treatment protocol that included the following:

- Preservation of normal colloidal-absorbing force
- A decease in intracapillary pressure by antihypertensive therapy using clonidine and metoprolol
- A simultaneous moderate constriction of the precapillary resistance vessels with low-dose thiopentone and dihydroergotamine
- Optimal general intensive care – fluids to maintain normovolaemia, monitoring of lung function, nutrition and electrolyte supplementation.

They compared 53 patients managed according to this protocol with historic controls and found mortality to be significantly lower in the protocol group (8 per cent) and the ratio of patients with vegetative or severe disability about the same (13 per cent), resulting in a higher ratio of patients having a favourable outcome. Further studies have been performed using this protocol, with similar results. However, there are no randomized controlled trials of this protocol compared to CPP management, and many neurointensive care physicians remain wary of the Lund protocol.

As stated already, the maintenance of cerebral perfusion pressure remains the most commonly followed protocol, and an algorithm for the management of a patient with a severe traumatic brain injury based on this is shown in Figure 11.9. This combines many of the principles discussed above. The rationale for the options used to manage an increased ICP is discussed below.

Management options for increased ICP

Whatever the protocol being used to manage the severely head-injured patient it is generally agreed that the higher the ICP, the worse the outcome. The Brain Trauma Foundation guidelines suggest that the ICP should be maintained below 20 mmHg.[7] A number of algorithms may be used to achieve this, commonly including the following medical and surgical practices.

MEDICAL

- **Positioning** The patient should be nursed in a head-up (approximately 30°) position to improve venous drainage and reduce ICP. In order to do this clearance of the integrity of the spine is essential, and good working protocols for early clearance should be in place

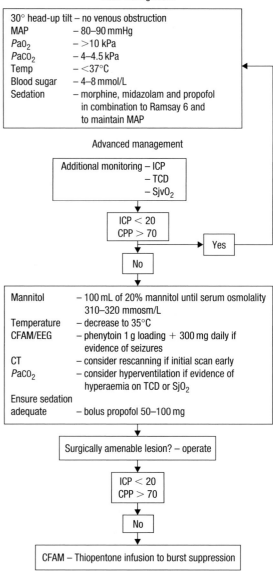

Figure 11.9 Algorithm for the management of the severely head-injured patient

- **Sedation and neuromuscular blockade** Deep sedation (to Ramsay score of 6 or equivalent) is used to reduce cerebral metabolism. In some units neuromuscular blockers are used as standard, whereas in others they are used when ICP remains difficult to control, all other medical measures are in place, and there is a concern that muscle activity may be contributing to the pressure. If the ICP remains difficult to control a thiopentone infusion may be used in conjunction with electroencephalogram (EEG) monitoring to bring about burst suppression. Once this is achieved other sedation agents can be withdrawn

- **Ventilation and carbon dioxide control** The objective of mechanical ventilation is to maintain $PaCO_2$ at 4–4.5 kPa. If ICP becomes dramatically raised, short-term hyperventilation may be used to gain control while other measures (e.g. mannitol) take effect
- **Mannitol and osmolality management** An increase in serum osmolality will result in a tendency to reduce brain tissue water and hence ICP. A serum osmolality of 300–310 mmol is targeted in the authors' unit, achieved by incremental 100 mL doses of mannitol 20 per cent
- **Seizure control** Both clinical and subclinical seizures may have dramatic effects on cerebral metabolism and ICP and should be prevented. In patients receiving neuromuscular blocking drugs or in whom subclinical seizures are suspected, EEG monitoring may aid detection of the fits
- **Temperature control and induced hypothermia** For reasons given above an increase in body temperature to >37°C should be actively avoided. Induced hypothermia remains contentious and there is conflicting evidence as to whether it affects outcome. There is some evidence that below 35°C brain tissue oxygenation may be impaired, but generally there is agreement that cooling will result in a reduction in intracranial pressure.

SURGICAL

- **CSF drainage** If hydrocephalus is demonstrated on CT scan in a patient with raised ICP, CSF drainage will usually decrease this pressure. In situations in which hydrocephalus is not demonstrated, great care must be exercised. In many patients the ventricles will be flattened and further supratentorial CSF drainage is not possible. Lumbar drainage of CSF may be dangerous and should only be performed following neurosurgical advice
- **Craniectomy** A bifrontal decompressive craniectomy may be performed to allow the brain tissue to expand and reduce the intracranial pressure. This technique has not been studied in a randomized trial, although scattered reports in the literature suggest that it may be beneficial
- **Lobectomy/removal of contusion** Either may be possible surgically, depending on the nature and location of the brain injury and whether there is midline shift that may be exacerbated by removing non-dominant tissue. Again, there is little evidence in terms of improved outcome to support this.

CEREBROVASCULAR DISEASE

The acute manifestations of cerebrovascular disease are known as stroke. Stroke is defined as an acute focal neurological deficit caused by cerebrovascular disease which lasts for more than 24 hours or causes death before 24 hours. Transient ischaemic attack (TIA) also causes focal neurology, but this resolves within 24 hours. In the UK stroke is responsible for 12 per cent of all deaths and is the most common cause of physical disability in adults.[16] The main causes of stroke are cerebral infarction due to thromboembolism and spontaneous intracranial haemorrhage, which may be intracerebral or subarachnoid, causing about 85 per cent and 15 per cent of strokes, respectively. The main risk factors are increasing age, hypertension, ischaemic heart disease, atrial fibrillation, smoking, obesity, some oral contraceptives, and raised cholesterol or haematocrit.[17] Stroke is a medical emergency and is a 'brain attack' as opposed to a 'heart attack', so that early aggressive treatment may result in improved outcome.[18,19]

Cerebral thrombosis and embolism

Thrombosis secondary to atherosclerosis is the major cause of occlusion in large cerebral arteries, and progressive plaque formation causes vessel narrowing, creating a nidus for platelet aggregation and thrombus formation. Ulceration and rupture of the plaque exposes its thrombogenic lipid core, thereby activating the clotting cascade. Hypertension and diabetes mellitus are common causes of smaller arterial thrombosis. Rarer causes include any disease resulting in vasculitis, vertebral or carotid artery dissection (either spontaneous or post-traumatic), or carotid occlusion by strangulation or systemic hypotension after cardiac arrest. Cerebral venous thrombosis, responsible for less than 1 per cent of strokes, may occur in hypercoagulable states such as dehydration, polycythaemia, thrombocythaemia, some oral contraceptive pills, protein C or S deficiency or antithrombin III deficiency, or vessel occlusion by tumour or abscess.

Embolism commonly occurs from thrombus or platelet aggregations overlying arterial atherosclerotic plaques, but 30 per cent of cerebral emboli will arise from thrombus in the left atrium or ventricle of the heart. This is commonly because of atrial fibrillation, left-sided valvular disease, recent myocardial infarction, chronic atrial enlargement or ventricular aneurysm. The presence of a patent foramen ovale or septal defects allows paradoxical embolism to occur. It may also occur as a complication of attempted coil embolization of cerebral aneurysms after subarachnoid haemorrhage.

Cerebral embolism may be characterized by sudden onset and the rapid development of complete neurological deficit, whereas in cerebral thrombosis there is initially no loss of consciousness or headache and the initial neurological deficit develops over several hours. There is no single clinical sign or symptom that can reliably distinguish between a thrombotic and an embolic event. The precise diagnosis requires a brain CT scan. The precise clinical presentation depends on the size of the infarcted area and its position in the brain.

Ideally, treatment for stroke patients should be coordinated within a Stroke Unit, as there is a 28 per cent reduction in mortality and disability at 3 months compared to patients treated on general medical wards.[20] In general only those patients with a compromised airway due to depressed conscious level or life-threatening cardiorespiratory disturbances require admission to medical or neurosurgical ICU. The immediate management goals relate to the prevention of progression of brain injury by preventing hypoxaemia and hypotension, and resuscitating the 'ABCs':

AIRWAY AND BREATHING

- Patients with GCS of 8 or less or those with absent gag will require intubation to preserve their airway and prevent aspiration. Where this requirement is likely to be prolonged, early tracheostomy should be considered
- Adequate oxygenation and ventilation should be confirmed by arterial blood gas analysis, and supplemental oxygen prescribed if there is any evidence of hypoxia
- If hypercarbia occurs then ventilatory support to achieve normocarbia is necessary to prevent exacerbation of cerebral oedema. Ventilatory support in such cases has been shown to result in improved prognosis.[21]

CIRCULATORY SUPPORT

- Some patients will have raised blood pressure on admission, presumably as an attempt by the vasomotor centre to improve cerebral perfusion. Hypertensive patients may have impaired autoregulation, and regional cerebral perfusion may be very dependent on blood pressure
- Too high a blood pressure may cause rebleeding, and too low a blood pressure may result in more ischaemic infarction
- Cardiac output should be maintained and any underlying cardiac pathology, such as failure, infarction and atrial fibrillation, treated appropriately.

METABOLIC SUPPORT

- Both hypo- and hyperglycaemia have been shown to worsen prognosis after acute stroke, and blood sugar levels should be maintained in the normal range[22]
- Nutritional support is essential, with early enteral feeding via a nasogastric tube. If bulbar dysfunction is prolonged then percutaneous gastrostomy may be necessary.

ANTICOAGULATION

- In theory, the use of anticoagulation reduces the propagation of thrombus and should prevent further embolism. In practice, the reduction in risk of further thromboembolic stroke is offset by a similar number of patients dying from cerebral or systemic haemorrhage as a result of anticoagulation[23]
- Anticoagulation can only be recommended in individuals where there is a high risk of recurrence, such as those with prosthetic heart valves, atrial fibrillation with thrombus, or those with thrombophilic disorders
- A brain CT scan must be obtained to exclude haemorrhage prior to commencing therapy. In patients with large infarcts there is always the risk of haemorrhage (haemorrhagic transformation) into the infarct, and early heparinization is best avoided
- Thrombolysis. The National Institute of Neurological Disorders and Stroke (NINDS) trial[24] showed a significant improvement in those patients given alteplase rather than placebo within 3 hours of acute stroke. However, this benefit was not found to be statistically significant in two European trials,[25,26] and the ATLANTIS trial[27] showed no significant benefit at 90 days in the alteplase group, together with an increased risk of intracranial haemorrhage. Currently thrombolysis cannot be recommended for acute ischaemic stroke in routine clinical practice, and further trials are required to identify those patients most likely to benefit
- Decompressive craniotomy is an option in young patients with large middle cerebral artery territory infarcts in the non-dominant hemisphere. Untreated these normally have a mortality of 80 per cent, and it is suggested that this procedure can reduce mortality to around 30 per cent but with residual neurological deficit. Other forms of surgical intervention proven to be effective are drainage of secondary hydrocephalus, and evacuation of haemorrhage into infarcted areas resulting in new compressive symptoms, especially in the posterior fossa.

Cerebral haemorrhage (Figure 11.10)

The most common cause is chronic systemic hypertension, although vessel rupture may also occur in malignant tumour neovasculature, vasculitic disease, mycotic aneurysms, amyloidosis, sarcoidosis, malignant hypertension, primary haemorrhagic disorders, and as a result of over-anticoagulation. Occasionally cerebral aneurysms or arteriovenous malformations (AVMs) may cause intracerebral haemorrhage without subarachnoid haemorrhage. Haemorrhage is usually due to rupture of a single vessel, and the size of the haemorrhage is

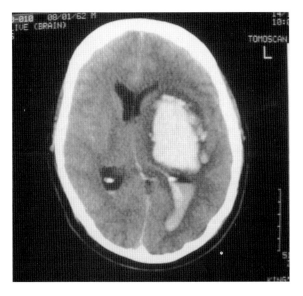

Figure 11.10 CT scan of intracerebral haematoma

influenced by the anatomical resistance of the site into which it occurs. The clinical signs are determined by the area of brain that is damaged. Usually there are no prodromal symptoms and there is a sudden onset of focal neurology or depressed level of consciousness. Headache and neck stiffness will occur in conscious patients if there is subarachnoid extension of the haemorrhage into the ventricles.

The management principles are identical to those for ischaemic stroke, but in addition a full coagulation screen must be performed and the administration of vitamin K, fresh frozen plasma, cryoprecipitate or other clotting factors directed by the results. Operative decompression[28] of the haematoma should be undertaken only in neurosurgical centres, and safe transfer must be assured if this is considered. The administration of mannitol prior to transfer should be discussed with the neurosurgical unit. There is no place for steroids, and hyperventilation to $PaCO_2$ of 3.5 or less to control raised intracranial pressure will have detrimental effects on blood flow in other areas of the brain. Ideally, clot evacuation within 6 hours maximum should be the goal. Not all intracerebral haematomata are amenable to surgery, and the CT scans should be reviewed by the neurosurgical unit, preferably via digital image link, prior to patient transfer.

Subarachnoid haemorrhage (SAH)[29,30]

This is bleeding into the subarachnoid space (Figure 11.11) and not into the brain parenchyma. Risk factors are the same as for stroke, but SAH patients are usually younger, the incidence peaking in the sixth decade, with a female to male ratio

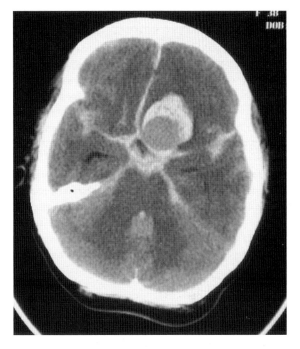

Figure 11.11 CT scan of large aneurysm of the left internal carotid artery and subarachnoid haemorrhage

of 1.6:1. Black people have twice the risk for SAH as whites. Between 5 and 20 per cent of patients with SAH have a positive family history, with first-degree relatives having a 3–7-fold risk whereas second-degree relatives have the same degree of risk as the general population. Specific inheritable disorders are rare and account for only a minority of all patients with SAH. Overall mortality is 50 per cent; 15 per cent of these die before reaching hospital, and up to 30 per cent of survivors have a residual deficit producing dependency.

The majority of cases of SAH (85 per cent) are caused by ruptured saccular (berry) aneurysms. The remainder are caused by non-aneurysmal perimesencephalic haemorrhage (10 per cent) and rarer causes such as arterial dissection, cerebral or dural arteriovenous malformations, mycotic aneurysm, pituitary apoplexy, vascular lesions at the top of the spinal cord, and cocaine abuse. Saccular aneurysms are not congenital, almost never occur in neonates and young children, and develop during later life. Classically there is a 'thunderclap' headache that develops in seconds, with half of patients describing its onset as instantaneous. This is followed by a period of depressed consciousness for less than an hour in 50 per cent of patients, with focal neurology in about 30 per cent. About a fifth of patients recall similar headaches, and these may have been due to 'warning leaks'. The degree of depression of consciousness depends upon the site and extent of the haemorrhage. Meningism – neck stiffness, photophobia,

Table 11.2 *World Federation of Neurological Surgeons (WFNS) grading*

WFNS grade	GCS	Motor deficit
I	15	Absent
II	14–13	Absent
III	14–13	Present
IV	12–7	Present or absent
V	3–6	Present or absent

vomiting and a positive Kernig's sign – are common signs in those patients with higher GCS. The clinical severity of SAH is often described by a grade, the most widely used being that developed by the World Federation of Neurological Surgeons (WFNS) (Table 11.2).[31] This, together with the extent of the haemorrhage and the age of the patient, gives some indication of the prognosis. The worse the grade and the older the patient, the worse the prognosis.

COMPLICATIONS

Acute hydrocephalus

- This may occur within the first 24 hours and should be suspected if there is a 1-point drop in GCS, sluggish pupillary responses, or bilateral downward deviation of the eyes ('sunset eyes'). If these signs occur the CT scan should be repeated, and if hydrocephalus is confirmed, or there is a large amount of intraventricular blood, then a ventricular drain may be inserted. This may provoke more bleeding and introduce infection

- Rebleeding may occur within the first few hours after admission and 15 per cent of patients may deteriorate from their admission status. They may require urgent intubation and resuscitation, but not all rebleeds are unsurvivable and such deterioration should be treated. The chance of rebleeding is dependent on the site of the aneurysm, the presence of clot, the degree of vasospasm, and the age and sex of the patient

- Cerebral vasospasm[32] is the narrowing of the cerebral blood vessels seen on angiography in response to SAH. It occurs in up to 70 per cent of patients, but not all of them will have symptoms. The use of transcranial Doppler (TCD) to estimate middle cerebral artery blood velocity has shown that a velocity of >120 cm/s correlates with angiographic evidence of vasospasm. Not all patients who have angiographic vasospasm or high Doppler velocities have symptoms

- Parenchymal haematoma may occur in up to 30 per cent of SAH following aneurysm rupture, and has a much worse prognosis than SAH alone. If there is mass effect with compressive symptoms then evacuation of the haematoma

and simultaneous clipping of the aneurysm may improve outcome

- Medical complications are very common (40 per cent)[33] and the mortality due to complications is almost the same as that due to the combined effects of the initial bleed, rebleeds and vasospasm. Medical complications include arrhythmias, neurogenic pulmonary oedema, liver dysfunction, pneumonia, renal failure, and syndrome of inappropriate ADH secretion (SIADH).

Early brain CT may enable localization of the arterial territory involved. Very rarely a false positive diagnosis may be made if there is severe generalized oedema resulting in venous congestion in the subarachnoid space. Small amounts of blood may not be detected and the incidence of false negative reports is around 2 per cent. It may be difficult to distinguish between post-traumatic SAH and primary aneurysmal SAH, which precipitates a fall in the level of consciousness that provokes an accident or fall. MRI scanning is particularly effective for localizing the bleed after 48 hours, when extravasated blood is denatured and provides a good signal on MRI.

Lumbar puncture is only necessary in those patients where the suspicion of SAH is high despite negative CT, or there is a need to exclude infection. There must be no raised intracranial pressure and at least 6 hours should have passed to give time for the blood in the CSF to lyse, enabling xanthochromia to develop.

Angiography enables identification of the aneurysm or other vascular abnormality. It is generally performed on patients who remain, or become, conscious after SAH. It is not without risk, as aneurysms may rupture during the procedure, and a meta-analysis has shown a complication rate of 1.8 per cent.

Intracranial pressure monitoring is of limited use in SAH patients, except those in whom hydrocephalus or parenchymal haematoma is present, and early detection of pressure increases may be the trigger for drainage or decompressive surgery.

MANAGEMENT

- General care of SAH is influenced by the grading, medical comorbidity or complications, and the timing or need for surgery. Patients with reduced GCS may need early intubation and ventilation simply for airway protection, whereas those with less severe symptoms require regular neurological observation, analgesia for headache, and bed rest prior to investigation and surgery

- Stress ulcer prophylaxis with sucralfate and DVT prophylaxis using compression stockings or boots should be used

- Seizures should be controlled with phenytoin or barbiturates, and if the patient is sedated and ventilated the use of an analysing cerebral function monitor should be considered to detect subclinical fitting
- Hyponatraemia should be treated with normal saline to keep electrolyte levels maintained in the normal range
- Blood pressure control is important to prevent hypertensive rebleeding and hypotensive infarction. If blood pressure exceeds 200 mmHg systolic or 100 mmHg diastolic, then empirically it would seem wise to reduce this pressure in SAH patients who have unclipped aneurysms. β-adrenergic blockers or calcium antagonists are the most widely used agents, as drugs producing cerebral vasodilation may increase ICP
- Vasospasm may be seen in about 70 per cent of SAH patients on angiography, but only about 30 per cent develop cerebral symptoms. Symptoms tend to occur between 4 and 14 days post bleed, which is the period when cerebral blood flow is decreased after SAH. One method of pre-empting vasospasm is the prescription of oral nimodipine 60 mg 4-hourly for 21 days, which has been shown to achieve a reduction in the risk of ischaemic stroke of 34 per cent.[34] Intravenous nimodipine should be used in patients who are not absorbing, but must be titrated against blood pressure to avoid hypotension. Low cerebral blood flow is known to worsen the outcome, and this results in the development of prophylactic hypertensive hypervolaemic haemodilution – so-called 'Triple-H Therapy'.[35] This involves fluid loading to achieve *hypervolaemia, haemodilution*, and vasopressor therapy to achieve *hypertension*. Very few centres use the strict protocol as originally described, but fluid loading rather than fluid restriction is the norm, and inotropes or vasopressors are used subsequently if neurological function decreases. Despite its widespread use, there remains no prospective randomized trial that demonstrates its utility. Where symptoms develop it is important to exclude other causes, such as rebleeding, hydrocephalus, hypoxaemia, hypercarbia or metabolic disorder
- Definitive treatment is by intravascular coiling during interventional radiology or by surgical clipping of the aneurysm. Intravascular coiling has a better outcome than surgery.[36] Not all aneurysms are amenable to coiling because of their size, position and shape. Complications include rupture, coil embolization, adjacent vessel occlusion and vasospasm
- Therapy of medical complications is obviously specific to the type of complication. Pneumonia may require CPAP or ventilatory support, together with directed antimicrobial therapy. ARDS requires lung protective/recruitment ventilatory strategies, and renal failure an appropriate means of renal replacement therapy. Arrhythmias require correction of trigger factors such as hypovolaemia and electrolyte or acid–base disturbances prior to use of the appropriate antiarrhythmic drug or DC cardioversion. Neurogenic pulmonary oedema may be associated with severe cardiogenic shock, which may require inotropic support or even temporary intra-aortic balloon counterpulsation. Where SIADH has been established for some time, then correction of low sodium must be slow to prevent central pontine myelinosis.

BRAINSTEM DEATH[37]

Brainstem death is defined as complete, irreversible loss of brainstem function, and in the UK the diagnosis is made according to well defined criteria and preconditions. Before such a diagnosis can be made certain preconditions must be met, reversible causes of apnoeic coma must be excluded, and brainstem areflexia and persistent apnoea must be confirmed.

Essential preconditions

- The patient must be in apnoeic coma (i.e. unresponsive and on a mandatory ventilation mode).
- There must be a positive diagnosis of coma and no doubt that there has been irreversible structural brain damage.

Essential exclusions

- No suspicion that the coma could be due to a reversible cause, e.g. the effects of drugs, metabolic or endocrine disturbance, or hypothermia (temperature $<35°C$)
- If the patient has received neuromuscular blocking drugs then neuromuscular function must be shown to have returned to normal by using a nerve stimulator.

Once these criteria have been met then the diagnosis of brainstem death can be considered. Brainstem death is a clinical diagnosis based on the absence of brainstem reflexes and apnoea despite a $PaCO_2 > 6.5$ kPa. Brainstem reflexes are absent if there is:

- No pupillary response to light (both direct and consensual) – cranial nerves II and III
- No corneal reflexes – cranial nerves V and VII
- No vestibulo-ocular reflex – cranial nerves III, VI and VIII. This reflex is examined by caloric testing. Otoscopy is performed to confirm that there is no obstruction of the external auditory canals, and ice-cold water is instilled into

each canal in turn while the eyelids are held open. There should be no eye movement of any kind

- No grimacing or motor response within the cranial nerve distribution on firm supraorbital pressure – cranial nerves V and VII. Peripheral responses to peripheral stimuli can occur at a reflex spinal level and do not preclude the diagnosis of brainstem death

- No gag and cough reflex in response to deep tracheal suction via the endotracheal tube – cranial nerves IX and X.

The oculocephalic reflex (doll's eye response) does not form an essential part of brainstem reflex testing as described in the original UK code. This reflex may only be tested if there is certainty that there is no biomechanical instability of the cervical spine. The head is rotated swiftly to one side and then the other from the midline, with the eyelids held open. If the eyes remain fixed centrally and move in tandem with the head (like the painted eyes on a china doll) then this brainstem reflex is absent.

Apnoea testing

This is done by preoxygenating the patient to avoid hypoxia and then disconnecting the ventilator. In addition, oxygen is insufflated into the trachea at 6–10 L/min. The chest and abdomen are then observed for signs of activity for at least 5 minutes. Difficulties may be encountered in patients with chronic pulmonary disease who run a higher than normal $PaCO_2$, in whom the starting $PaCO_2$ should be set at the upper end of their normal range or until they are mildly acidotic. For patients with a normal metabolic rate the $PaCO_2$ should rise at 3 mmHg/min, or just over 1 kPa every 3 minutes.

Testing for brainstem death should be performed by two doctors trained in the technique on two separate occasions to ensure that there is no observer error.

SPINAL CORD INJURY

Although spinal cord trauma affects central neurological tissue in a similar way to traumatic brain injury, the management principles are much simpler. In the UK there are 10–20 new cases of spinal cord injury per million population each year, of which 50–70 per cent are due to road traffic accidents.

If spinal trauma has resulted in damage to the spinal cord with neurological involvement, neurological recovery is extremely uncommon. Surgical fixation may be required to prevent further extension of cord damage. Spinal cord oedema may resolve to the extent that the level of the cord injury is decreased, but cord damage is likely to persist.

If the bones or ligaments of the spine are damaged, resulting in instability without clinical neurological compromise, urgent surgery is required to stabilize the spine and prevent cord damage occurring.

The use of glucocorticoids to limit spinal cord damage has been the subject of many studies; however, overall there is no evidence of benefit and their use remains controversial.[38] Thus, critical care management tends to focus on the respiratory and cardiovascular effects of spinal cord injury and less on the injury itself.

Respiratory effects

If the spinal cord is injured above the level of C5 (lower limit of diaphragmatic innervation) immediate ventilatory support is required. If the cord is injured below the level of T12 ventilatory support is rarely required, and if between C5 and T12 ventilation may be substantially compromised, requiring mechanical support. If ventilatory function depends on diaphragmatic function alone, there may be an acute decrease in forced vital capacity and maximal inspiratory force by about 70 per cent. The contribution of the abdominal muscles to expiration is also compromised, reducing expiratory force and the ability to cough and clear secretions. As spinal shock resolves and the paralysis of the intercostal muscles becomes spastic, the chest wall becomes rigid and no longer moves paradoxically with inspiration. Thus, ventilatory function improves, and by 5 months after the injury forced vital capacity and maximal inspiratory force may be 60 per cent of predicted preinjury levels. However, expiratory force is less affected by these long-term changes and remains at 33 per cent of the preinjury level.

In patients with spinal cord injuries who require tracheal intubation and ventilation, ventilator-associated pneumonia becomes a leading cause of death. Close attention must be paid to diagnosing and treating these infections, particularly in the early postinjury period. The majority of these patients will require ventilation for a significant period, but because of the chest wall changes that occur, as described above, many of those with a C4 injury or below will be weaned from mechanical ventilation in time. Factors that aid weaning in these patients include a tracheostomy, abdominal binders or the supine position and a weaning programme that includes periods of complete rest rather than continuously decreasing pressure support ventilation.

Cardiovascular effects

Loss of sympathetic outflow from the spinal cord results in hypotension, and if the high thoracic region is compromised cardiac arrhythmias may also occur. The first line of treatment for hypotension is volume resuscitation. However, if cardiac accelerator fibres have been interrupted, the heart may only be able to increase cardiac output by increasing stroke volume. If this is not attainable because of cardiac disease, congestive cardiac failure may ensue. Thus, if there is a likelihood of cardiac compromise, due to either ischaemic disease or traumatic contusion, cardiac output monitoring may be essential in guiding fluid and vasopressor therapy.

These patients are all at extremely high risk of thromboembolic disease. Prophylaxis should be started acutely and a combination of mechanical devices, compression stockings and pneumatic compression devices and anticoagulants should be used. Once they are over the acute stage patients will require long-term warfarin therapy.

ACUTE NEUROLOGICAL EMERGENCIES

These medical conditions can be divided into neuromuscular diseases, epilepsy and infective conditions. In this chapter only a brief summary will be given of the critical care management options for neuromuscular diseases and epilepsy: a neurological text should be consulted for detailed description of management. A recent resurgence of infective conditions, particularly in intravenous drug users, necessitates a brief description of the critical care management of those conditions that have been reported in recent months.

Neuromuscular diseases

MYASTHENIA GRAVIS

A myasthenic crisis – an exacerbation of myasthenia gravis with impairment of ventilation – occurs in approximately 15–20 per cent of patients with this condition, and this is associated with 4 per cent mortality. Endotracheal intubation may be required for respiratory failure due to ventilatory failure (vital capacity <15 mL/kg) or bulbar weakness resulting in failure to protect the airway. The standard medical treatment for a crisis is to start oral prednisone at a low dose, increasing over a few days. However, around half the patients managed in this way will deteriorate within the first week of treatment, necessitating ventilation. Maintenance of the cholinesterase inhibitors during treatment with glucocorticoids is controversial, because despite the potential benefit of increased muscle strength the altered, unpredictable metabolism during critical illness makes correct dosing very difficult. In addition, once adequate steroid doses are achieved there is potentially little extra gain from anticholinesterases.

Two other treatments are available, plasma exchange and intravenous immunoglobulin (IVIg) administration. Plasma exchange is effective when administered as five exchanges on alternate days. The standard course of IVIg is three to five administrations of 0.4 g/kg. One comparative clinical trial has shown no difference in outcome when the two treatment options were compared. However, IVIg does expose the patient to the risk of hepatitis B and C, as well as a theoretical risk of exposure to human immunodeficiency virus (HIV).

GUILLAIN–BARRÉ SYNDROME

This syndrome of muscle weakness is usually associated with infections that include campylobacter, cytomegalovirus and the Epstein–Barr virus. Two forms exist, the more common demyelinating, and axonal. As for myasthenia gravis, critical care management is usually associated with ventilatory failure requiring mechanical support, or to providing plasma exchange. In this condition, IVIg and plasma exchange have been shown to have similar efficacy, and combining the two treatments has not been shown to have any added benefit. Autonomic instability may also be a feature requiring careful use of fluid and vasoactive therapies.

EPILEPSY

Epilepsy only requires critical care management during periods of status epilepticus. This may be because of the nature of the treatment required to stop the seizure activity, or the effects of the medication given on conscious level and airway protection. Typically, epileptiform convulsions are treated with benzodiazepines, phenytoin and, if these fail, with barbiturates administered intravenously. There is some evidence to suggest that lorazepam should be the benzodiazepine used, although midazolam has also been used successfully. Phenytoin needs to be administered as a loading dose, normally 1 g, followed by 300 g daily. The therapeutic level for phenytoin is 10–20 mg/L, and this should be measured in critically ill patients, particularly because of the effects of other drugs that may be coadministered on liver cell function and drug metabolism. If the phenytoin level is within the therapeutic range and seizure activity continues an intravenous thiopentone infusion may be effective. However, this should only be administered in the presence of CFAM (cerebral function analyser monitor)/EEG monitoring, and the infusion should be titrated to eliminate seizure activity. The prolonged elimination half-life of thiopentone may mean that after a 48-hour infusion resulting in burst suppression, thiopentone levels only decrease to subsedation levels after 5–7 days.

Infective conditions

Infective conditions affecting neurological function to an extent that requires admission to critical care have been relatively rare in the UK in last few decades. However, very recently, intravenous drug users in particular have presented with two infective conditions, tetanus and botulism, which have required critical care admission on a number of occasions.

TETANUS

In the 6-month period from July 2003 20 cases of tetanus were reported in England, Scotland and Wales in intravenous drug users. All but two of these were graded as severe, defined as severe trismus and general spasticity, severe dysphagia and respiratory difficulties, and severe prolonged spasms, and required critical care admission.

Tetanus is caused by a neurotoxin produced by *Clostridium tetani,* which has an incubation period of between 3 and 21 days. Patients present with local fixed muscle rigidity and painful spasms confined to the area close to the site of injury, and usually progress to generalized tetanus in about 2 weeks. Generalized tetanus presents with symptoms ranging from mild trismus, neck stiffness and/or abdominal rigidity through to general spasticity, severe dysphagia, respiratory difficulties, severe painful spasm, opisthotonus and autonomic dysfunction. Laboratory confirmation of the disease may be with detection of tetanus toxin in a serum sample, isolation of tetanus bacillus from an infection site, or low or absent tetanus toxin antibodies in serum. However, none of these may be conclusive and the diagnosis may remain clinical.

The principles of management include intravenous tetanus immunoglobulin administration, wound debridement, antimicrobial agents, and vaccination following recovery. Tetanus immunoglobulin should be administered in a dose of 5000–10 000 IU units intravenously.

Airway management, if required, should be with a definitive airway. Although patients present with trismus, mouth opening is not usually impeded following induction of anaesthesia and the administration of a muscle relaxant drug. Management of generalized spasm may be difficult and a number of agents have been suggested, including intravenous magnesium infusion, intravenous dantrolene and intravenous sodium valproate.

BOTULISM

Botulism is a rare paralytic illness caused by *Clostridium botulinum.* It may be caused by eating foods containing the toxin, or by a wound being infected. The latter is the cause of the botulism that has been seen in drug users. Patients present with blurred vision, ptosis, slurred speech, dysphagia and muscle weakness. Ventilatory paralysis may occur if the early symptoms are untreated. Administration of antitoxin may prevent further deterioration, and wounds should be debrided surgically. The remainder of the treatment is supportive and, as for tetanus, this may require several weeks of critical care management.

SUMMARY

Neurologic critical care encompasses a wide range of pathologies, including surgical and medical conditions. The management of these conditions is dependent on an understanding of the appropriate physiology and pathophysiology. Recent advances in monitoring and clinical measurement have resulted in significant developments in the care of patients with neurological conditions, and these are likely to continue to progress swiftly in the next few years.

REFERENCES

1. National Institute of Clinical Excellence. *Triage, assessment, investigation: an early management of head injury in infants, children and adults. Clinical guideline 4, 2003.* London: Oaktree Press, 2003.
2. Teasdale G, Jennet B. Assessment of coma and impaired consciousness. *Lancet* 1974; **ii**: 81–4.
3. Choi SC, Muizelaar JP, Barnes TY, *et al.* Prediction tree for severely head-injured patients. *J Neurosurg* 1991; **75**: 251–5.
4. Jennet B, Snoeck J, Bond MR, *et al.* Disability after severe head injury: Observations on the use of the use of Glasgow Outcome Scale. *J Neurol Neurosurg Psychiatry* 1981; **44**: 285–93.
5. Thornhill S, Teasdale GM, Murray GD, *et al.* Disability in young people and adults one year after head injury: prospective cohort study. *BMJ* 2000; **320**: 1631–5.
6. Patel HC, Menon DK, Tebbs S, *et al.* Specialist neurocritical care and outcome from head injury. *Intensive Care Med* 2002; **28**: 547–53.
7. Brain Trauma Foundation and the American Association of Neurological Surgeons. *Management and prognosis of severe traumatic brain injury.* New York: Brain Trauma Foundation and the American Association of Neurological Surgeons, 2000.
8. Lindegaard KF, Nornes H, Bakke SJ, *et al.* Cerebral vasospasm diagnosis by means of angiography and blood velocity measurements. *Acta Neurochir* 1989; **100**: 12–24.
9. Czosnyka M, Matta BF, Smielewski P, *et al.* Cerebral perfusion pressure in head-injured patients: a noninvasive assessment using transcranial Doppler ultrasonography. *J Neurosurg* 1998; **88**: 802–8.
10. Cruz J. The first decade of continuous monitoring of jugular bulb oxyhaemoglobin saturation. *Crit Care Med* 1998; **26**: 344–51.
11. van Santbrink H, vd Brink WA, Steyerberg EW, *et al.* Brain tissue oxygen response in severe traumatic brain injury. *Acta Neurochir* 2003; **145**: 429–38.

12. Vespa PM, McArthur D, O'Phelan K, *et al.* Persistently low extracellular glucose correlates with poor outcome 6 months after human traumatic brain injury despite a lack of increased lactate: a microdialysis study. *J Cereb Blood Flow Metab* 2003; **23**: 865–77.

13. Reinert M, Barth A, Rothen HU, *et al.* Effects of cerebral perfusion pressure and increased fraction of inspired oxygen on brain tissue oxygen, lactate and glucose in patients with severe head injury. *Acta Neurochir* 2003; **145**: 341–9.

14. Rosner M, Rosner S, Johnson A. Cerebral perfusion pressure: management protocol and clinical results. *J Neurosurg* 1995; **83**: 949–62.

15. Eker C, Asgeirsson B, Grande PO, *et al.* Improved outcome after severe head injury with a new therapy based on principles for brain volume regulation and preserved microcirculation. *Crit Care Med* 1998; **26**: 1881–6.

16. Wolfe CDA. The impact of stroke. *Br Med Bull* 2000; **56**: 275–86.

17. Bonita R. Epidemiology of stroke. *Lancet* 1992; **339**: 342–4.

18. Treib J, Grauer MT, Woessner R, Morgenthaler M. Treatment of stroke on an intensive stroke unit: a novel concept. *Intensive Care Med* 2000; **26**: 1598–611.

19. Wolfe C, Rudd A, Dennis M, *et al.* Taking acute stroke care seriously. *BMJ* 2001; **323**: 5–6.

20. Stroke Trialists Collaboration. Collective systematic review of the randomised trials of organised inpatient (stroke unit) care after stroke. *BMJ* 1997; **314**: 1151–9.

21. Steiner T, Mendoza G, De Gorgia M, *et al.* Prognosis of stroke patients requiring mechanical ventilation in a neurological critical care unit. *Stroke* 1997; **28**: 711–15.

22. Jorgensen HS, Nakayam H, Raaschon HO, *et al.* Effect of blood pressure and diabetes on stroke in progression. *Lancet* 1994; **344**: 156–9.

23. International Stroke Trial Collaborative Group. The International Stroke Trial (IST): a randomised trial of aspirin, subcutaneous heparin, both or neither among 19435 patients with acute ischaemic stroke. *Lancet* 1997; **349**: 1564–5.

24. National Institute of Neurological Disorders and Stroke rt-PA Stroke Study Group. Tissue plasminogen activator for acute ischaemic stroke. *N Engl J Med* 1996; **333**: 1–7.

25. Hacke W, Kaste M, Fieschi C, *et al.* Intravenous thrombolysis with recombinant tissue plasminogen activator for acute hemispheric stroke. The European Co-Operative Acute Stroke Study (ECASS). *JAMA* 1995; **274**: 1017–25.

26. Hacke W, Kaste M, Fieschi C, *et al.* For the Second European–Australasian Acute Stroke Study Investigators. Randomised double blind placebo-controlled trial of thrombolytic therapy with intravenous alteplase in acute ischaemic stroke (ECASS II). *Lancet* 1998; **352**: 1245–51.

27. Clark WM, Wissman S, Albers GW, *et al.* Recombinant tissue type plasminogen activator (alteplase) for ischaemic stroke 3 to 5 hours after symptom onset. The ATLANTIS study: a randomised controlled trial. Alteplase thrombolysis for acute non-interventional therapy in ischaemic stroke. *JAMA* 1999; **282**: 2019–26.

28. Siddique MS, Mendelow AD. Surgical treatment of intracerebral haemorrhage. *Br M Bull* 2000; **56**: 444–56.

29. Van Gijn J, Rinkel GJE. Subarachnoid haemorrhage: diagnosis, causes and management. *Brain* 2001; **124**: 249–78.

30. Teunissen LL, Rinkel GJE, Algra A, *et al.* Risk factors for subarachnoid haemorrhage – a systematic review. *Stroke* 1996; **27**: 544–9.

31. Drake CG, Hunt WE, Kassell NF, *et al.* Report of the World Federation of Neurological Surgeons Committee on a universal subarachnoid haemorrhage grading scale. *J Neurosurg* 1996; **84**: 985–6.

32. Weir B, MacDonald L. Cerebral vasospasm. *Clin Neurosurg* 1992; **40**: 40–55.

33. Solenski NJ, Haley EC, Kassell NF, *et al.* Medical complications of aneurysmal subarachnoid haemorrhage: a report of the multicenter cooperative aneurysm study. *Crit Care Med* 1995; **25**: 1007–17.

34. Pickard JD, Murray GD, Illingworth R, *et al.* Effect of oral nimodipine on cerebral infarction and outcome after subarachnoid haemorrhage: British Aneurysm Nimodipine Trial (BRANT). *BMJ* 1989; **298**: 636–42.

35. Origatano TC, Wascher TM, Reichman OU, Anderson DE. Sustained increased cerebral blood flow with prophylactic hypertensive hemodilution ('triple-H' therapy) after subarachnoid haemorrhage. *Neurosurg* 1990; **27**: 729–40.

36. Brilstra EH, Hop JW, van der Graaf Y, *et al.* Treatment of intracranial aneurysms by embolisation with coils: a systematic review. *Stroke* 1999; **30**: 470–6.

37. Pallis C. *ABC of brain stem death.* London: BMJ Books, 1989.

38. Molloy S, Price M, Casey AT. Questionnaire survey of the views of the delegates at the European Cervical Spine Research Society meeting on the administration of methylprednisolone for acute traumatic spinal cord injury. *Spine* 2001; **26**: E562–4.

12 Pain management in critical care

JOHN WILLIAMS & JONATHAN THOMPSON

Viva topics

- Describe the methods available for managing pain in critically ill patients.
- What are the potential complications associated with epidural analgesia?
- What are the physical signs of local anaesthetic toxicity?

INTRODUCTION

Pain is reported by up to 79 per cent of hospital inpatients and is a significant problem in the intensive care unit (ICU). In a large multicentre investigation of over 5000 patients from five US teaching hospitals (the SUPPORT study), almost 50 per cent of ICU patients overall and over 60 per cent of those with colonic cancer or liver failure complained of pain.[1] Fifteen per cent of patients had 'moderate' or 'severe' pain at least half the time. Surprisingly, however, less than 15 per cent were unhappy with the pain relief offered, although patients suffering from anxiety, depression or more severe pain were less satisfied with their pain control overall.

Pain is common in ICU patients for several reasons. It may arise from the acute condition causing ICU admission, for example surgery, trauma, or painful medical conditions associated with inflammatory processes. Pain may also be caused by coexisting chronic disease. Prolonged immobility is common in the critically ill; this can cause musculoskeletal stiffness and pain, or lead to pressure sores, particularly in the elderly or debilitated. Pain may also be caused directly by the institution of monitoring procedures, medical or nursing interventions. The Thunder Project II examined pain scores for six standard interventions performed in 6000 adult ICU patients: patient turning, wound drain removal, tracheal suctioning, femoral catheter removal, central venous catheter placement and non-burn wound dressing change.[2] Patient turning and wound drain removal were rated as being most painful (with pain scores of 4–5 on an 11-point rating scale). Despite all the interventions being described as painful to a greater or lesser extent, only 17.4 per cent of patients were given any opioid analgesia prior to a procedure. Less than 5 per cent received analgesia before tracheal suctioning, despite evidence that both the procedure is painful and the memory of it long-lived.[2]

The situation may be exacerbated by difficulties of pain perception and communication. Most nursing and medical procedures performed on critically ill patients are perceived by health professionals as being potentially quick, simple, and requiring little analgesia. Conversely, patients often perceive them as being slow and painful. Communication and vocalization may be difficult for critical care patients, for example in the presence of an endotracheal or tracheostomy tube, and patients may be unable to report their pain. Sedative drugs, patient confusion or agitation may exacerbate this problem. In addition, the provision of effective vital organ support may be afforded a higher priority by carers than effective analgesia. There is a potential conflict if the adverse effects of analgesic techniques (e.g. hypotension associated with epidural analgesia, or respiratory depression with opioids) are seen as potentially exacerbating organ dysfunction, even though such problems are usually easily remedied. So, despite the wide range of analgesic drugs and strategies available, misunderstanding of these issues by nursing and medical staff can lead to inadequate provision of pain relief.

CONSEQUENCES OF PAIN IN CRITICAL CARE PATIENTS

Pain is often associated with tissue damage. This may cause reflex activation of neuroendocrine stress responses, coordinated via the autonomic nervous system. Although a number of inflammatory mediators associated with tissue damage are involved, pain itself is a potent trigger for this cascade, which has widespread effects on different organs.

Pain causes reflex local vasoconstriction and muscle spasm, coordinated at a segmental level in the spinal cord.

Pain limits mobility and can cause pulmonary and psychological dysfunction.

It is well established that inadequate analgesia in situations of acute pain can cause changes in the central nervous system pain pathways, which exacerbate pain in the short term and in some cases lead to the development of chronic pain states.[3] There is also evidence that the provision of good analgesia can improve outcome in a variety of clinical situations.[4]

Neuroendocrine stress response

The 'stress response' comprises a number of physiological and neuroendocrine responses to noxious stimuli, coordinated by the autonomic nervous system (Table 12.1). These responses are no longer considered an 'all or nothing' phenomenon, but act broadly to conserve circulating blood volume and body water, and increase the delivery of oxygen and energy substrates to vital organs and tissues.

These homeostatic mechanisms are not intrinsically harmful but can be detrimental, particularly in patients with coexisting medical disease, where they can cause tachycardia and increase myocardial oxygen demand. If myocardial oxygen supply does not increase in parallel (e.g. in elderly patients or those with cardiorespiratory disease), myocardial ischaemia, arrhythmias and myocardial infarction may occur.[5] The increased tendency to blood coagulation increases the risk of coronary or deep venous thrombosis and pulmonary emboli. Excessive sodium and water retention can precipitate tissue or pulmonary oedema.

Pulmonary dysfunction

Many of the conditions that require critical care admission and are associated with pain also cause cardiopulmonary

Table 12.1 *Components of the stress response*

CVS	Increased heart rate
	Increased cardiac contractility
	Increased cardiac output
	Coronary vessel vasodilatation
GI	Splanchnic vasoconstriction
Hormones	Increase in epinephrine, cortisol, glucagons, AVP, renin/angiotensin
Metabolic	Hyperglycaemia
	Lipolysis
	Protein catabolism
Haematological	Increased fibrinogen
	Platelet aggregation
	Decreased fibrinolysis

dysfunction as part of the pathophysiological process (e.g. acute pancreatitis, burns, trauma etc.). In other conditions pulmonary dysfunction occurs as a secondary consequence of pain, for example after abdominal or thoracic surgery. Overt postoperative pulmonary complications requiring some type of medical intervention occur in only 1–3 per cent of patients after elective surgical procedures, or up to 10 per cent of patients after emergency surgery. However, after cardiac and abdominal surgery, pulmonary atelectasis and radiographic changes are much more frequent, with incidences of 90 per cent and 75 per cent, respectively.[6] Pulmonary dysfunction after abdominal surgery may be caused by peritoneal inflammation and abdominal muscle spasm. The abdominal muscles (rectus, transversus abdominis, internal and external oblique) normally aid in forced expiration, and continuous contraction restricts diaphragmatic and chest wall movement, causing reduction of lung volumes and functional residual capacity (FRC) by up to 50 per cent. This renders some areas of the lung vulnerable to atelectasis, and increases venous admixture or shunt by reducing the V/Q ratio, causing hypoxaemia. Reductions in FRC and forced vital capacity (FVC) lead to inability to cough and clear bronchial secretions, thereby increasing the likelihood of pulmonary infection. Lung volumes and PaO_2 are at their lowest on the first postoperative day, and it may take up to 12–14 days for FRC and FVC to return to preoperative values. These pulmonary changes vary depending on the site and extent of surgery, and their effects depend on pre-existing medical disease and subsequent management.

Effective analgesia improves lung function after abdominal surgery. In one study, epidural local anaesthetic or opioid increased FEV_1 from 45 per cent to 67 per cent of preoperative figures,[7] and patient-controlled analgesia has been shown to reduce postoperative pulmonary atelectasis after coronary artery bypass grafting. Early mobilization, facilitated by effective analgesia, can help reduce the risk of deep vein thrombosis and pulmonary embolism, which is the most common cause of sudden death in the first 10 days after surgery. However, it should be noted that the *excessive* use of sedative analgesic drugs may *prolong* the duration of ventilatory support and *increase* the likelihood of pulmonary complications, and high epidural blockade can compromise respiratory muscle function and the ability to cough.

Psychological aspects

Persistent anxiety and depression are being increasingly recognized following discharge from ICU, and recent research has improved the appreciation of the physiological and psychological processes involved.[8] In one small study 38 per cent of respondents to a postal questionnaire reported psychological symptoms consistent with those occurring as a part of post-traumatic stress disorder (PTSD). Symptoms were more severe in young adults and women, and 15 per cent warranted a formal diagnosis of PTSD.[9] In a study of 80 survivors of ARDS, the chances of developing PTSD were increased significantly in those who recalled pain during their ICU stay. Conversely, others propose that PTSD is related to recall of delusional thoughts or memories, with memory of real events, even if unpleasant, providing some protection.[10] The situation is therefore unclear. Although poorly treated pain undoubtedly affects subsequent memories of ICU stay, there is little evidence that effective pain relief per se improves long-term psychological outcome, and further research is required.

Effects on outcome

As pain contributes to immobility, decreased pulmonary function, stress responses and possibly to a poor psychological outcome after critical care stay, it is tempting to assume that effective analgesia improves overall ICU outcome. However, direct evidence is limited.

Nevertheless, some studies have indicated that effective epidural analgesia improves cardiovascular and respiratory function following major surgery compared to intravenous opioids, and the incidence of thromboembolic events is reduced.[11–14] Perioperative epidural analgesia may also reduce the incidence of postoperative myocardial infarction and gastrointestinal stasis. After coronary artery bypass grafting, high-dose opioid regimens are associated with less postoperative ischaemia than low-dose regimens. However, in one study blood pressure and heart rate were similar with the two regimens.[15] Patient-controlled analgesia can provide better pain control and is associated with less postoperative pulmonary atelectasis than nurse-administered analgesia.[16] The precise method of administration may be less important than the quality of pain control achieved. A recent large multicentre randomized trial comparing epidural analgesia with intravenous opioids showed no difference in postoperative mortality following major surgery.[11]

EVALUATION OF PAIN IN THE INTENSIVE CARE PATIENT

Pain relief is often inadequate in ICU because of misconceptions of both patients and staff, as outlined above. However, a major contributory factor is poor communication, which leads to poor estimation by carers of patients' requirements for analgesia. Indirect measures (e.g. autonomic signs or grimacing) are non-specific, and self-reporting of pain is by far the most accurate way of assessing pain and analgesic requirements. However, there are wide variations between individuals in their perception of pain.

Pain perception

Pain is a subjective experience, with many features altering its individual perception, including psychological factors (anxiety, fear, depression and fatigue), educational and social status, ethnic and cultural background, prior expectations and understanding. Age and sex are also important: elderly patients frequently complain of less postoperative pain and require lower doses of analgesics than younger patients undergoing equivalent surgical procedures.[17] Confused patients or those who have obtunded higher mental functions may find it difficult to understand the nature of their discomfort. Systemic opioid analgesics may increase sedation and confusion, but can be impractical in the uncooperative patient. Optimal analgesia for these patients is difficult, and involves a balance between effective analgesia and excessive sedation.

Assessment of pain in ICU

Pain can be assessed and evaluated in a variety of ways, including subjective and objective assessment or one-dimensional and multidimensional measurements.[18,19] Any ICU scoring system should be simple to understand and use, and provide accurate and reproducible information. The site and severity of pain should be evaluated with regard to expectations and coexisting disease, including chronic painful conditions. If pain is unduly severe or in a site unrelated to known pathology, the possibility of other unrecognized sources of pain should be considered.

SUBJECTIVE SCORING SYSTEMS

Subjective assessments rely upon the patient providing medical staff with information about their pain. Commonly used examples include the visual analogue scale (VAS), numeric rating scale (NRS), adjective rating scale (ARS) and McGill Pain Questionnaire (MPQ).

Visual analogue score (Figure 12.1)

Patients mark on the line the point they feel correlates to their pain at that particular moment. Measuring the distance of each mark along the original 100 mm line allows a

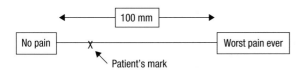

Figure 12.1 Visual analogue score

quantification of pain. The VAS is simple and widely used, although it has a failure rate of around 7 per cent in adults.

Numeric rating scale

The NRS works in a similar way to VAS, but the patient chooses a number from 0 to 10 or 0 to 100 which reflects the degree of pain they feel. This is also simple and easily administered, and may have advantages over a VAS in patients with communication difficulties.

Adjective rating scale

Adjective rating scales (ARS) comprise a list of words corresponding to increasing levels of pain, and patients choose the word that best fits their experience.

The VAS, NRS and ARS are all one-dimensional scoring systems, and although they are simple to understand and perform in critically ill patients they focus only upon pain intensity, which tends to oversimplify the patient's experience of pain. The McGill Pain Questionnaire (MPQ) is probably the most widely used multidimensional assessment tool available. In addition to assessing pain intensity (on a scoring system of 0–5), patients have to choose descriptive words from four different groupings: sensory, affective, evaluative and miscellaneous. The words chosen by the patient are then scored and collated with the subjective pain scores to give an overall pain-rating index.

Objective scoring systems

However simple the method of pain assessment, many patients may be confused, sedated, or have difficulty in communication, so an objective system of pain measurement is required.

Sympathetic nervous system activation causes increases in heart rate, arterial pressure, respiratory rate, intracranial pressure, pupil size and amplitude of the light reflex. Lacrimation, grimacing or reflex movements may also occur. However, all these changes are non-specific and are affected by many other factors, including circulating blood volume, body temperature, levels of arousal and CNS pathology. In addition, patients may be receiving sedative or opioid drugs or other medications that act directly or indirectly on the autonomic nervous system. Indirect physiological signs are therefore too inaccurate to be interpreted in a scientific or systematic way and are of limited use.

The ability to move, cough or breathe deeply has pragmatic value but depends on motivation and other factors.

An objective observer may assess subjective scales. Nurses have used VAS to estimate patients' pain, but they underestimate between 35 and 55 per cent of the time. Similarly, in a large subgroup of the SUPPORT study family members assessed the degree of pain accurately only 53 per cent of the time.[1,20]

Although several objective pain-related measures are available, no single system has gained universal favour.

Even though pain assessment is difficult in the critically ill, carers should remember that pain potentially occurs in the vast majority of ICU patients. Attempts to quantify pain and its source should always be made in order to enable adequate rapid diagnosis and treatment.

THE PHYSIOLOGY OF PAIN TRANSMISSION

In order to treat pain effectively it is necessary to have a basic understanding of the physiology of pain transmission. This is illustrated in Figure 12.2.

Pain sensation is modified physiologically in a number of ways. Tissue damage leads to a decrease in local pH and changes in nociceptor function, which then amplify the transmission of painful impulses to the spinal cord (primary hyperalgesia). This also permits previously non-noxious stimuli to be perceived as painful (allodynia), and the reflex release of 5-hydroxytryptamine (5HT), histamine and substance P leads to widening of the receptive field so that impulses from adjacent non-injured tissue are also perceived as painful (secondary hyperalgesia). Repeated transmission of noxious impulses to the spinal cord increases its responsiveness to further noxious stimuli (the wind-up phenomenon), thereby facilitating the transmission of pain signals to the brain. The neurotransmitters involved in these phenomena include glutamate, N-methyl-D-aspartate (NMDA), kinins and substance P. If allowed to persist, permanent changes in spinal cord neurons and impulse transmission occur (long-term potentiation) to exacerbate pain sensation.

A number of descending impulses inhibit transmission through lamina II of the dorsal horn (the substantia gelatinosa), including stimulation of large-diameter afferent fibres and descending pathways from the periaqueductal grey area via the nucleus raphe magnus. These are affected by opioid and α_2-adrenergic pathways. In particular, the substantia gelatinosa and periaqueductal grey are rich in endogenous opioids (β-endorphins and enkephalins) and opioid receptors.

The complexity of pain physiology means that pain can be treated using a number of different strategies (Figure 12.3 and Table 12.2).

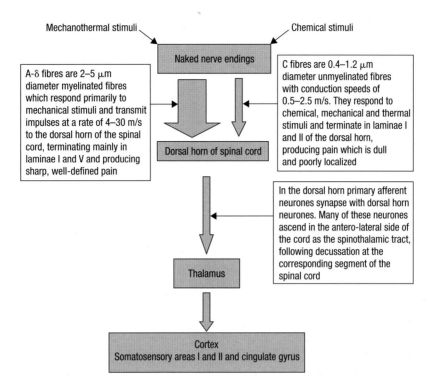

Figure 12.2 Physiology of pain transmission

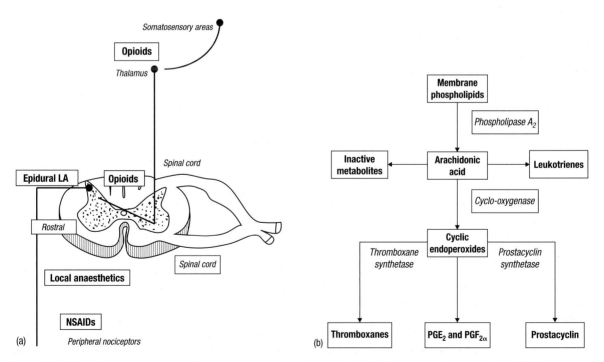

Figure 12.3 (a) Sites of action of some commonly used analgesic agents (b) Prostaglandin metabolisms and mechanism of action of NSAIDs. Membrane phospholipid is converted to arachidonic acid via the action of phospholipase A_2. This is then converted to cyclic endoperoxides by the enzyme cyclooxygenase, and subsequently to a variety of other prostaglandins. NSAIDs inhibit the action of cyclooxygenase and so reduce the production of the prostaglandins shown

Table 12.2 *Sites of action of some commonly used classes of analgesics*

Class	Site of action
NSAIDs	Decrease PG production at site of injury
Local anaesthetics	Block peripheral afferent nerve transmission
Opioids	Centrally mediated action at spinal and supraspinal CNS opioid receptors

Several other agents have also been used in ICU (e.g. clonidine, ketamine, tricyclic antidepressants etc.) for their analgesic properties, and may be useful as adjunctive therapy or in particular scenarios as they act at specific sites in the pain pathway.

ANALGESIA STRATEGIES IN CRITICAL CARE

General pharmacokinetic and pharmacodynamic considerations in ICU patients

Almost all normal pharmacokinetic processes (drug absorption, distribution, metabolism and elimination) are disturbed in the critically ill and the usual assumptions may not apply (Table 12.3).

ABSORPTION

The generally preferred route of drug administration is gastrointestinal (GI), but GI function in critical care patients is frequently impaired even in the absence of overt intra-abdominal disease. Gastric emptying is delayed by many physiological factors (including pain, stress or trauma), pharmacological factors (opioids, dopamine, sympathomimetic or anticholinergic drugs) or by extra-abdominal disease (diabetes, head injuries, systemic sepsis, acid–base or electrolyte disturbances). In addition, intra-abdominal pathology (e.g. perforated viscus, intra-abdominal sepsis, post surgery, actual obstruction or idiopathic pseudo-obstruction) causes delayed gastric emptying. Even if gastric emptying is normal, intestinal function may be impaired by mucosal oedema or hypoperfusion; mucosal integrity is diminished within days by the effects of starvation.

Consequently, absorption of drugs from the GI tract is often unpredictable, and even if the ICU patient has a gastric tube or is able to swallow, other routes of drug administration may be preferred. Similarly, peripheral tissue perfusion is frequently decreased (because of tissue oedema, shock, sympathetic stimulation, or the administration of vasoconstrictor drugs), or may be increased in the septic or burned patient. Therefore subcutaneous, intramuscular

Table 12.3 *Important factors influencing drug efficacy in ICU patients*

Process	Consequence in ICU patient
Variable tissue blood flow	Unpredictable absorption of subcutaneous or intramuscular drugs
Variations in plasma protein	Changes in free drug concentration
Renal impairment	Impaired excretion of metabolites, prolonged drug effect
Variations in cardiac output	Possible major alterations in drug delivery to site of action, drug metabolism and excretion. Assumptions regarding drug volumes of distribution, metabolism and clearance should be interpreted with caution
Hepatic impairment	Reduced drug metabolism and clearance for some compounds, reduced clinical effect for prodrugs
Gastric emptying delayed	Delayed drug absorption
Polypharmacy	Drug interactions possible
Genetic differences	Differences in drug metabolism and drug efficacy
Age	Variations in organ function, drug metabolism and excretion

and transdermal routes of delivery are unpredictable and usually unsuitable for use in ICU patients. Certain drugs may be nebulized or inhaled, but systemic absorption depends on pulmonary function, which is frequently impaired, and this route is usually reserved for drugs acting directly on the respiratory system (e.g. bronchodilators). Consequently, most drugs in ICU are delivered by the intravenous route.

DISTRIBUTION

Following absorption into the circulation, most drugs bind to transport proteins for transport to their site of action. The two most important transport proteins in this regard are albumin and α_1 acid glycoprotein (AAG). Plasma albumin concentrations often decrease in critical illness, whereas AAG concentrations increase in response to physiological stress. The reduction in albumin concentrations may increase free drug concentrations and produce enhanced drug effects (e.g. NSAIDs, which bind to albumin). NSAIDs may also increase free drug levels of oral anticoagulants by displacing warfarin from albumin. Opioids are basic compounds predominately bound to AAG, and it would be expected that with the increase in binding protein the amount of free drug would be decreased. This is not seen, however, and it is thought that this may be because there are different isoforms of AAG that change independently of each other.

The delivery of drug to its site of action also depends on the cardiac output, circulating blood volume, the integrity of capillary membranes and body composition, all of which may be abnormal. Analgesic drugs differ in their distribution throughout the body, but most act in the central nervous system (CNS). The clinical effects of drugs acting in the CNS (e.g. opioids, intravenous sedative or hypnotic drugs) depend on the concentration achieved. Therefore, cerebral blood flow and the integrity or otherwise of the blood–brain barrier are also important. In general, it may be assumed that the clinical effects of opioids or other CNS-acting drugs are enhanced in all ICU patients, and initial doses are reduced accordingly. For example, in hypovolaemic ICU patients or those with impaired cardiac function, the proportion of cardiac output being delivered to the CNS may actually be increased, so the effective CNS drug concentrations and clinical effect are higher. In addition, such patients are more sensitive to the cardiodepressant effects of opioids, so that the administered dose should be reduced. Elderly ICU patients also show increased pharmacodynamic sensitivity to many drugs, so that a greater drug effect is observed after a given dose, irrespective of alterations in protein binding, distribution volumes or organ-dependent elimination. However, in all cases the dose should be titrated to clinical effect.

METABOLISM

The aim of metabolism is to change lipid-soluble drugs into water-soluble compounds that may easily be excreted by the kidney and so eliminated from the body. The majority of drugs are metabolized in the liver, though extrahepatic sites of metabolism do exist (e.g. the volatile anaesthetic halothane is metabolized within the gut wall as well as in the liver; remifentanil is metabolized by plasma and tissue esterases). Hepatic metabolism occurs in two phases. Most phase I reactions (e.g. oxidation, reduction and hydroxylation) are performed by the cytochrome P450 superfamily, a non-specific enzyme system of over 150 related enzymes. In phase II synthetic reactions, drugs or the products of phase I reactions are conjugated with one of a variety of differing groups (glucuronide, methyl, acetate, sulphate) which render the compound water soluble. These processes are highly variable and are affected by temperature, stress, inflammatory mediators, endocrine disease, racial origin, sex and diet. In addition, drugs that share a common cytochrome P450 isoenzyme may compete for binding sites. The activity of enzymes involved in both phase I and phase II reactions can be induced or inhibited by other drugs, alcohol or cigarette smoking.

Hepatic drug metabolism can be impaired by two main mechanisms. Hepatocellular dysfunction directly decreases the activity of phase I and II enzymatic pathways. In addition, drug metabolism may be affected by changes in hepatic blood flow. Hepatic blood flow normally comprises approximately 30 per cent of cardiac output, but decreases in response to haemorrhage or decreased cardiac output, when sympathetically mediated splanchnic vasoconstriction occurs. The effect on drug metabolism of alterations in hepatic blood flow or hepatocellular function depends on the individual drug, but is more prominent for drugs with high hepatic extraction ratios. In ICU patients both considerations apply, and over 50 per cent of such patients display some degree of hepatic dysfunction. The consequences depend on the individual drug, but include drug accumulation and enhanced effects or toxicity, particularly after prolonged infusions.

Most opioids used in clinical practice are metabolized predominantly by glucuronidation. This metabolic process is very effective, with opioids displaying flow-limited clearance, i.e. the clearance of drug is determined by blood flow to the liver and not by enzyme function. For this reason hepatic function must become quite severely impaired before opioid metabolism decreases, but alterations in hepatic blood flow may delay clearance. Alfentanil is metabolized primarily by oxidative phase I systems, and its half-life is increased and clearance markedly reduced in patients with liver cirrhosis. Age also has important effects on opioid metabolism. Morphine is metabolized by glucuronidation to morphine-3-glucuronide (M3G) and morphine-6-glucuronide (M6G). The enzyme systems responsible are immature in neonates and premature infants, and so morphine and its two metabolites may accumulate. In the elderly population hepatic blood flow is reduced by up to 50 per cent and enzyme function reduced, leading to enhanced sensitivity to opioids or prolonged drug effects. The elderly also have higher levels of AAG, which binds several compounds including bupivacaine and opioids. Hence the proportion of bound to free drug may be altered in elderly patients.

Drug administration itself may alter metabolism, with certain compounds inhibiting and others inducing metabolic pathways. This is particularly important in critical care patients, who may be receiving a variety of drugs. For example, morphine suppresses its own metabolism by inhibiting desmethylation, but its main metabolic pathway, glucuronidation, is unaffected. Likewise, propofol has also been shown to reduce the metabolism of alfentanil and midazolam by the inhibition of cytochrome P450 in laboratory models.[21]

Genetic factors may also be important. Morphine-3-glucuronide is known to have antanalgesic properties, whereas M6G is 40 times more potent an analgesic than morphine. Two different types of UDP-glucuronyl transferase are responsible for the production of these two metabolites; some people lack the enzyme responsible for M6G production and consequently experience poor analgesia from morphine.[21]

Codeine is effectively a prodrug, being metabolized to morphine by the enzyme CYP 2D6. Codeine is ineffective in up to 10 per cent of the population who lack a functioning form of this enzyme. Remifentanil differs from the other opioids used in clinical practice as it is metabolized by a wide range of esterases found in the blood and tissues. For this reason, disease states and genetic variations have little or no effect upon its pharmacokinetics.

ELIMINATION

The renal elimination of water-soluble drugs and metabolites from the body is governed by three processes: glomerular filtration, tubular secretion and tubular reabsorption. Although renal blood flow and glomerular filtration rate (GFR) are autoregulated, renal function is frequently impaired in ICU patients, usually as a consequence of reduced circulating volume or arterial pressure compounded by the effects of sepsis or nephrotoxic drugs. GFR is usually decreased, so drugs filtered at the glomerulus will tend to accumulate. The physiological response to oliguria is to increase tubular reabsorption, enhancing the reabsorption of certain drugs or their metabolites, which if the metabolites are pharmacologically active may accumulate and cause adverse effects. The active metabolites of morphine include M6G and morphine-3-glucuronide (M3G), both of which are μ-opioid receptor agonists which can cause sedation, respiratory depression, analgesia etc. Norpethidine, a metabolite of pethidine, accumulates in renal failure and has been associated with neuroexcitatory phenomena (tremors, myoclonus and seizures).

From the above it is clear that many physiological and pharmacological factors influence both the sensation of pain and analgesic requirements. Even in healthy volunteers analgesic requirements may vary 10-fold between individuals. Furthermore, the pharmacokinetic and dynamic principles that are applied to the hospital population at large may not hold true in critically ill patients. It is therefore important to recognize that different patients have great variations in analgesic requirements, and all analgesics drugs should be titrated. In addition, drugs administered in ICU may easily accumulate, particularly after prolonged infusions, and all sedative and analgesic infusions should be stopped daily to assess their clinical effect.

Routes of administration of analgesic agents in the critical care unit

Analgesic drugs may be administered by a variety of different routes to ICU patients: intravenous, intramuscular, transdermal, intrathecal, epidural, oral, inhalational, sublingual, intranasal, rectal and subcutaneous routes have all been used. A number of different dosing regimens can be employed, e.g. on a prn basis (i.e. as needed), as patient-controlled analgesia, or as a continuous infusion (most commonly seen with opioids in ICU patients). The problems of unpredictable absorption and elimination in ICU patients are described above, but all these routes are associated with their own advantages and disadvantages. Intravenous administration is most commonly used in ICU, because it is associated with a rapid onset, flexibility of dosage allowing titration, and consistent drug delivery. Disadvantages of intravenous administration include the potential for a rapid onset of adverse as well as therapeutic effects, and the requirements for indwelling cannulae, infusion devices, staff expertise and monitoring equipment. Most of these can be overcome in a critical care environment, but other routes are occasionally used. Systemic effects of drugs administered intravenously may also be significant, so regional or local anaesthetic techniques are also widely employed. Epidural analgesia is described in detail below. Patient-controlled analgesia (PCA) allows the patient access to an electronic pump which is programmed to deliver an intravenous bolus of analgesic drug on demand. The prescriber determines the bolus dose and the minimum lockout period. For morphine used through a PCA a common regimen would be the use of a 1 mg bolus with a 5-minute lockout period. PCA allows some degree of patient autonomy and reassurance, avoids intermittent intramuscular injections, and can be used on general wards provided nursing resources are adequate. However, to be successful it requires the patient to be alert and cooperative, and can cause respiratory depression, particularly in the elderly or those with impaired organ function. It is intrinsic to the safety of the equipment that only the patient (not well-intentioned relatives or health professionals) may activate the device.

Pharmacology of systemic analgesics

Three groups of analgesic drug are in common use in ICU patients: opioids, non-steroidal anti-inflammatory agents and local anaesthetic agents.

OPIOIDS

Opioids are potent analgesics but also have a wide range of adverse effects (Table 12.4). Many newer semisynthetic and synthetic opioid analgesics have been manufactured, in an attempt to produce drugs with fewer adverse effects. All opioids act at endogenous opioid receptors, which are distributed throughout the CNS (e.g. in the caudate nucleus, putamen, neocortex, thalamus, nucleus accumbens, peri-aqueductal grey area and dorsal horn of the spinal cord, and in some peripheral sites). Opioid receptors are G-protein coupled systems that reduce neuronal excitability via reductions in intracellular cAMP in response to binding of an opioid agonist. Opioid receptor subtypes were originally classified as μ, δ and κ, but a new opioid-like receptor (the nociceptin receptor) has recently been discovered. Some sources describe multiple isoforms of specific opioid receptors (e.g. μ, and μ_2), but there is no evidence from molecular biology that separate isoforms exist. Different opioid drugs vary in their pharmacokinetic and physicochemical properties, but all the opioid drugs in common use are μ (μ opioid peptide, MOP) receptor agonists with very similar pharmacodynamic effects. Cardiovascular effects are caused by inhibition of central sympathetic activity, as well as direct effects on the heart and vascular smooth muscle and vagal stimulation causing bradycardia. Histamine release contributes to vasodilatation and may lead to allergic reactions. In critical care patients reduced gut motility and gastric emptying may delay the institution of enteral nutrition and increase the risk of aspiration of gastric contents. Morphine, pethidine, fentanyl, alfentanil and remifentanil are the opioids used most commonly in anaesthesia and ICU practice in the UK (Table 12.5). All have a relatively rapid onset of effect after IV injection, but all except remifentanil tend to accumulate after prolonged (>24 hours) IV infusions. In

these circumstances the offset of effect is not reflected by their terminal half-lives, and can be several days.

Morphine

Morphine is usually administered either as a continuous intravenous infusion or in bolus doses of 2–10 mg, producing its peak effect after approximately 15–20 minutes. As it is hydrophilic and comparatively lipid insoluble, its onset of action is slower than that of other opioid drugs. The main metabolites (M6G and M3G) are pharmacologically active. They are excreted via the kidney and their effect may be prolonged in renal failure. Morphine may be administered via the epidural or spinal routes. Like other opioids, after epidural or spinal administration morphine spreads via the CSF to act at a supraspinal level. Morphine is relatively lipid insoluble (about 1/500th that of fentanyl) and so has a slow onset of action after epidural administration, and adverse effects (e.g. respiratory depression) may be delayed for up to 16 hours after the last epidural dose. Morphine is the most widespread opioid used for PCA, as described above.

Pethidine

Pethidine is a synthetic phenylpiperidine derivative which was first investigated as an anticholinergic but was found to have analgesic properties. Pethidine 75 mg is equivalent to 10 mg of morphine. Pethidine is more lipophilic than morphine, but has a similar onset of action. It may produce tachycardia and slightly less pupillary constriction than morphine. Pethidine has been advocated for use in pancreatitis or biliary colic, where choledochoduodenal sphincter tone may be of importance. However, the use of pethidine is limited in renal failure by the accumulation of its metabolite norpethidine.

Fentanyl

Fentanyl is used infrequently in UK ICU practice but is used commonly in the USA. It is a phenylpiperidine and is highly

Table 12.4 *Adverse effects of opioid analgesics*

Respiratory depression	Histamine release
Gastric stasis	Smooth muscle spasm
Bradycardia	Urinary retention
Nausea	Muscle rigidity
Vomiting	Euphoria
Pruritus	Dysphoria
Sedation	Tolerance

Table 12.5 *Pharmacokinetic data for opioid analgesics*

Drug	Relative lipid solubility Vd (L/kg)	Half-life (hr)	Onset of action IV (min)	Peak effect IV (min)	Duration of action of a bolus (hr)	Intermittent bolus dose	Adult
Morphine	1	2.5–3.5	2–3	5	20–30	2–7	IV: 0.05–0.1 mg/kg Epi: 100–200 μg
Fentanyl	580	6.5–10	4–8	1–2	5–15	0.5–1	IV: 1–2 μg/kg Epi: 25–100 μg
Alfentanil	90	0.5–1	1–2	1	1.5	0.1–0.2	2–5 μg/kg
Pethidine	28	4–5	3–5	5	20–60	2–4	25–100 mg
Remifentanil	13	0.3	0.1–0.2	1	1–2	0.1	0.05–0.25 μg/kg

lipid soluble, with a rapid onset of action and large volume of distribution. A transdermal preparation is available but fentanyl has a slow onset and offset of action by this route. Epidural opioids act synergistically with local anaesthetic agents. Fentanyl has a higher lipid solubility than morphine, leading to a more rapid onset of action and less rostral spread when administered via an epidural, making it a common choice in epidural infusions. As with other opioids, delayed respiratory depression, pruritus, sedation and urinary retention can occur with epidural fentanyl. Continued intravenous infusions lead to prolonged effects because fentanyl has a very high volume of distribution, and accumulation occurs in the tissues.

Alfentanil

Alfentanil is less lipid soluble than fentanyl but has a faster onset of action, because it is predominantly non-ionized at body pH (alfentanil 89 per cent vs fentanyl 9 per cent), enabling rapid penetration of the blood–brain barrier. Its duration of action after a bolus dose is brief (2–3 min) because offset is related to redistribution of the drug, but after a prolonged infusion its effect may persist because clearance is low.

Sufentanil

Sufentanil is a phenylpiperidine derivative which is potent, highly lipid soluble, and has broadly similar pharmacokinetic properties to fentanyl. It is not available in the UK but is commonly used in Europe.

Remifentanil

Remifentanil is a phenylpiperidine derivative introduced into clinical anaesthetic practice in the UK in 1996, but only recently licensed for use as an analgesic or sedative adjunct in ICU, and experience here is limited. Its pharmacodynamic effects are similar to those of fentanyl and alfentanil, but remifentanil is metabolized rapidly by non-specific esterase enzymes in tissues and plasma to remifentanil acid, which is excreted via the kidneys. Remifentanil acid is pharmacologically active, but is less than 1/300 times as potent as remifentanil, and although it accumulates in patients with renal failure it has negligible clinical effects. Metabolism is also independent of hepatic function, and therefore offset of effect is rapid and predictable, irrespective of the duration of the infusion. It is 20–40 times more potent than alfentanil and is best administered by continuous intravenous infusion because of the possibility of bradycardia or respiratory depression after bolus administration. Remifentanil is currently formulated in glycine as a chemical buffer. Glycine is

Table 12.6 *Main actions of prostaglandins, thromboxanes and leukotrienes*

Thromboxanes	Platelet aggregation
	Vasoconstriction
Prostacyclin (PGI$_2$)	Vasodilatation
	Opposes platelet aggregation
PGE$_2$	Arteriolar vasodilatation
	Renal vasodilatation
	Bronchodilator
	Sensitizes nerve endings to bradykinins
	Pyretic
PGF$_2$	Bronchoconstriction
	Variable effects on vasculature
Leukotrienes	Mediators of inflammation
	Vasoconstriction
	Bronchoconstriction
	Increased vascular permeability
	Chemotactic agent for inflammatory cells

potentially neurotoxic, and the spinal or epidural administration of remifentanil is contraindicated.

NON-STEROIDAL ANTI-INFLAMMATORY DRUGS (NSAIDs)

NSAIDs are indicated in the treatment of mild or moderate pain and may be used in ICU patients as an adjunct to opioids (to reduce opioid requirements), or as first-line analgesics for pains of musculoskeletal origin. They act by inhibiting the enzyme cyclooxygenase, which is involved in the pathway of prostaglandin production throughout the body (see Figure 12.3). Prostaglandins have a variety of effects, including modulation of inflammatory processes, vascular reactivity, renal and platelet function, and bronchial and other smooth muscle activity (Table 12.6). They do not cause pain per se, but sensitize nerve endings to stimulation by bradykinin (a polypeptide rapidly produced following tissue damage). One advantage of NSAIDs in clinical ICU practice is that they do not cause respiratory depression and have useful opioid-sparing effects.

Common adverse effects include gastric erosions and haemorrhage, renal impairment and inhibition of platelet function. Bronchospasm may occur, especially in atopic individuals with a history of aspirin sensitivity and nasal polyps. In conditions of reduced renal blood flow (e.g. caused by a reduction in cardiac output, haemorrhage, septic shock or anaesthesia) renal vasoconstriction occurs. In response to this, vasodilator prostaglandins (prostaglandin E$_2$ or prostacyclin) maintain GFR by compensatory intrarenal vasodilatation. NSAIDs inhibit this compensatory vasodilatation and can therefore cause renal dysfunction. Conditions associated with decreased renal blood flow are common in seriously ill patients, and the risks may be exacerbated in the elderly or those with pre-existing renal disease. The American College of Critical Care Medicine therefore recommends limiting the use of the NSAID ketorolac to 5 days in the critically ill,[22] and renal function should be carefully monitored during therapy.

Cyclooxygenase has two isoforms, COX-1, a constitutive form produced constantly, and COX-2, an inducible form produced after tissue injury. The newer specific COX-2 inhibitors have no effect on COX-1 and therefore have several potential advantages in ICU patients, including potentially less nephrotoxicity, although few data are available. Currently, however, the most commonly used NSAIDs in ICU are diclofenac (usually administered orally or rectally) and ketorolac (intravenous infusion), neither of which is COX-2 specific.

LOCAL ANAESTHETICS

Local anaesthetic drugs (LAs) cause reversible inhibition of the excitation–conduction process in peripheral nerves and nerve endings by blocking voltage-dependent sodium, potassium and calcium channels. Most local anaesthetics are tertiary amine bases, which must be un-ionized to penetrate through the nerve sheath, perineuronal tissue and neuronal membrane. Within the axoplasm the local anaesthetic molecule acquires a proton to become positively charged; this charged local anaesthetic enters the voltage-gated ion channel from the intracellular portion to bind with a receptor within the channel and cause it to close. Sodium channels are mainly affected, and so depolarization and hence conduction are prevented, but potassium and calcium channels are also blocked. Blockade of nerve transmission depends on the fibre size. Small unmyelinated fibres are blocked more easily than larger myelinated ones, and so pain fibres are blocked before touch and motor fibres. The speed of onset, potency and duration of block are related to the physicochemical properties, dissociation constant (pKa), lipid solubility, protein binding and the pH of the environment into which the LA is injected. Compounds with a low pKa and high lipid solubility tend to enter the nerve more rapidly and so act more quickly, whereas highly protein-bound drugs have a longer duration of action (Table 12.7).

Local anaesthetics stabilize the membranes of all excitable tissues. They are therefore administered close to the intended site of action, but in significant systemic concentrations can cause cardiovascular and CNS toxicity.

The progression of local anaesthetic toxicity is as follows:

- Perioral paraesthesiae
- Lightheadedness

Table 12.7 *Physicochemical properties of local anaesthetics*

Agent	pK$_a$	Per cent protein bound	Recommended maximum safe dose (mg/kg)	Duration of action
Amethocaine	8.5	76	1.5	Long
Procaine	8.9	6	12	Short
Bupivacaine	8.1	96	2	Long
Lidocaine	7.9	64	3–7	Moderate
Mepivacaine	7.6	78	5	Moderate
Prilocaine	7.9	55	5–8	Moderate
Ropivacaine	8.1	94	3.5	Long

- Tremor
- Unconsciousness
- Convulsions
- Hypotension
- Central apnoea
- Myocardial depression.

Most local anaesthetics have a narrow therapeutic margin and maximum doses should always be respected. Factors affecting toxicity include the site of injection and local vascularity (such that intercostal or intrapleural injection may lead to rapid uptake of local anaesthetic into the bloodstream, owing to high tissue vascularity, and subcutaneous infiltration will produce only slowly rising plasma concentrations of local anaesthetic). To reduce the toxicity local anaesthetics are often coadministered with vasoconstrictors (e.g. epinephrine) to limit systemic uptake. In critical care local anaesthetics are used for local infiltration (for placement of intravascular catheters or drains or wound infiltration), or for regional or neuroaxial blockade (see later). Lidocaine, bupivacaine and ropivacaine are the most commonly used local anaesthetics in the UK.

Lidocaine

Lidocaine has an onset of action of 2–20 minutes, depending upon route of administration, and a duration of action of 200–400 minutes. A toxic dose of 3 mg/kg is frequently quoted, or 7 mg/kg if epinephrine is added to the local anaesthetic mixture. Although its therapeutic index is relatively narrow, causing cardiovascular compromise in toxic doses, lidocaine has been used to treat ventricular tachyarrhythmias.

Bupivacaine

Bupivacaine is highly protein bound and has a terminal half-life of approximately 160 minutes. It has a slower onset and longer duration of action than lidocaine. Maximum dose is 2 mg/kg (with or without epinephrine). Bupivacaine cardiotoxicity is caused partly by its effect on cardiac calcium and potassium channels, but is often refractory to treatment. Bupivacaine is traditionally presented as a racemic mixture of two stereoisomers. The S configuration L-bupivacaine is now commercially available on its own, and is potentially less cardiotoxic, allowing a similar dose to the racemic mixture to be used but with a reduced likelihood of adverse events.

Ropivacaine

Ropivacaine has a similar pharmacokinetic and clinical profile to bupivacaine; it is, though, slightly less potent and may produce less motor blockade. Ropivacaine is also an enantiomer, but is available commercially as the S isomer, with less cardiotoxicity than bupivacaine. Ropivacaine also has some vasoconstrictor capabilities. The maximum safe dose is approximately 3.5 mg/kg.

OTHER DRUGS

Several other analgesic drugs with a variety of modes of action may be useful.

Tramadol is a weak opioid agonist which also inhibits neuronal reuptake of epinephrine and increases serotonin release. It has a similar potency to pethidine but has a favourable side-effect profile, although it may cause nausea, dizziness, sedation and dependence. It is claimed that tramadol produces less respiratory depression than the other opioid agonists. Tramadol may be administered intravenously, intramuscularly or orally in a dose of 50–100 mg every 4–6 hours.

Inhaled **nitrous oxide** is widely used in anaesthetic practice and has been used (in the form of entonox, a 50:50 mixture of N_2O and oxygen) to provide analgesia on the ICU. It is rarely used in the UK apart from in the treatment of burns, when its rapid onset and offset are advantageous.

Ketamine is a phencyclidine derivative usually used to produce dissociative anaesthesia. It possesses potent analgesic properties via its non-competitive antagonism of NMDA receptors in the CNS, limiting the passage of calcium ions. Ketamine maintains cardiac output and blood pressure by increasing sympathetic tone, and it also causes mild respiratory stimulation and bronchodilatation; importantly, airway reflexes are relatively preserved. A typical intravenous dose of 1–2 mg/kg produces intense sedation and analgesia lasting 5–10 minutes; 10 mg/kg intramuscular injection has a duration of action of up to 20 minutes. Lower doses (e.g. 0.15–0.5 mg/kg intravenously) may produce adequate analgesia with less sedative effects. Common indications include dressing changes in burns patients, or orthopaedic manipulations. Adverse effects, including hallucinations, catalepsy, salivation, tachycardia and hypertension, limit the use of

ketamine, but these may be reduced by combining it with benzodiazepines. Psychological phenomena occur less frequently in the young; one study of paediatric burns victims administered ketamine as the sole anaesthetic agent found that, when questioned at a later date, less than 0.5 per cent of the children experienced nightmares.[23] Ketamine is a racemic mixture of two optical isomers: the S (+) isomer is a more potent analgesic and may produce fewer psychotomimetic effects than the D (−) isomer or the racemic mixture. Preservative-free S-ketamine is available for epidural administration and has been used with no evidence of toxicity. In an adult patient a usual epidural dose is 10 mg.

Clonidine is an α_2-adrenergic agonist which provides analgesia after epidural administration by spinal and supraspinal mechanisms, inhibiting central transmission of painful signals up the spinal cord. It combines synergistically with epidural local anaesthetic or opioid, but does not provide surgical anaesthesia when administered alone. It may be useful as an adjunct where epidural analgesia is patchy or incomplete, although it is limited by adverse effects of hypotension, bradycardia and sedation. Typical adult epidural doses are 10–50 μg/h or bolus doses of 0.5–1.0 μg/kg.

Oral **tricyclic antidepressants** and **antiepileptic** drugs are commonly used for patients suffering from neuropathic pain not remediable by conventional analgesics. Their mechanism of action is not precisely known, but it probably involves modification of ion channel function. **Gabapentin** has few side effects and so is often chosen in preference to other drugs with action against neuropathic pains.

Regional anaesthetic techniques

Regional techniques provide analgesia that is targeted to an anatomical site, and can minimize systemic drug effects. However, these techniques require experience and may produce adverse effects, e.g. sympathetic blockade, and patients should be closely monitored.

EPIDURAL ANAESTHESIA

In experienced hands epidural anaesthesia can produce excellent analgesia for thoracic, abdominal, pelvic or lower limb trauma or surgery, with minimal systemic effects. After abdominal surgery, perioperative epidural analgesia is associated with improved bowel and respiratory function and may reduce the incidence of thromboembolic events in high-risk surgical patients.[5] However, it is not without certain adverse effects and possible complications. Epidural local anaesthetic drugs block sympathetic and motor nerves as well as sensory afferents. The sympathetic chain runs from T1 to L2; epidural local anaesthesia sufficient to provide adequate analgesia for abdominal or thoracic surgery will cause some degree of autonomic blockade, with possible loss of sympathetic vascular tone and hypotension. Higher blocks in the region of the cardioaccelerator nerves (T1–T5) may cause bradycardia and decreased cardiac contractility. The extent of cardiovascular effects depends on several factors, including pre-existing cardiovascular function, circulating volume, concentration and total dose of local anaesthetic, and the concomitant administration of other vasoactive drugs. Loss of sympathetic tone may also occur even when sensory blockade is patchy. Hypotension associated with epidural analgesia can usually be overcome by careful dose titration of local anaesthetic, timely fluid replacement and vasopressors, e.g. a low-dose norepinephrine infusion or intermittent boluses of ephedrine. Bradycardia may be treated with positive chronotropic drugs such as atropine, ephedrine or epinephrine.

Respiratory compromise can occur after epidural administration of local anaesthetic if the block progresses high enough to involve the muscles of respiration, or if an epidural dose is inadvertently administered as a subarachnoid injection. Neurological complications associated with epidural anaesthesia are rare, but include dural puncture, direct nerve damage, and epidural haematoma or abscess.[2] Careful technique, close observation and documentation of the patient's cardiovascular and respiratory status, combined with frequent assessment of the height of sensory and motor blockade by means of response to cold and pinprick, will reduce the incidence of many of these untoward events.

Practical aspects of epidural anaesthesia

Epidural anaesthesia may be provided as a 'one-shot' technique, but more commonly a catheter is placed within the epidural space for prolonged use. Epidural catheterization is a routine procedure for the majority of anaesthetists, and many postoperative patients arrive in the ICU or high-dependency unit with an epidural catheter already in situ. Detailed descriptions of the techniques of epidural anaesthesia are available in specialized texts, but the epidural space is commonly identified using a loss of resistance technique which is performed 'blind'. This partly explains the incidence of associated complications, such as vascular or subarachnoid perforation, haematoma formation, ectopic catheter placement and nerve damage. Some of these risks may be reduced if the patient is awake during catheter insertion. However, this is often not feasible in ICU because of intercurrent illness, or the use of sedative drugs. In addition, correct positioning may be impossible in patients already in pain after surgery or trauma. Therefore, most epidural catheters sited in ICU are performed on patients who are

Table 12.8 *Contraindications to the placement of an epidural catheter*

Absolute epidural contraindications	Relative epidural contraindications
Sepsis	Anticoagulation – see text
Coagulopathy	Systemic sepsis
Increased intracranial pressure	Previous spinal surgery
Local infection at the site of insertion	Planned ITU sedation

sedated and unable to communicate pain or discomfort adequately. Only a physician trained in performing the technique and aware of the risks involved should undertake placement of the epidural under these conditions.

Indications and contraindications

Epidural anaesthesia is widely used in ICU after trauma or major surgery to the thorax, abdomen, pelvis or lower limbs. However, there are a number of absolute and relative contraindications to the placement of an epidural catheter (Table 12.8).

The administration of anticoagulants can be timed to minimize the risk of vascular trauma on insertion leading to haematoma formation. Most clinicians wait for 4 hours following the administration of unfractionated heparins and a minimum of 12 hours after prophylactic low-dose heparin before epidural insertion or removal. Low molecular weight heparins are often prescribed for evening administration, allowing epidural catheter insertion to be undertaken electively the following day. Ideally, platelet counts should be above 100×10^9/L, and INR and APTT ratios below 1.5. There is no evidence that aspirin at normal doses increases the risk of haemorrhagic complications with epidural catheterization. Epidural anaesthesia should be used with great caution in patients suffering from fixed cardiac output disorders (e.g. aortic or mitral stenosis) because of the risks of cardiovascular collapse. Likewise, it should be borne in mind that respiratory function can be compromised as progressively more intercostal muscles become paralysed.

Drugs administered via the epidural route

The drugs most frequently administered via the epidural route are local anaesthetics and opioids. When administered concomitantly, opioids act synergistically with local anaesthetics to improve analgesia and decrease both the local anaesthetic requirements and the associated cardiovascular effects of sympathetic blockade. Many ICUs administer the local anaesthetic by continuous infusion (e.g. bupivacaine 0.05–0.25 per cent or 0.1–0.2 per cent ropivacaine), although an initial bolus dose is preferable for rapid effect. Local anaesthetics block autonomic nerves as well as sensory and motor nerves, and some degree of vasodilatation may occur, depending on the concentration of drug used. The degree of sensory and motor blockade also depends on the concentration of local anaesthetic used. Higher concentrations (e.g. ≥0.375 per cent bupivacaine) can provide sensory blockade sufficient for surgical anaesthesia, but at the expense of profound autonomic and motor blockade. In contrast, 0.1 per cent bupivacaine rarely, if ever, produces significant motor blockade. Larger volumes may be administered with less risk of exceeding the toxic dose (see above), and therefore dilute solutions are preferable in ICU.

After epidural catheter insertion, a test dose of local anaesthetic is administered via the catheter (e.g. 3–5 mL 1–2 per cent lidocaine or 0.5 per cent bupivacaine). If the catheter has been inadvertently sited in the intrathecal space, profound hypotension develops within minutes and spinal anaesthesia soon follows. Some anaesthetists advocate the addition of epinephrine (concentration 1 in 200 000) to the test dose because an increase in heart rate within a minute signifies intravascular injection.

The spread of block depends primarily on the dose of local anaesthetic administered and the volume in which it is carried. The mass of drug is the main determinant of this, but an equivalent dose of local anaesthetic may give more widespread sensory blockade when administered in a larger rather than a smaller volume. Weight and height have little effect on the extent of epidural block, though the epidural space is smaller in the morbidly obese and the elderly. In these patients block height may be greater and initial doses decreased. As a rule of thumb 1–2 mL of local anaesthetic blocks approximately one spinal segment, although the size of the epidural space varies considerably between individuals. The site of block is also important and it is preferable to site an epidural catheter as closely as possible to the intended target site for optimal analgesia. Therefore, in order to provide analgesia for a 'rooftop' incision the catheter should be sited in the midthoracic region. If the surgery is above this the epidural should be placed in the upper thoracic region etc.

Epidural or spinal opioids are thought to produce analgesia primarily by effects at the dorsal horn of the spinal cord, although rostral spread to the brain does occur, particularly with the less lipid-soluble opioids such as morphine. In addition, spread into the systemic circulation occurs. CNS spread increases the problems of respiratory depression, sedation and pruritus. Epidural opioids can cause respiratory depression either early (within 1 hour of administration) as systemic absorption occurs, or later (8–24 hours) because of rostral opioid spread. Late respiratory depression occurs most commonly with morphine as it moves slowly

from the epidural space into the subarachnoid space. The duration of action of opioids with low lipid solubility will also be considerably longer than that of the lipid-soluble compounds. Fentanyl is highly lipid-soluble and rapidly penetrates the dura mater after administration.[25] Fentanyl, therefore, has a lower potential for rostral spread and is widely used for epidural administration in the UK. Fentanyl is often mixed in a concentration of 2 μg/mL with 0.1 per cent bupivacaine for epidural administration at an infusion rate of 0–15 mL/h. The lipid solubility of diamorphine is between that of fentanyl and morphine, and it is commonly used to provide prolonged epidural analgesia, typically in doses of 2.5–5 mg.

Clonidine (see above) is a useful alternative to opioids as an adjunct to decrease epidural local anaesthetic requirements. The use of clonidine may be limited by sedation, bradycardia and hypotension. Typical adult epidural doses are 10–50 μg/h or bolus doses of 0.5–1.0 μg/kg. Epidural preservative free S-ketamine can provide useful analgesia. It is rapidly absorbed into the systemic circulation, where it displays its normal pharmacological profile. S-ketamine is available and has been used with no evidence of toxicity.

Troubleshooting epidurals

Epidural techniques can provide excellent analgesia, although they may be associated with a number of practical difficulties. Many of these are simply remedied, but can create problems for the inexperienced.

Hypotension

Hypotension often accompanies epidural anaesthesia. It can usually be treated with fluid replacement and/or vasopressors.

Motor weakness

This is particularly likely if higher concentrations of local anaesthetic are used. However, the use of lower concentrations may compromise effective analgesia.

Pruritus

Naloxone may reverse the pruritus accompanying the use of epidural and spinal opiates, but often pain relief is moderated at the same time. Naloxone can also be used to reverse opiate-induced respiratory depression, which occurs more commonly with longer-acting, less lipid-soluble opiates (e.g. morphine).

Infection

A high index of suspicion should be maintained for epidural infection as this can rapidly progress to an epidural abscess, with devastating neurological consequences. There must be a low threshold for the removal of the catheter if there is local erythema or tenderness. Some units routinely remove all epidural catheters after 5 days to guard against this complication.

Systemic toxicity

Signs of systemic toxicity are the same as for intravascular injection or absorption of toxic amounts of local anaesthetic, and should be treated in a similar manner. However, rapid development of the signs of toxicity should raise the suspicion of intravascular catheter placement.

Incomplete block

If more than 4 cm of catheter is left within the epidural space migration out of an intervertebral foramen or into a dural sleeve can occur. This may result in poor distribution of local anaesthetic and produce patchy or unilateral analgesia. The problem can usually be rectified by withdrawing the catheter by 1–2 cm, or by positioning the patient on the opposite (unblocked) side. Segmental sparing may also occur for less obvious reasons, e.g. uneven distribution of local anaesthetic in the epidural space. Altering the position of the patient or the catheter, increasing the overall volume of epidural local anaesthetic, or the addition of other epidural drugs may all be effective, but it may be necessary to resite the epidural.

Occasionally intravenous opioids may be administered in ICU in conjunction with an imperfect epidural, but adverse effects (e.g. hypotension, respiratory depression) are more common. The sacral nerves are particularly large, and low-dose local anaesthetic regimens may fail adequately to block transmission through them. A higher local anaesthetic concentration will provide better analgesia for the lower leg if this happens. Some lower abdominal structures, such as the inguinal ligament and spermatic cord, take their nervous supply from a higher spinal level, so it may be necessary to block a higher thoracic region to provide adequate pain relief.

A common scenario is the problem of ineffective analgesia when an effective epidural is being titrated downwards to convert to alternative (usually oral) analgesia. The use of simple analgesia with an epidural enhances pain relief and allows reduction of the epidural rate during weaning; all patients receiving epidural analgesia should also receive simple analgesia. This should be prescribed as regular rather than prn medication, and should be administered orally as soon as the patient can tolerate fluids. Alternatively, rectal analgesia can be used if the patient has not had surgery in the anal/rectal region. An algorithm to address this is presented in Figure 12.4.

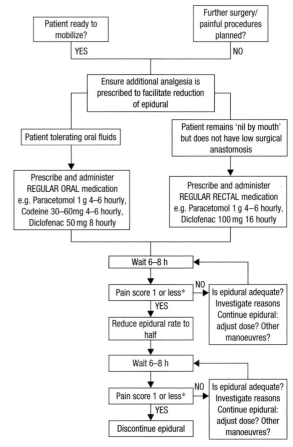

RECORD ALL ACTION TAKEN ON EPIDURAL OBSERVATION FORM

Figure 12.4 Algorithm for decreasing the infusion rate of an effective epidural

Other types of regional analgesia

A variety of other regional techniques can be used in ICU to provide analgesia, either alone or in combination with other drugs (Table 12.9).[26,27] As with epidural anaesthesia, many regional procedures need some experience, and adverse effects can limit their usage. However, they may be useful in particular circumstances. For example, intercostal nerve blocks or interpleural catheters can be used to provide analgesia after surgery or injuries to the chest or upper abdomen, particularly when epidural anaesthesia is contraindicated or impractical. They are usually performed as unilateral blocks and may be particularly useful for surface analgesia, e.g. after rib fractures or before chest drain insertion, as they block pain from somatic rather than visceral afferents. Alternatively, catheters can be inserted under direct vision by surgeons during thoracotomy. Bilateral blocks can be performed, but systemic absorption from these proximal sites is rapid and

Table 12.9 *Advantages and disadvantages of some commonly used regional techniques*

Technique	Advantages	Disadvantages
Epidural	Effective analgesia with potentially minimal systemic drug effects Reduced stress response ?Improved outcome after surgery	Widespread analgesia May be technically difficult Unsuitable if coagulopathy Sympathetic blockade in ICU patients Potential for major neurological damage Close monitoring required
Intercostal block	Technically easy Useful if epidural contraindicated Low risk pneumothorax ($<$0.5 per cent) Less invasive than epidural	Usually unilateral Limited anatomical range Potentially rapid systemic absorption and toxicity Little effect on visceral pain
Interpleural catheter	Technically easy Useful if epidural contraindicated Continuous infusion possible Less invasive than epidural	Usually unilateral Little effect on visceral pain Pneumothorax (up to 2 per cent) Potentially rapid systemic absorption and LA toxicity Risk of infection
Paravertebral block	Fewer cardiovascular effects than epidural Continuous infusion possible Low-risk pneumothorax ($<$0.5 per cent)	Usually unilateral Technically more difficult Little effect on visceral pain Epidural spread of LA usually occurs: toxicity possible Sympathetic block may occur, especially if bilateral blocks
Brachial plexus techniques	Continuous infusion via catheter possible Analgesia provided to relatively large area	Technically more difficult LA toxicity with continuous infusion Missed sensory area may occur
Femoral nerve block	Good for fractures of the femur or burns to anterior thigh	Limited anatomical range Vascular damage (femoral artery)

local anaesthetic toxicity may occur, particularly if epinephrine is not used. Paravertebral blockade with needle or catheter techniques is a useful alternative to epidural analgesia, but unilateral sympathetic blockade and spread of local anaesthetic into the epidural space are frequent; the risks of cardiovascular complications are increased if bilateral blocks are performed.

PRACTICAL ASPECTS OF ANALGESIC ADMINISTRATION

It is good (evidence-based) practice to allow a daily rest period from opioid and sedative infusions in order to reduce accumulation of the drugs and their metabolites, particularly in patient groups who are most sensitive to their effects. Likewise, PCA doses may need to be reduced for certain patients or the dosing interval increased.

Epidural analgesia can be delivered via PCEA (patient-controlled epidural analgesia), with similar considerations

to PCA. PCA can also be used to complement an existing epidural infusion, but only under strict supervision. Typically systemic and epidural opioids are not co-administered.

In the days following surgery, epidural infusion rates are normally decreased gradually. Before doing this it is important to provide simple regular analgesia, depending on local practice and clinical appropriateness, to supplement pain relief. Commonly oral or rectal preparations of NSAIDs, codeine or paracetamol are used.

SUMMARY

Pain in critically ill patients is a significant problem which is frequently under-recognized. Not only is it unpleasant, it can also have marked effects on morbidity and mortality in higher-risk patients. Although critical care provides an environment in which medical expertise and close supervision allow for a range of therapies and analgesic techniques to be more easily employed than on the ward, problems of communication, polypharmacy and coexisting organ dysfunction make effective pain control difficult. Only with a sound understanding of pain physiology, the pharmacology of the medications used and the techniques available can effective analgesia be consistently provided.

REFERENCES

1. Desbiens NA, Wu AW, Broste SK, *et al.* Pain and satisfaction with pain control in seriously ill hospitalized adults: Findings from the SUPPORT research investigations. *Crit Care Med* 1996; **24**: 1953–61.
2. Puntillo KA, White C, Morris AB, *et al.* Patients' perceptions and responses to procedural pain: results from thunder project II. *Am J Crit Care* 2001; **10**: 238–51.
3. Williams M, Kowaluk EA, Americ SP. Emerging molecular approaches to pain therapy. *J Med Chem* 1999; **42**: 1481–500.
4. Lang JD. Pain. A prelude. *Crit Care Clin* 1999; **15**: 1–15.
5. Epstein J, Breslow MJ. The stress response of critical illness. *Crit Care Clin* 1999; **15**: 17–33.
6. Desai PM. Pain management and pulmonary dysfunction. *Crit Care Clin* 1999; **15**: 151–66.
7. Bromage PR, Camporesi E, Chestnut D. Epidural narcotics for postoperative analgesia. *Anesth Analg* 1980; **59**: 473–80.
8. Cammarano WB, Pittet JF, Weitz S, *et al.* Acute withdrawal syndrome related to the administration of analgesic and sedative medications in adult intensive care unit patients. *Crit Care Med* 1998; **26**: 676–84.
9. Scragg P, Jones A, Fauvel N. Psychological problems following ICU treatment. *Anaesthesia* 2001; **56**: 9–14.
10. Jones C, Griffiths RD, Humphris G, Skirrow PM. Memory delusions and the development of acute post-traumatic stress disorder-related symptoms after intensive care. *Crit Care Med* 2001; **29**: 573–80.
11. Rigg JRA, Jamrozik K, Myles PS, *et al.* Epidural anaesthesia and analgesia and outcome of major surgery: a randomised trial. *Lancet* 2002; **359**: 1276–82.
12. Rodgers A, Walker N, Schug S, *et al.* Reduction of postoperative mortality and morbidity with epidural or spinal anaesthesia: results from overview of randomised trials. *BMJ* 2000; **321**: 1493–7.
13. Beattie WS, Badner NH, Choi P. Epidural analgesia reduces postoperative myocardial infarction: A meta-analysis. *Anesth Analg* 2001; **93**: 853–8.
14. Atanassoff PG. Effects of regional anesthesia on perioperative outcome. *J Clin Anesthesiol* 1996; **8**: 446–55.
15. Mangano DT, Siliciano D, Hollenberg M, *et al.* Post operative myocardial ischaemia: Therapeutic trials using intensive analgesia following surgery. *Anesthesiology* 1992; **76**: 342–53.
16. Gust R, Pecher S, Gust A, *et al.* Effect of patient controlled analgesia on pulmonary complications after coronary artery bypass grafting. *Crit Care Med* 1999; **27**: 2218–23.
17. Macintyre PE, Jarvis DA. Age is the best predictor of postoperative morphine requirements. *Pain* 1995; **64**: 357–64.
18. Hamill-Ruth RJ, Marohn ML. Evaluation of pain in the critically ill patient. *Crit Care Clin* 1999; **15**: 35–54.
19. Payen J, Bru O, Bosson JL, *et al.* Assessing pain in critically ill sedated patients by using a behavioural pain scale. *Crit Care Med* 2001; **29**: 2258–63.
20. Desbiens NA, Mueller-Rizner N. How well do surrogates assess the pain of seriously ill patients? *Crit Care Med* 2000; **28**: 1347–52.
21. Park GR. Molecular mechanisms of drug metabolism in the critically ill. *Br J Anaesth* 1996; **77**: 32–49.
22. Nasraway SA Jr, Jacobi J, Murray MJ, Lumb PD; Task Force of the American College of Critical Care Medicine of the Society of Critical Care Medicine and the American Society of Health-System Pharmacists, American College of Chest Physicians. Sedation, analgesia and neuromuscular blockade of the critically ill adult: Revised clinical practical guidelines for 2002. *Crit Care Med* 2002; **30**: 117–41.
23. McArdle P. Perspectives in pain management: Intravenous analgesia. *Crit Care Clin* 1999; **15**: 89–104.
24. Auroy Y, Narchi P, Messiah A, *et al.* Serious complications related to regional anesthesia. *Anesthesiology* 1997; **87**: 479–86.
25. Coda BA, Brown MC, Schaffer R, *et al.* Pharmacology of epidural fentanyl, alfentanil and sufentanil in volunteers. *Anesthesiology* 1994; **81**: 1149–61.
26. Burton AW, Eappen S. Regional anesthesia techniques for pain control in the intensive care unit. *Crit Care Clin* 1999; **15**: 77–88
27. Clark F, Gilbert HC. Regional analgesia in the intensive care unit. *Crit Care Clin* 2001; **17**: 943–66.

KEY ARTICLES

Desbiens NA *et al.* Pain and satisfaction with pain control in seriously ill hospitalized adults: Findings from the SUPPORT research investigations. *Critical Care Medicine* 1996; **24**: 1953–61.

A large multicentre study from five US teaching hospitals, interviewing over 9000 patients about their experiences of pain while in ICU. Nearly 50 per cent of patients reported pain during their ICU stay, with 15 per cent reporting extreme or moderate pain at least half the time; 15 per cent of patients were dissatisfied with their pain control.

Nasraway SA *et al.* Sedation, analgesia and neuromuscular blockade of the critically ill adult: Revised clinical practical guiudelines for 2002. *Critical Care Medicine* 2002; **30**: 117–41.

Guidelines for the use of sedatives and analgesics in ICU from the American College of Critical Care Medicine. Fentanyl, hydromorphone and morphine are the recommended opiates. Fentanyl or hydromorphone are preferred for patients with haemodynamic instability or renal insufficiency. Ketorolac should be limited to 5 days of use.

Rigg JRA *et al.* Epidural anaesthesia and analgesia and outcome of major surgery: A randomized trial. *Lancet* 2002; **359**: 1276–82.

Large multicentre trial comparing mortality and major morbidity endpoints with epidural or conventional analgesia following major surgery. Found no improvement in mortality with epidural analgesia, and only an improvement in respiratory morbidity.

Puntillo KA *et al.* Patients' perceptions and responses to procedural pain: results from Thunder II project. *American Journal of Critical Care* 2001; **10**: 238–51.

Data from over 6000 acutely and critically ill patients, assessing their responses to six commonly performed procedures on the ICU (wound care, wound drain removal, tracheal suctioning, turning, femoral sheath removal and placement of a central venous catheter).

Rodgers A *et al.* Reduction of postoperative mortality and morbidity with epidural or spinal anaesthesia: Results from overview of randomized trials. *British Medical Journal* 2000; **321**: 1493.

Meta-analysis of 141 trials, suggesting overall mortality reduced by one-third with the use of neuroaxial blockade. Significant reductions in DVT, PE, pneumonia and respiratory depression also shown.

13 Ethics in critical care medicine

ROBERT WINTER

Viva topics

- What are the four basic principles underpinning ethical medical practice?
- What governs a patient's ability to give informed consent?
- You have to decide which patient to transfer to another intensive care unit to accommodate a new admission from the accident and emergency department. Should you move the most stable patient or the most recent admission?

This chapter will attempt to introduce the reader to the basic principles of medical ethics, address the topic of futility, and lead on to cover the withdrawal of life-sustaining treatment, and withdrawal vs withholding treatment. Four basic principles are said to govern ethical medical practice:

- **Autonomy**: the right to individual self-determination (given the correct information in a way the individual can understand)
- **Benificence**: any action must be in **that** patient's best interests
- **Non-malificence**: avoiding harm to the patient
- **Justice**: maximum benefit for the most patients.[1]

BASIC PRINCIPLES

The two main basic ethical theories relevant to medical practice are *consequence based* (utilitarian) and *duty based* (Kantian, based on the writings of Immanuel Kant (1724–1804)). Other theories include *rights-based, community-based* and *care-based theories*.

The origins of the consequence-based theories are derived from the writings of Bentham (1748–1832) and Mill (1806–1873).

Utilitarianism/consequentialism holds that actions are right or wrong based on the balance of good and bad consequences they produce. This appears at first sight a very useful and pragmatic approach, and utilitarians can offer many supportive examples. Bentham and Mill were hedonistic

utilitarians who thought of 'utility' in terms of happiness/pleasure, so the correct action is the one that leads to the greatest sum of human happiness. Recent utilitarians have argued that other values of 'utility', such as health, friendship or autonomy, are important. Whatever the list of values, 'utility' should be considered in terms of the underlying principle that any action should be assessed in terms of the greatest good it produces, i.e. the consequence of that action.

Criticisms of consequence-based theory include the apparent sanctioning of (generally considered) immoral actions if the overall consequence appears to benefit the majority. For example, if an elderly person becomes frail and requires increasing resources to maintain their independence, a utilitarian could argue that that person has a duty to die, to allow the resources to be used to benefit younger and more productive members of society. Utilitarian theories could also be used to defend the practice of interventional ventilation of patients with severe intracerebral bleeds, purely to obtain their organs for the benefit of up to seven other patients on transplant waiting lists (this is discussed further below).

Duty-based/Kantian theory states that features of an action rather than just its consequences make that action right or wrong. The features of an action that make it worthy depend upon the *morally* valid reason that justifies that action.

If a doctor tells the truth to a patient while obtaining consent purely to avoid the threat of a lawsuit, the act of telling the truth in this case has no particular moral worth despite being the correct course of action. If another doctor takes precisely the same course of action out of respect for the personal dignity of the patient, then the action has moral value.

Duty-based theories are founded on respect for reason, autonomy, individual worth and equality. People must be regarded as ends in themselves, and not as means to an end. This approach leads to what are termed *deontological constraints* on how we can treat others. In the example of the frail elderly person above, that individual's worth as a person would forbid us from killing them for the greater good of the community.

Duty-based theory can be criticized as it does not allow for moral conflicts or conflicting obligations, as the moral rules proposed are categorical. If two conflicting obligations coincide (staying late at work to complete a vital job vs taking the children to the cinema as promised), duty-based theory implies that both must be done, although this is clearly impossible.

None of the ethical/moral theories outlined above provides a complete understanding, but most would support the four general principles mentioned at the start of this chapter: *autonomy* from the duty-based end of the ethical theoretical spectrum, and *justice* from the consequence-based end.

NORMATIVE VS NON-NORMATIVE ETHICS

Ethics can be described as normative or non-normative. Normative ethics is based on the generally or community-specific norms of moral behaviour which govern how we *ought* to behave. Non-normative ethics is either descriptive – the factual investigation of how people reason and react – or meta-ethics, analysis of the language methods of reasoning and concepts in ethics. In summary, non-normative ethics tries to establish what *is* the case, whereas normative ethics tries to establish what *ought* to be the case. Professional codes of conduct are a form of non-normative (descriptive) ethics, but the question of whether these codes are justifiable is a normative issue. Although norms of moral behaviour may be generally accepted, they are not absolute.

Most people would regard lying as unacceptable but would also regard it as acceptable to lie to prevent a murder. Sometimes clearly enunciated professional codes of ethics or behaviour may be breached in the greater public good. This was judged to be the case in an example where a psychiatrist learnt that a patient was intending to kill an individual who was not a patient of that psychiatrist. Following consultation, the psychiatrist decided that to reveal this information was a breach of patient confidentiality but, unfortunately, the patient carried out his threat. Judges hearing the resulting civil case made a majority ruling that the greater public good overrode the individual's right to confidentiality. A minority, however, felt that respecting the patient's confidentiality was ethically correct, as there was a risk that future patients would not come forward for treatment if they felt that their confidentiality would not be protected.

This conflict is sometimes referred to as the *relative weight of norms*. If this principle is used, it is important that the infringement of the overridden norm is necessary (no morally preferable alternative can be substituted), the least possible infringement is selected, and any negative effects of the infringement are minimized. An example of this might be the decision to transfer a critically ill patient from one intensive care unit to another in a nearby hospital to accommodate a new admission.

It would clearly be preferable not to transfer any patient and thereby put them at risk. It could also be argued that transferring a patient already in a critical care bed is taking a course of action that does not benefit that individual patient, and indeed exposes them to an unjustifiable potential harm. If it is assumed, however, that the new admission is more likely to be more physiologically unstable than the most stable patient suitable for transfer already on the unit, the greater harm would be produced by transferring the more unstable patient at greater risk from the transfer (this problem can also be examined using the four ethical principles mentioned above and discussed below).

THE FOUR ETHICAL PRINCIPLES

Autonomy

Autonomy is the principle of respect for an individual's right to determine their own treatment. This is the opposite of *paternalism*, as in 'the doctor knows best'. Many (if not most) patients in intensive care units lack the ability to express their right to autonomy, either because of the effects of their underlying illness or because of the administration of sedative and analgesic drugs.

This has a bearing on consent to treatment options, especially in patients who may lack the capacity to make an informed choice. *Capacity* is the key issue when obtaining consent. There are three preconditions that must be fulfilled before an individual may be regarded as having the capacity to make a choice, i.e. is *competent*. They are described in the judgment on a schizophrenic patient detained under the Mental Health Act (re C 1994 1 All ER 819). The individual must *retain* and *comprehend* the relevant information, they must *believe* the information, and they must have the *ability* to weigh the information and make a decision. As for civil cases, capacity is assessed on the balance of probability.

Because a decision seems unwise to the medical professional this does not mean that it is invalid. Equally, just because a belief system appears to be irrational to the medical profession, it does not mean that it can be considered invalid and overruled by the profession. The largest single group of patients for whom a valid decision that seems unwise to the majority of medical practitioners are the Jehovah's Witnesses. Their refusal of blood transfusion is based on a biblical interpretation that is not accepted by other religious groups and although this may seem irrational to the doctors looking after the patient this refusal must be respected.

In the case of an *incompetent* patient the medical staff looking after them should act in the patient's best interests using the Bolam standard as a guide, where the decision taken should be in accordance with that of a responsible body of medical opinion.

There is no place in current English law for surrogacy of decision making, such as proxy consent (consent from a relative, for instance). In Scotland the appointment of a medical surrogate is possible, and in other countries surrogates may be ranked according to their blood ties to the patient. Equally, under English law a relative cannot refuse permission for a procedure such as blood transfusion, but may make the doctors aware of the patient's allegedly previously stated wishes. These wishes might be used to make a decision for the patient based on the principle of *substituted judgment*, i.e. the decision the patient would *probably* have made if competent, based on previously stated wishes and general values. If the patient has made an advance directive (living will) this may also be used as a basis for decision making. However, advance directives are often open to interpretation and may not have considered the situation the patient is currently in, in sufficient detail. A Jehovah's Witness who is brought in unconscious *without* an advance directive available could therefore be treated in his medical best interests whatever representations are made by the relatives.

A competent patient can refuse even life-saving treatment if they have the capacity to understand the decision and believe in its consequences. This also means that a clearly expressed refusal of blood transfusion expressed when a patient has the capacity cannot be overruled if that patient becomes unconscious at a later date, unless the patient himself has reversed the decision.

Benificence and non-malificence

Benificence can be thought of as the principle that we must always 'do good' to our patients and any action must have a positive risk–benefit ratio. Non-malificence is the duty to all not to do harm, but only to be beneficent to our patients.

To think about these two principles, let us re-examine the suggestion of interventional ventilation of patients with severe intracerebral bleeds normally expected to die. Traditionally such patients would be placed in a quiet area of a general ward and nature be allowed to take its course. However, many of these patients are relatively young, and if intubated, ventilated and given circulatory support, would not die of apnoea and cardiac arrest, but develop brainstem death. Once this diagnosis had been made they could be considered suitable to donate organs for transplantation. Ignoring the resource constraints on critical care beds, the increased yield of organs seems to make good medical, economic and humanitarian sense. It would also seem to accord with utilitarian ethical principles. An examination using the principles outlined above, however, throws up some problems.

These patients would be in no position to give or refuse consent for such a protocol, as they would by the nature of their disease be incompetent. In the UK, relative proxy consent has no legal standing, so relatives could not give legal consent to the patient's ongoing management. Operative removal of organs would be non-consensual contact (not governed by the Doctrine of Necessity and Bolam) and thus, in law, constitute *battery*. This intervention clearly is not in *this* patient's best interests and therefore fails the test of beneficence. In addition, some would argue that prolonging death and the dying process does the patient harm, thus failing the test of non-malificence.

The argument has been put forward that the moment of apnoea is the moment of death, and that by intubating the patient at that point it is merely the timing of the diagnosis that is altered (by waiting to perform brainstem death tests). Most medical practitioners, however, have seen patients who have been intubated at the point of apnoea and survived. Apnoea, of itself, cannot therefore be a reliable sign of death unless untreated. If there is, therefore, the potential for the patient not to die (remaining terribly neurologically damaged), then the potential to do harm seems very real. In a UK pilot of such a scheme no patient remained in a persistent vegetative state during the trial, but this seems as likely to have been fortuitous as inevitable.

Another way of examining these principles would be to re-evaluate the problem of what to do if there are more patients than intensive care beds. One argument could be that it is unethical to transfer a patient already in a bed to another unit, as the transfer is not in that patient's best interests but in the best interests of the 'extra' patient. We are therefore putting the patient in the bed at risk (maleficence) for the benefit of a third party. A counter argument to this is that there are $n + 1$ patients requiring intensive care and n intensive care beds, but that the underlying principle is that all $n + 1$ patients *must* have access to a bed. The argument then runs that the patient from the ICU to be transferred requires an intensive care bed and being transferred to a bed elsewhere is clearly in their best interests, if the alternative is not to be in an intensive care bed at all. This implies that the intensive care staff owe a duty of care to all patients requiring intensive care, and not just those actually already in a bed.

Justice

The principle of justice is essentially that of fairness. Individual patients should have access to the same treatments based on need. That is not to say that all treatments are always available, as resource constraints limit treatment availability in many healthcare systems. Which treatments are available has to be assessed on the basis of local population need and the availability of resources. This is a utilitarian principle that the consequence of any action should result in the greatest good for the greatest number.

Instruments such as the Quality Adjusted Life Year (QALY) gain for a given treatment can be used to make comparative judgments. To calculate QALYs it is assumed that 1 year of healthy life is worth one QALY, being dead is worth 0, and 1 year of unhealthy life is worth less than 1. QALYs allow a calculation to take into account both the gain in life years and the quality of health gain. As an example, assume that a patient has a life expectancy without an operation of 10 years and a quality of life of 0.6 (6 QALYs), and that with an operation they live 15 years and have a quality of life of 0.9 (13.5 QALYs). The gain from the operation is therefore 13.5 − 6 = 7.5 QALYs, and a cost per QALY based on the gain and the cost of the operation (less the costs of conservative treatment) can be derived. A cost-effective treatment is one with a low cost per QALY.

One criticism of the use of QALYs is that they are intrinsically ageist, as they discriminate in favour of patients with a longer life expectancy. They also discriminate against patients with a lower initial apparent quality of life, such as the disabled, because the possible gain is less, and also take no account of life-saving rather than life-enhancing treatment. This is addressed at least in part by using *needs-based assessment*, which in turn has the limitation that it would be possible to spend huge amounts of resource on small numbers of patients with large needs, ignoring the resource requirements of the larger population.

The largest social experiment of this type is the Oregon Medicaid programme. In 1989, the Oregon legislature decided to cover all people eligible for Medicaid to 100 per cent rather than 67 per cent. In order to manage the budgetary consequences of this, access to certain treatments was not funded. The list of available treatments was initially derived from a series of condition treatment pairs (a diagnosis linked to a number of treatment choices), with the benefit from each treatment assessed by professional societies. This medical benefit was used to derive a quality of life scale (quality of wellbeing) using a telephone survey of 1001 Oregon citizens. The attempt to modify Medicaid was turned down by the Bush and then the Clinton administrations until references to quality of life were removed, and the end result was a prioritization system based on the ability of a treatment to prevent death. This would have adhered to the principle of justice if the treatments that were offered were available to all on the basis of need.

End of life decisions

Currently up to 20 per cent of US citizens die in intensive care units.[2] Attitudes towards decisions at the end of life vary from country to country and institution to institution. It is possible to view treatment decisions at the end of life as a continuum, from preserving life at all costs at one end through to active euthanasia ('mercy killing') at the other, with withholding life-sustaining treatments, withdrawing life-sustaining treatments and assisted suicide as steps along the way.

The vast majority of people (medical and non-medical in this country) would hold the view that there are states of life that are worse than death, and that it would be unethical to sustain life in these circumstances. Preservation of life at all costs is therefore an uncommonly held view at the present time.

At the other end of the spectrum lies the moral distinction between killing and letting die. It has been argued that there is little moral distinction between the two. An example is the case of someone (Smith) with a large potential inheritance based on the death of his 6-year-old cousin. If Smith finds his cousin in the bath and drowns him by holding his head under water, or sees him slip in the bath, hit his head, and then watches him drown without intervening, most people would regard both courses of action as morally wrong. It can be argued that this is the same moral argument as between active killing of a patient and passively letting them die. Euthanasia is a direct act performed with the primary intention of causing death. The withdrawal of life-sustaining treatment is not euthanasia, as there is no direct act where the primary intention is to cause death. We are allowing people to die who would have died of the consequences of their underlying disease in any event. We are more logically just avoiding prolonging the dying process by continuing treatment.

In order for this to be logically consistent, treatment limitation decisions must be made on the basis of *futility* of treatment, i.e. a treatment which has no prospect of succeeding. The majority of treatment withdrawal decisions are taken as a consequence of continued deterioration in the face of maximal appropriate supportive therapy. This has been termed *imminent demise futility*. The concept of medical futility may be further subdivided, as follows:

- **Physiological futility**, in which the degree of injury is such that treatment will not succeed, e.g. performing a thoracotomy on a patient who has sustained asystolic cardiac arrest following blunt chest trauma.
- **Interactive futility**, in which the medical intervention will preserve physiological function but will not restore the individual's ability to interact, e.g. persisting vegetative state.

- **Qualitative futility** In such patients the treatment proposed will sustain life but at a cost that the medical staff consider to be unacceptable. Such decisions are subjective and based on opinion formed by experience on the balance of probability. Medical and paramedical staff tend to make quality-of-life judgments based on their own perceptions and experience, and may differ widely from what the patient would regard as a wholly acceptable quality of life.

If death is felt to be inevitable then providing treatment that merely prolongs the process of dying could be regarded as futile (no beneficence), and we are under no obligation to provide futile treatment. Indeed, it could be regarded as unethical, as the treatment would be doing harm (malificence) and depriving other patients of needed resources (justice). Even if a competent patient demands a treatment felt not to be in their best interests by the medical staff, we are under no obligation to provide it. In the case of an incompetent patient, the medical staff should act in that patient's best interests, as outlined above.

Many doctors and other staff find it easier (both emotionally and practically) to withhold or not increase a treatment than to withdraw one. This is especially true of a treatment such as ventilation, where the temporal link between the intervention and death is so clear. Logically, however, there is no difference between withdrawing ventilation, where death occurs in minutes to hours, and withdrawing haemofiltration or haemodialysis, where death occurs in hours to days. In some countries it is illegal to withdraw a treatment but not illegal to withhold or not escalate. This holds the risk that doctors might be reluctant to initiate potentially beneficial treatment for fear of being 'stuck with it' if it fails and death becomes inevitable. It is common practice in some UK intensive care units to offer a trial of up to 48 h of aggressive therapy, with withdrawal if there is no response to therapy. Most would be unwilling to offer this if there was no prospect of reducing the level of support in the face of deterioration after the 48-h window.

Process of withdrawal of life-sustaining treatment

Most patients ventilated on intensive care units are receiving opiates as sedative analgesics, and it is entirely reasonable to continue these even if ventilation is discontinued on the grounds of futility. Although the morphine will depress ventilation and may hasten death, this is not the intention of its prescription. The intention of the morphine is to relieve pain and suffering, which is clearly not futile. Ventilatory depression can be considered an accepted side effect. This idea is known as the doctrine of *double effect*: the good effect is intended and outweighs the bad effect, which is permitted or tolerated.

The case of a man in his 40s with multiple organ failure following pancreatitis is illustrative. The patient in question has cardiovascular failure requiring high-dose pressor and inotrope infusions, adult respiratory distress syndrome requiring pressure-controlled inverse ratio ventilation with high levels of positive end-expiratory pressure and 100 per cent oxygen, renal failure requiring renal replacement therapy, hepatic failure, gut failure requiring total parenteral nutrition, and haematological failure requiring repeated transfusions of platelets and red cells. He has had three laparotomies for pancreatic necrosectomy and now has an open abdomen. In addition to antibiotics, he is receiving a high-dose opiate infusion to control his pain. He has been in this condition for more than a week (and so the morphine has gradually been increased to 60 mg/h) and his death is considered inevitable by the entire clinical team. The first step in the process of withdrawal of life-sustaining treatment is the implementation of a 'Do Not Resuscitate' order.

The patient's condition is continuing to deteriorate despite maximal therapy, and continuation of treatment is *futile*. The whole team are entirely happy with discontinuing the renal replacement therapy, transfusions, parenteral nutrition and antibiotics. Most people in the team are also comfortable with withdrawing the inotropes and pressors, and with reducing the ventilatory support by ventilating him on air without positive end-expiratory pressure. Some in the team are uncomfortable about withdrawing ventilation altogether, as the high doses of morphine required for analgesia mean that he will die shortly afterwards.

Logically and ethically, however, there is no distinction between the withdrawal of the renal support (artificially normalizing biochemistry) and respiratory support (artificially normalizing blood gases). The proximity of the withdrawal to death may make us uncomfortable, but the ethical or logical distinction does not exist as both are futile treatments in the face of inevitable death. In practice, ventilation is often continued at a reduced level to manage the dying process for the emotional comfort of relatives and staff, but it could be argued that this is unethical treatment as it inevitably prolongs the death, which may not be in the best interests of the patient. The continued use of morphine in such circumstances is clearly not futile, as it prevents pain and suffering despite the respiratory depression that will ensue.

Guidance to medical staff regarding these matters has been published by both the GMC[3] and the BMA.[4] This states that: 'Developments in technology have led to a misconception in society that death can almost always be postponed. There needs to be a recognition that there comes a point in all lives where no more can reasonably or helpfully be done to benefit patients other than keeping them comfortable and free from pain.' Neither organization has published specific guidance for ICU patients, but the principles are transferable. The acceptance of the concept of futility is very variable between cultures, and there is an increasing tendency in some sections of the community to seek an injunction regarding withdrawal of treatment.

Where such decisions are made, the reasoning behind them should be discussed with medical and nursing colleagues, a full explanation given to relatives, and their assent obtained. ICU staff aim for the assent of relatives in all such cases, and the discussions should be fully documented. Palliative, compassionate care should be continued on the ICU if death is imminent, but where death is inevitable but likely to be delayed, the patient should be transferred to a non-ICU/HDU area for terminal care.

CONCLUSION

Medical ethics in critical care revolves around moral thinking and behaviour concerning what is right and what is wrong. Although aimed primarily at ensuring ethical care of patients, it is impossible to separate this from the ethical and moral behaviour of the critical care staff. Ethical decision making in critical care is always challenging and rarely simple. Discussion with and advice from all members of the multidisciplinary team is essential. Some units may refer complex problems to a Clinical Ethics Committee, or in extreme cases to the Courts.

REFERENCES

1. Beauchamp TL, Childress JF. *Principles of biomedical ethics.* Oxford: Oxford University Press, 2001.
2. Prendergast TJ, Luce JM. Increasing incidence of withholding and withdrawal of life support from the critically ill. *Am J Resp Crit Care Med* 1997; **155**: 1–2.
3. http://www.gmc-uk.org/index.htm
4. British Medical Association. *Withholding and withdrawing life-prolonging medical treatment.* London: BMJ Books, 2001.

Index